T0226560

Biologics in Inflammatory Bowel Disease

Editor

EDWARD V. LOFTUS Jr

GASTROENTEROLOGY CLINICS OF NORTH AMERICA

www.gastro.theclinics.com

Consulting Editor
GARY W. FALK

September 2014 • Volume 43 • Number 3

ELSEVIER

1600 John F. Kennedy Boulevard • Suite 1800 • Philadelphia, Pennsylvania, 19103-2899
http://www.theclinics.com

GASTROENTEROLOGY CLINICS OF NORTH AMERICA Volume 43, Number 3
September 2014 ISSN 0889-8553, ISBN-13: 978-0-323-32325-3

Editor: Kerry Holland
Developmental Editor: Susan Showalter

Gastroenterology Clinics of North America (ISSN 0889-8553) is published quarterly by Elsevier Inc., 360 Park Avenue South, New York, NY 10010-1710. Months of issue are March, June, September, and December. Business and Editorial Offices: 1600 John F. Kennedy Blvd., Suite 1800, Philadelphia, PA 19103-2899. Customer Service Office: 6277 Sea Harbor Drive, Orlando, FL 32887-4800. Periodicals postage paid at New York, NY and additional mailing offices. Subscription prices are $320.00 per year (US individuals), $160.00 per year (US students), $530.00 per year (US institutions), $350.00 per year (Canadian individuals), $651.00 per year (Canadian institutions), $445.00 per year (international individuals), $220.00 per year (international students), and $651.00 per year (international institutions). Foreign air speed delivery is included in all *Clinics* subscription prices. All prices are subject to change without notice. **POSTMASTER**: Send address changes to *Gastroenterology Clinics of North America*, Elsevier Health Sciences Division, Subscription Customer Service, 3251 Riverport Lane, Maryland Heights, MO 63043. Telephone: 1-800-654-2452 (U.S. and Canada); 314-447-8871 (outside U.S. and Canada). Fax: 314-447-8029. E-mail: journalscustomerservice-usa@elsevier.com (for print support); journalsonlinesupport-usa@elsevier.com (for online support).

Reprints. For copies of 100 or more, of articles in this publication, please contact the Commercial Reprints Department, Elsevier Inc., 360 Part Avenue South, New York, New York 10010-1710. Tel. 212-633-3874, Fax: 212-633-3820, E-mail: reprints@elsevier.com.

Gastroenterology Clinics of North America is also published in Italian by Il Pensiero Scientifico Editore, Rome, Italy; and in Portuguese by Interlivros Edicoes Ltda., Rua Commandante Coelho 1085, 21250 Cordovil, Rio de Janeiro, Brazil.

Gastroenterology Clinics of North America is covered in *MEDLINE/PubMed (Index Medicus)*, *Excerpta Medica*, *Current Contents/Clinical Medicine*, *Science Citation Index*, *ISI/BIOMED*, and *BIOSIS*.

Contributors

CONSULTING EDITOR

GARY W. FALK, MD, MS
Professor of Medicine, Division of Gastroenterology, Hospital of the University of Pennsylvania, University of Pennsylvania Perelman School of Medicine, Philadelphia, Pennsylvania

EDITOR

EDWARD V. LOFTUS Jr, MD
Professor of Medicine, Mayo Clinic College of Medicine; Director, Inflammatory Bowel Disease Interest Group, Division of Gastroenterology and Hepatology, Mayo Clinic, Rochester, Minnesota

AUTHORS

WAQQAS AFIF, MD
Assistant Professor of Medicine, Division of Gastroenterology, McGill University Health Center, Montreal, Quebec, Canada

PREET BAGI, MD
Division of Gastroenterology, University of California, San Diego, La Jolla, California

BRIGID S. BOLAND, MD
Division of Gastroenterology, Department of Medicine, Inflammatory Bowel Disease Center, University of California San Diego; Digestive Diseases Research Development Center, University of California San Diego, La Jolla, California

NIELS VANDE CASTEELE, PharmD, PhD
Robarts Clinical Trials Inc., London, Ontario, Canada; Division of Gastroenterology, University of California, San Diego, La Jolla, California; Department of Pharmaceutical and Pharmacological Sciences, KU Leuven, Leuven, Belgium

JOHN T. CHANG, MD
Division of Gastroenterology, Department of Medicine, Inflammatory Bowel Disease Center, University of California San Diego; Digestive Diseases Research Development Center, University of California San Diego, La Jolla, California

ADAM S. CHEIFETZ, MD
Director and Associate Professor of Medicine, Division of Gastroenterology, Department of Medicine, Center for Inflammatory Bowel Diseases, Beth Israel Deaconess Medical Center, Harvard Medical School, Boston, Massachusetts

MANEESH DAVE, MBBS, MPH
Instructor in Medicine, Division of Gastroenterology and Hepatology, Mayo Clinic, Rochester, Minnesota

GEERT R. D'HAENS, MD, PhD
Robarts Clinical Trials Inc., London, Ontario, Canada; Department of Gastroenterology, Academic Medical Centre, Amsterdam, The Netherlands

PARAMBIR S. DULAI, MBBS
Inflammatory Bowel Disease Center, Dartmouth-Hitchcock Medical Center, Lebanon, New Hampshire

WILLIAM A. FAUBION Jr, MD
Associate Professor of Immunology, Medicine and Pediatrics, Division of Gastroenterology and Hepatology, Mayo Clinic, Rochester, Minnesota

JOSEPH D. FEUERSTEIN, MD
Clinical instructor of Medicine, Division of Gastroenterology, Department of Medicine, Center for Inflammatory Bowel Diseases, Beth Israel Deaconess Medical Center, Harvard Medical School, Boston, Massachusetts

SARA HORST, MD
Assistant Professor of Medicine, Vanderbilt University Medical Center, Nashville, Tennessee

JENNIFER JONES, MD, MSc, FRCPC
Department of Medicine, University of Saskatchewan, Saskatoon, Saskatchewan, Canada

SUNANDA KANE, MD, MSPH
Professor of Medicine, Mayo Clinic, Rochester, Minnesota

URI KOPYLOV, MD
IBD Fellow, Division of Gastroenterology, McGill University Health Center, Montreal, Quebec, Canada

YVETTE LEUNG, MD
Assistant Clinical Professor, Division of Gastroenterology, Department of Medicine, University of Calgary, Calgary, Alberta, Canada

BARRETT G. LEVESQUE, MS, MD
Robarts Clinical Trials Inc., London, Ontario, Canada; Division of Gastroenterology, University of California, San Diego, La Jolla, California

KIRK LIN, MD, MA
Gastroenterology Fellow, UCSF Center for Colitis and Crohn's Disease, Division of Gastroenterology, Department of Medicine, University of California, San Francisco, San Francisco, California

UMA MAHADEVAN, MD
Professor of Medicine, UCSF Center for Colitis and Crohn's Disease, Division of Gastroenterology, Department of Medicine, University of California, San Francisco, San Francisco, California

REMO PANACCIONE, MD
Professor, Division of Gastroenterology, Department of Medicine, University of Calgary, Calgary, Alberta, Canada

KONSTANTINOS A. PAPADAKIS, MD, PhD
Professor of Medicine, Division of Gastroenterology and Hepatology, Mayo Clinic, Rochester, Minnesota

DARRELL S. PARDI, MD, MS
Professor of Medicine, Inflammatory Bowel Disease Clinic, Division of Gastroenterology and Hepatology, Department of Internal Medicine, Mayo Clinic, Rochester, Minnesota

JUAN NICOLÁS PEÑA-SÁNCHEZ, MD, MPH, PhD(c)
Department of Medicine, School of Public Health, University of Saskatchewan, Saskatoon, Saskatchewan, Canada

LAURENT PEYRIN-BIROULET, MD, PhD
Inserm U954, Department of Hepato-Gastroenterology, Université de Lorraine, Vandoeuvre-lès-Nancy, France

MARK A. SAMAAN, MBBS
Robarts Clinical Trials Inc., London, Ontario, Canada; Department of Gastroenterology, Academic Medical Centre, Amsterdam, The Netherlands

WILLIAM J. SANDBORN, MD
Digestive Diseases Research Development Center, University of California San Diego; Division of Gastroenterology, Department of Medicine, Inflammatory Bowel Disease Center, University of California San Diego, La Jolla, California

MASAYUKI SARUTA, MD, PhD
Assistant Professor of Medicine, Division of Gastroenterology and Hepatology, Department of Internal Medicine, The Jikei University School of Medicine, Tokyo, Japan

COREY A. SIEGEL, MD, MS
Inflammatory Bowel Disease Center, Dartmouth-Hitchcock Medical Center, Lebanon, New Hampshire

SIDDHARTH SINGH, MD
Fellow, Inflammatory Bowel Disease Clinic, Division of Gastroenterology and Hepatology, Department of Internal Medicine, Mayo Clinic, Rochester, Minnesota

Contents

> Inflammatory bowel disease (IBD) is an immune-mediated disease and involves a complex interplay of host genetics and environmental influences. Recent advances in the field, including data from genome-wide association studies and microbiome analysis, have started to unravel the complex interaction between host genetics and environmental influences in the pathogenesis of IBD. A drawback of current clinical trials is inadequate or lack of immune phenotyping of patients. However, recent advances in high-throughput technologies provide an opportunity to monitor the dynamic and complex immune system, which may to lead to a more personalized treatment approach in IBD.

> The therapeutic approach in inflammatory bowel disease has evolved to target end-organ inflammation to heal intestinal mucosa and avoid structural damage. Objective therapeutic monitoring is required to achieve this goal. Earlier intervention with biologic therapy has been shown, indirectly, to be associated with higher clinical response and remission rates. A personalized approach to risk stratification with consideration of key clinical factors and inflammatory biomarker concentrations is recommended when deciding whether or not to start a patient on biologic therapy.

> Inflammatory bowel disease (IBD) treatment has progressed significantly over the past decade with the advent of biologics. Anti-tumor necrosis factor (anti-TNF) agents are the most widely available biologics, but the optimal approach when using them remains unclear. In this review, we highlight the currently available evidence regarding the use of anti-TNF monotherapy versus combination therapy with an immunomodulator. We focus on those patients at greatest risk for adverse events and outline the clinical approach when considering the use of combination therapy. We review the available tools through which providers may efficiently communicate these data to patients in the clinical setting.

Anti-tumor necrosis factor-α (TNF) agents, including infliximab, adalimumab, and certolizumab pegol, are effective medications for the management of moderate to severe Crohn disease (CD). They are effective in inducing and maintaining clinical remission, inducing mucosal healing, improving quality of life, and reducing the risk of hospitalization and surgery in adult and pediatric patients with CD. Future research into comparative effectiveness of different agents, as well as better understanding of predictors of response, is warranted to allow optimization of therapeutic response.

Anti-tumor necrosis factor-α agents are key therapeutic options for the treatment of ulcerative colitis. Their efficacy and safety have been shown in large randomized controlled trials. The key evidence gained from these trials of infliximab, adalimumab, and golimumab is reviewed along with their effect on mucosal healing and long-term outcomes. Also reviewed are methods for optimizing their effectiveness, including therapeutic drug monitoring and treat-to-target strategies. Finally, remaining unresolved questions regarding their role and effectiveness are considered including how these may be addressed in future clinical trials.

Biologic therapies, including anti–tumor necrosis factor antibody therapy and anti-integrin antibodies, are currently approved for the treatment of and are increasingly being used in patients with moderate to severe inflammatory bowel disease, including Crohn disease and ulcerative colitis. Because patients who require these medications are often in their childbearing years, knowledge of the safety of these medications before and after pregnancy is imperative. This article summarizes the available data regarding the use of biologic therapy during and after pregnancy, highlighting such issues as safety for mother and newborn, length of medication use during pregnancy, and breastfeeding after pregnancy while on biologic therapy.

An increasing proportion of patients with inflammatory bowel disease (IBD) are treated with biological medications. The risk of infectious complications remains a significant concern in patients treated with biologics. Treatment with biological agents in IBD is generally safe, but there may be an increased risk of certain opportunistic infections. Some of the infectious risks are class specific, whereas others are a common concern for all biologics. A careful screening, surveillance, and immunization program, in accordance with available guidelines, is important to minimize any risk of infectious complications.

In this review, the available data regarding the risk of lymphoma, skin cancers, and other malignancies associated with biological agents that are approved and those under investigation for use in inflammatory bowel disease (IBD) are highlighted. How providers may approach the use of these agents in various clinical scenarios is discussed. This review may help providers better understand the true risk of malignancy associated with these agents, thereby leading to an enhanced communication process with patients with IBD when therapeutic decisions are being made.

Anti-tumor necrosis factor-α (anti-TNF) agents are frequently used in the treatment of inflammatory bowel disease (IBD). Currently, there are 4 anti-TNF therapies that are Food and Drug Administration–approved for moderate to severe IBD: infliximab, adalimumab, golimumab, and certolizumab pegol. For most noninfectious, nonmalignant adverse events, cessation of anti-TNF therapy typically leads to improvement or resolution of drug-induced complications. In this article, the current knowledge regarding the noninfectious and nonmalignant toxicities associated with anti-TNF agents is summarized.

Biologic therapies, including the anti–tumor necrosis factor-α and cell adhesion molecule inhibitor drugs, have revolutionized the treatment of moderate-to-severe inflammatory bowel disease. Since the introduction of anti–tumor necrosis factor therapies, the strategy of empiric dose-escalation, either increasing the dose or frequency of administration, has been used to recapture clinical response in inflammatory bowel disease. Disparate clinical outcomes have been linked to serum drug and antidrug antibody levels. Therapeutic drug monitoring has emerged as a framework for understanding and responding to the variability in clinical response and remission.

Lymphocyte homing antagonists represent promising therapeutic agents for the treatment of idiopathic inflammatory bowel disease (IBD). Several critical molecules involved in the recruitment of inflammatory cells in the intestine, including integrins and chemokine receptors, have been successfully targeted for the treatment of IBD. These agents have shown great promise for the induction and maintenance of remission for both Crohn disease and ulcerative colitis. This article discusses currently approved prototypic agents for the treatment of IBD (natalizumab, anti-α4 integrin; vedolizumab, anti-α4β7 integrin), and several other agents in the same class currently under development.

Janus kinase (JAK) inhibitors have emerged as a novel orally administered small-molecule therapy for the treatment of ulcerative colitis and possibly Crohn disease. These molecules are designed to selectively target the activity of specific JAKs and to offer a targeted mechanism of action without risk of immunogenicity. Based on data from clinical trials in rheumatoid arthritis and phase 2 studies in inflammatory bowel disease, tofacitinib and other JAK inhibitors are likely to become a new form of medical therapy for the treatment of inflammatory bowel disease.

Despite the success of antitumor necrosis factor (TNF) therapy in Crohn's disease, there remains a need for biologic therapy that targets other immune pathways of disease. Ustekinumab is a fully human monoclonal immunoglobulin antibody that targets the interleukin (IL)-12 and IL-23 shared P40 subunit. It has been studied in 2 phase 2 randomized, double-blind, placebo-controlled trials in Crohn's disease. This article reviews the clinical efficacy and safety data of ustekinumab in Crohn's disease in anticipation of the final results of the phase III development program in moderate to severe Crohn's disease.

GASTROENTEROLOGY
CLINICS OF NORTH AMERICA

DOWNLOAD
Free App!

Review Articles
THE CLINICS

NOW AVAILABLE FOR YOUR iPhone and iPad

Foreword

Biologics of IBD

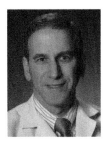

Gary W. Falk, MD, MS
Consulting Editor

The therapy of inflammatory bowel disease has changed dramatically in recent years with the advent of biologic therapy. Whereas therapy of inflammatory bowel disease once involved a simple menu of choices, such as corticosteroids, 5-ASA compounds, azathioprine, and surgery, the introduction of biologics has altered clinical practice. Current questions for both patients and physicians include the following:

1. When should biologic therapy be commenced?
2. What biologic is optimal?
3. What is the correct dosing?
4. How should therapy be monitored?
5. What are the risks of therapy including infection and neoplasia?
6. Are there new and better options on the horizon?

Ed Loftus from the Mayo Clinic has brought together an outstanding group of contributing authors to address these and other questions related to biologics in inflammatory bowel disease. These state-of-the-art articles will provide practical guidance for you as you navigate the rapidly changing world of inflammatory bowel disease therapy.

Gary W. Falk, MD, MS
Division of Gastroenterology
Hospital of the University of Pennsylvania
University of Pennsylvania Perelman School of Medicine
9 Penn Tower
One Convention Avenue
Philadelphia, PA 19104, USA

E-mail address:
gary.falk@uphs.upenn.edu

http://dx.doi.org/10.1016/j.gtc.2014.07.001
0889-8553/14/$ – see front matter © 2014 Elsevier Inc. All rights reserved.
gastro.theclinics.com

Preface

Biologic Therapy in Inflammatory Bowel Disease

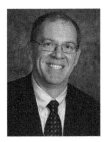

Edward V. Loftus Jr, MD
Editor

By the time this issue of *Gastroenterology Clinics of North America* is released, it will have been 16 years since infliximab was approved by the US Food and Drug Administration for the treatment of moderate to severe Crohn disease. Not only have we come a long way in understanding the efficacy and safety of infliximab, we are beginning to understand how and when to use the drug. Furthermore, as of this writing, we have five other biologic agents approved for either Crohn disease or ulcerative colitis, and there are many more molecules currently in drug development for these indications. In this issue, we have assembled a collection of experts to provide us the most cutting-edge information on the status of biologic therapy for inflammatory bowel disease (IBD).

In their article, Drs Maneesh Dave, Konstantinos Papadakis, and William Faubion of Mayo Clinic review what is known about perturbations in the epithelial barrier, the innate immune system, and the adaptive immune system in patients with IBD. Although this basic work may seem a bit esoteric to the practicing clinician, these back-breaking efforts have led to the identification of multiple useful drug targets, such as tumor necrosis factor-α (TNF-α), other cytokines (both pro-inflammatory and anti-inflammatory), integrins, adhesion molecules, and kinases.

Drs Jennifer Jones and Juan-Nicholas Pena-Sanchez of the University of Saskatchewan then review our current thinking about which IBD patients are eligible for biologic therapy. In general, we are using biologic agents earlier in the disease course, especially in patients deemed to be at high risk of intestinal complications. They nicely document our shift from a reactive, symptom-based therapeutic approach to a more proactive one based on objective markers of inflammation such as endoscopy. In the following article, Drs Parambir Dulai and Corey Siegel from Dartmouth-Hitchcock Medical Center and Dr Laurent Peyrin-Biroulet from the Université de Lorraine review the rationale for using anti-TNF drugs in combination with thiopurines or methotrexate in most cases. The combination of an anti-TNF agent and a thiopurine seems to be our

Gastroenterol Clin N Am 43 (2014) xv–xvii
http://dx.doi.org/10.1016/j.gtc.2014.06.001
0889-8553/14/$ – see front matter © 2014 Elsevier Inc. All rights reserved.

most efficacious combination of medication thus far. Most biologic agents are large protein molecules that are immunogenic, and it appears that combining them with a thiopurine reduces antidrug antibody formation and decreases clearance of the biologic. The authors remind us that we should be a little more wary of combination therapy in the elderly and in young men, but in certain high-risk patients in those demographics, combination therapy should still be considered.

In another article, Drs Siddarth Singh and Darrell Pardi of Mayo Clinic review the top-line efficacy results of infliximab, adalimumab, and certolizumab pegol in the treatment of Crohn disease. The authors also review data for secondary endpoints such as fistula healing, endoscopic improvement ("mucosal healing"), and health-related quality of life. Importantly, the use of these drugs is associated with statistically and clinically significant reductions in Crohn-related hospitalizations and surgeries. They also discuss the problems of primary nonresponse to anti-TNF therapy as well as secondary loss of response. Drs Mark Samaan, Preet Bagi, Niels Vande Casteele, and Geert D'Haens of the Amsterdam Medical Center and Dr Barrett Levesque of the University of California-San Diego review the efficacy of infliximab, adalimumab, and golimumab in the treatment of ulcerative colitis. The authors summarize not only the top-line efficacy data, such as clinical remission and response, but also important secondary endpoints, such as corticosteroid-free remission, mucosal healing, and reduction in ulcerative colitis–related hospitalizations and colectomies. The authors also compare the efficacy of infliximab and cyclosporine in the acute severe colitis setting. At the end of the article, the authors expand upon the concepts of "treat-to-target" and therapeutic drug monitoring, both of which are significantly altering the way we manage IBD patients.

Dr Sara Horst of Vanderbilt University Medical Center and Dr Sunanda Kane of Mayo Clinic provide an update on the use of biologic agents in pregnant women with IBD. They review how pregnancy impacts IBD and vice versa, the concept of placental transfer of biologic agents, and the safety of these agents in pregnant women with IBD and in mothers who are breastfeeding. The good news is that the anti-TNF agents appear to be safe for both the mother and the baby, and it may be wise to continue biologic therapy throughout the pregnancy.

Drs Uri Kopylov and Waqqas Afif of McGill University Health Center review infectious risks with biological agents, with specific emphasis on tuberculosis, granulomatous infections, fungal infections, and viral infections. The authors remind us of the small but real risk of progressive multifocal leukoencephalopathy in patients who are JC virus–positive and who have received the α-4 integrin antagonist, natalizumab, and that this serious neurologic complication has not been seen in patients treated with the gut-selective α-4 β-7 integrin antagonist, vedolizumab. They also discuss the role of keeping vaccinations up-to-date in our IBD patients, who are likely to receive immunosuppression at some point in their clinical course. In the article by Drs Dulai and Siegel of Dartmouth, they review what is known about the risk of cancer in IBD patients receiving biologic agents, with particular emphasis on the risk of lymphoma, nonmelanoma skin cancer, and melanoma. In contrast with the anti-TNF agents, no clearcut signal for increased malignancy risk has been detected with natalizumab or vedolizumab, but we probably need more person-years of observation on the drug to make any definite conclusions about this. Then, Drs Joseph Feuerstein and Adam Cheifetz of Beth Israel Deaconess Medical Center review what is known about other adverse events associated with these drugs, including infusion reactions (both acute and delayed), injection site reactions, autoimmune phenomena, such as drug-induced lupus, vasculitis, paradoxical arthritis, psoriasiform lesions, and demyelinating disorders.

Drs Kirk Lin and Uma Mahadevan of the University of California-San Francisco bring us up to speed on the current status of therapeutic drug monitoring of biologics. There are enormous interindividual differences in the pharmacokinetics of the biologics, and we can truly personalize our approach to each patient by periodically checking drug levels and the presence of antidrug antibodies and altering therapy accordingly. They present interesting data showing an inverse correlation between drug levels and objective markers of inflammation; in contrast, the presence of antidrug antibodies correlates with higher objective degrees of inflammation, loss of clinical response, and infusion reactions.

Dr Masayuki Saruta of the Jikei University School of Medicine and Dr Papadakis of Mayo Clinic review the lymphocyte trafficking pathway in intestinal inflammation and then provide us an update on drugs in this class, including the two already commercially available (natalizumab and vedolizumab), as well as a number of drugs in the development pipeline (including etrolizumab, PF-00547659, AMG181, and AJM300). Many of these drugs, including vedolizumab, etrolizumab, PF-00547659, and AMG181, appear to be gut-selective, and therefore, hold out the potential for a wider therapeutic window. Drs Brigid Boland, William Sandborn, and John Chang from the University of California-San Diego provide an update on Janus kinase inhibitors, including the one furthest along in drug development for IBD, tofacitinib. A phase 2 study of tofacitinib in ulcerative colitis was promising, leading to phase 3 trials. The authors also review potential side effects including opportunistic infections, dyslipidemia, and bone marrow suppression. In the final article, Drs Yvette Leung and Remo Panaccione of the University of Calgary review what is known about the efficacy and safety of the anti-IL-12/23 antibody, ustekinumab, for moderate to severe Crohn disease. Phase 2 trials of this drug in Crohn disease were promising, especially in the anti-TNF-exposed population, leading to ongoing phase 3 trials.

As you can see, considerable progress has been made in developing new therapies for our tough-to-treat IBD patients. We now have multiple drug targets and mechanisms of action. We are also beginning to better understand when to use the best drug in the best patient at the best time. More work needs to be done, however. We owe it to our patients.

Edward V. Loftus Jr, MD
Mayo Clinic College of Medicine
Inflammatory Bowel Disease Interest Group
Division of Gastroenterology and Hepatology
Mayo Clinic
200 First Street, South West
Rochester, MN 55905, USA

E-mail address:
loftus.edward@mayo.edu

Immunology of Inflammatory Bowel Disease and Molecular Targets for Biologics

CrossMark

Maneesh Dave, MBBS, MPH, Konstantinos A. Papadakis, MD, PhD,
William A. Faubion Jr, MD*

KEYWORDS

- Immunology • IBD • Biologics • Innate immunity • Adaptive immunity

KEY POINTS

- Most of the recent advances in inflammatory bowel disease (IBD) have resulted from studies of mucosal immunity in the normal and inflamed intestine.
- Both murine models of IBD and human studies have shown dysfunction of the epithelial barrier, innate immune cells, and adaptive T cells in the pathogenesis of IBD.
- The insight gained from the study of the aberrant immune system in IBD has led to the identification of molecular targets in the immune system for the design of drugs, some of which are already being used in clinical practice with many others in various phases of development.
- Despite the increased knowledge gained from animal and human studies, many aspects of mucosal immunity remain unclear in patients with IBD.
- Recently, significant progress has been made in high-throughput technologies like genomic sequencing and mass cytometry that provide multiparametric data which can be used to not just define the various immune cells states but also assess how these interact with each other in a variety of conditions.

INTRODUCTION

Inflammatory bowel disease (IBD), specifically Crohn disease (CD) and ulcerative colitis (UC), are autoimmune diseases whose incidence and prevalence are increasing worldwide.[1] Over the last few decades, substantial progress has been made in

Dr M. Dave is supported by an Inflammatory Bowel Disease Working Group research award. Dr W.A. Faubion's laboratory is supported by NIH (R01 AI089714). Dr K.A. Papadakis is supported by the Mayo Research Foundation.
Division of Gastroenterology and Hepatology, Mayo Clinic, 200 First Street Southwest, Rochester, MN 55905, USA
* Corresponding author.
E-mail address: faubion.william@mayo.edu

understanding the pathophysiology of IBD, which has been translated into newer, more effective therapies (biologics) that have reduced flares, brought more patients into remission, and improved the quality of life of patients with IBD.[2–4] IBD is considered to be an immune-mediated disease that involves a complex pattern/interplay of host genetics and environmental influences.[5] Our knowledge of the immune system and its homeostatic imbalance is derived from mouse models of colitis and human studies involving clinical and laboratory experiments.

The immune system evolved in multicellular organisms/metazoans as a defense mechanism against pathogens like bacteria, protozoa, parasites, and fungi.[6] The human immune system can be broadly categorized into innate and adaptive based on the differences in timing of the response and specificity. The immune system comes in contact with a foreign challenge, which could be food, commensal flora, microbial pathogens, and xenobiotics at different sites like the skin, mucous membrane of lungs, gastrointestinal tract, and so forth. The human gastrointestinal tract, with a total surface area roughly equal to that of a tennis court (400 m^2), serves as the largest area of interface with the external environment. The gut mucosal immune system, which interacts with this large antigenic load, thus, has the most varied immune cells in the body. In a disease-free host, there is a fine balance between a protective and deleterious response of the immune system, which becomes perturbed in patients with IBD. To understand these perturbations in IBD that produce a disease state, it is necessary to first understand how the intestinal immune system works. In this review, the authors divide their article into subsections of innate and adaptive immunity and link it with the currently identified abnormalities in these pathways in IBD. In addition, the authors have summarized in **Table 1** the current and emerging therapies for IBD that target specific molecules in the immune system.

INNATE INTESTINAL IMMUNITY
Epithelial Barrier

The gastrointestinal tract has a continuous layer of single epithelial cells that are derived from a common progenitor LGR5+ intestinal stem cell.[7] The epithelial cells comprise enterocytes (intestinal absorptive cells), goblet cells, neuroendocrine cells, Paneth cells, and microfold (M) cells.[7] The epithelial cells are sealed with intercellular tight junctions that serve a barrier function and regulate the trafficking of macromolecules between the luminal environment and the host.[8] The tight junctions are composed of a meshwork of proteins like occludin, claudin family members, and the junctional adhesion molecule,[8] with zonulin as one of the physiologic modulators (of tight junctions) that controls intestinal permeability.[9] The luminal surface is covered by a thick layer of mucus, which is produced by goblet cells. Mucus is rich in secreted immunoglobulin A (IgA) antibodies,[10] proteins with antibacterial activity (ie, α- and β-defensins),[11] and proteolytic and glycolytic enzymes[12] that form the first line of defense against invasion by foreign pathogens. In spite of this barrier, gut bacteria and luminal antigens do enter the subepithelial lamina propria (an extracellular matrix compartment that contains a variety of immune and nonimmune cells), with some entering through unwanted breaks but most through the specialized, follicle-associated epithelium (FAE) that overlies the organized lymphoid tissue of the gut (gut-associated lymphoid tissue [GALT]). GALT consists of organized lymphoid compartments (Peyer patches, mesenteric lymph nodes, isolated lymphoid follicles, cryptopatches) and dispersed lymphoid cells in lamina propria and intraepithelial spaces.[13] The FAE overlies the large lymphoid aggregates called Peyer patches and, compared with other parts of intestinal epithelium, is devoid of goblet cells and has a lower

Table 1
Some of the key biologic molecules in active use or under study for treatment of IBD

Biologic Target	Antibody/Drug	Mechanism of Action	CD, UC, or Both
CCR9	CCX282-B	Inhibition of CCR9	CD
	CCX 025	Inhibition of CCR9	CD
IL-21	PF 05230900	IL-21 receptor antagonist	CD
IL-13	QAX576	IL-13 antagonist	CD
	Anrukinzumab	IL-13 antagonist	UC
	Tralokinumab	IL-13 antagonist	UC
IL-17	Vidofludimus	Inhibitor of IL-17 A and IL-17F	Both
IL-12/23	Ustekinumab	Blockade of IL-12/23	CD
IL-18	GSK1070806	Blockade of soluble IL-18	CD
IL-6 and IL-6R	Tocilizumab	Inhibitor of IL -6	CD
	PF04236921	Inhibitor of IL -6	CD
IP-10	MDX 1100	Blockade of interferon-γ inducible protein (IP-10 or CXCL10)	UC
IRAK4/TRAF6/ MyD88	RDP58	Disrupts IRAK4/TRAF6/MyD88 signaling and reduces production of proinflammatory cytokines	Both
JAK3	Tofacitinib	Inhibition of JAK3	Both
MAdCAM-1	PF-547659	Blocks MAdCAM-1	Both
NF-κB	HE3286	Synthetic steroid that modulates NF-κB activity	UC
NKG2D	NN8555	Anti-NKG2D receptor monoclonal antibody	CD
PKC	AEB071/Sotrastaurin	PKC inhibitor	UC
T Cell	Laquinimod	Reduces IL-17 level and interferes with migration of T cells	CD
TLR	DIMS0150	Blockade of Toll-like receptor	UC
	BL-7040	Blockade of Toll-like receptor	UC
TNF-α	Infliximab	Neutralization of TNF-α	Both
	Adalimumab	Neutralization of TNF-α	Both
	Certolizumab pegol	Neutralization of TNF-α	CD
	Golimumab	Neutralization of TNF-α	UC
	Debiaerse	Vaccine against TNF-α consisting of a TNF-α derivative TNF-α kinoid	CD
Effector T cells, B cells	Antigen specific Type 1 regulatory cells (OvaSave)	Autologous ova expanded regulatory T cells injected	CD
α4 integrin	AJM-300	Blockade of α4 integrin	CD
α4 integrin	Natalizumab	Blockade of α4 integrin	Both
α4β7 integrin	Vedolizumab	Blockade of α4β7 integrin	Both
β7 integrin	Etrolizumab (aka rHuMab β7)	Anti-β7 integrin	UC

Abbreviations: aka, also known as; CCR9, chemokine receptor 9; IL, interleukin; IP, inducible protein; IRAK-4, interleukin-1 receptor-associated kinase 4; JAK3, Janus kinase 3; MAdCAM-1, human mucosal addressin cell adhesion molecule-1; MyD88, myeloid differentiation primary response 88; NF-κB, nuclear factor-κB; PKC, protein kinase C; TLR, Toll-like receptor; TNF-α, tumor necrosis factor-α; TRAF6, TNF receptor-associated factor 6, E3 ubiquitin protein ligase.

concentration of brush border enzymes. The FAE also contains unique highly specialized epithelial cells called M cells that actively pinocytose or endocytose selected luminal macromolecules into underlying lymphoid follicles, thus, facilitating transepithelial transport.[13] M cells, in comparison with enterocytes, have irregular microvilli, decreased alkaline phosphatase activity,[14] and no IgA secretory component.[15] Immediately below the FAE is the subepithelial dome region that overlies the lymphoid follicle containing large numbers of dendritic cells (DCs). The antigens and microorganisms transported through M cells are captured by these DCs, which then present antigenic peptides to interfollicular T cells or naïve T cells within the mesenteric lymph nodes (**Fig. 1**). Paneth cells are epithelial cells found at the base of the small intestinal crypt that can sense luminal microbiota and antigens to secrete antimicrobial peptides and contribute to innate host immunity.[16,17]

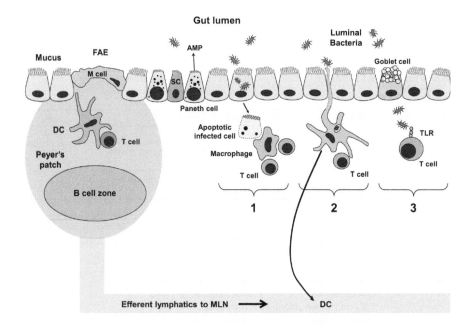

Fig. 1. Basic organizational structure of the small intestine mucosal immune system. On the left of the figure is FAE. The main functional component of the FAE is the M cell, which is specialized in transepithelial antigen transport. DCs and antigen-presenting cells (APC) take up these transported antigens and then present them to naïve T cells. A single layer of epithelial cells that are derived from a common progenitor LGR5+ intestinal stem cell (SC) act as a barrier against the pathogens and foreign antigens. The Paneth cells are found in base of small intestine crypts and secrete antimicrobial peptides (AMP). Goblet cells secrete mucus that limits exposure of intestinal epithelium to bacteria. Immune cells present in the mucosa include macrophages, DCs, T cells, intraepithelial lymphocytes, IgA-secreting plasma cells, atypical lymphocytes, B cells, and stromal cells. The right side of the figure depicts the likely pathways through which bacterial antigens can activate mucosal T cells: (1) apoptosis of infected epithelial cells; (2) luminal sampling and acquisition of bacteria by mucosal DCs; and (3) direct contact of translocated bacteria with T cells mediated by Toll-like receptor (TLR) recognition. APCs like the DC on activation migrate through the efferent lymphatics to the mesenteric lymph nodes, where they interact with naïve T cells and induce 2 surface molecules, $\alpha 4\beta 7$ integrin and the chemokine receptor CCR9, that induce homing of T cells back to the gut (site of activation of DC). MLN, mesenteric lymph node.

Innate Immune Cells

The cells of the innate immune system, in contrast to the adaptive immune system, have a rapid and less specific response to invading microorganisms or toxic macromolecules. This response is mediated by pathogen recognition receptors (PRR), which are membrane-bound (ie, Toll-like receptors [TLRs], C-type lectin receptor) or cytoplasmic (ie, nucleotide-binding oligomerization domain family members [NODs], retinoic acid–inducible gene 1–like receptor). These receptors are germ-line encoded, invariable, and predetermined to recognize a repertoire of bacterially/virally associated carbohydrate and lipid structures leading to the rapidity of response. The microbial molecules recognized by these receptors are called pathogen-associated molecular patterns (PAMPs) (eg, lipopolysaccharide and peptidoglycan). The PAMPs are highly conserved molecules on microbes as they are central to survival. These receptors also recognize endogenous or self-danger signals (eg, heat-shock proteins, uric acid), which are known as damage-associated molecular pattern molecules. The professional phagocytic cells (macrophages, dendritic cells and neutrophils), eosinophils, and lymphoid cells have immediate bactericidal activity; in the following paragraphs, the authors present data on these cells and their functions.

Macrophages

Macrophages are phagocytic cells present throughout the gastrointestinal mucosa, with the GALT containing the largest reservoir of macrophages within the adult mouse.[18] Macrophages are derived from peripheral blood monocytes and are recruited to the intestine by chemoattractants, chemokines, and bacterial degradation products. Macrophages mature after migrating to intestinal mucosa,[19] in contrast to neutrophils that are produced and lost in large numbers each day. In the noninflamed mucosa, macrophages differ from peripheral monocytes in their downregulated proinflammatory function, characterized by hyporesponsiveness to TLR ligands, diminished ability to prime adaptive immune responses, but still preserved capacity for phagocytosis and intracellular killing.[19] However, in the setting of pathogen invasion and inflammation, intestinal macrophages freshly recruited from blood monocytes rapidly convert to a proinflammatory phenotype by ligation of their PRR. This proinflammatory phenotype is marked by abundant cytokine production (interleukin [IL]-1, IL-6, IL-8 and tumor necrosis factor [TNF]-alpha) and accessory cell function, instead of a primarily scavenger function. Once activated, the macrophages express receptors specific for opsonized particles and pathogens, complement, and common bacterial proteins (ie, mannose receptor, TLR, NOD). Pathogens are recognized by these receptors, which lead to their phagocytosis and subsequent intracellular killing. In addition, the activated macrophages secrete cytokines, which are proteins that affect the function of other cells in the absence of cell contact. Transforming growth factor beta (TGF-β), a cytokine produced by activated macrophages, is a potent chemoattractant for other macrophages and neutrophils and, hence, augments the recruitment of these cells to sites of inflammation.[20] Cytokine secretion not only augments the phagocytic intracellular killing but also serves as a critical link between the 2 arms (ie, innate and adaptive of the immune system) and plays an important role in gut homeostasis and inflammation.[21] For simplicity, macrophages had been broadly divided into inflammatory M1 and wound-healing M2; but recently, this view is being replaced by one of considerable plasticity of macrophages wherein they acquire distinct functions of host defense, wound healing, and immune regulation based on environmental cues they encounter. So they are considered a highly heterogeneous population of cells with a continuum of activation states.[22,23]

DCs

DCs are phagocytic cells, which, like the macrophages, originate from blood mono-cytes or a common DC progenitor in the bone marrow. DCs have the most potent abil-ity to initiate adaptive immune responses against pathogens. Current evidence supports that intestinal DCs continuously migrate in an immature or tolerogenic state, form scavenging apoptotic cells, and acquire antigens sampled either directly from the lumen[24] or shuttled from the lumen through M cells (see **Fig. 1**).[25] After the acquisition of antigen, DCs process it within, load the antigenic peptide onto major histocompat-ibility complex (MHC) class II molecules, and display this complex on its cell surface. DCs then migrate to the draining mesenteric lymph nodes where they present a partic-ular MHC-peptide complex to T cells bearing the T cell receptor (TCR) specific for the antigen being presented. In a normal physiologic state, these antigen-loaded DCs (in-testinal DCs) express low levels of costimulatory molecules and cytokines and, on contact with T cells, preferentially stimulate their differentiation into T regulatory cells (Tregs) that produce antiinflammatory cytokines IL-4, IL-10, and TGF-β. In contrast, when intestinal DCs are activated in a proinflammatory microenvironment, they migrate to T cell areas of the GALT, where they induce effector rather than tolerogenic T-cell responses. The DCs isolated from these sites express high levels of costimula-tory molecules and adhesion molecules and produce large amounts of cytokines.[26] The intestinal DCs can then induce the mucosal homing receptor α4β7 and the che-mokine receptor CCR9 on T cells, suggesting that they can instruct a T cell to home back to the original site of the DC's activation.[27,28]

Atypical lymphocytes

The atypical lymphocytes γδT cells and natural killer T cells (NKT) are also a part of the innate immune response. T cells normally express alpha and beta TCR chains; but when they express gamma and delta TCR chains (γδT cells), they are considered atyp-ical lymphocytes.[29] These γδT cells only exist in significant numbers in the epithelial tissues and constitute greater than 10% of small intestinal intraepithelial lymphocytes, with the remaining majority being CD8+ T cells.[29] The γδT cells, unlike the conven-tional T cells, do not depend on the thymus for development[30] and do not recognize antigen in association with MHC class I or II.[31] The γδT cells perform different func-tions, including acting as effectors against pathogens and tumors and as professional antigen-presenting cells (APCs); but their role depends on tissue distribution and the local microenvironment.[32,33] NKT cells are a subset of T cells that mature in the thymus and recognize lipid antigen (presumably bacterial) presented on the MHC-like complex Cd1d.[34] On activation, they secrete large quantities of proinflammatory cytokines and readily kill infected cells or tumor cells. NKT cells that produce large amounts of proinflammatory cytokine IL-13 have been found in the intestine of pa-tients with UC[35] and are also the mediators of inflammation in the oxazolone-induced murine model of colitis, which resembles UC.[5]

EVIDENCE FOR INNATE IMMUNE CELLULAR DYSFUNCTION IN THE PATHOGENESIS OF IBD

There are multiple lines of evidence that indicate a major role for innate immune cells in the perpetuation of human chronic intestinal inflammation. The most recent meta-analysis of genome-wide association studies (GWAS) in IBD has implicated multiple susceptibility genes involved in innate mucosal defense (NOD2, CARD9, REL, SLC1A) and antigen presentation (ERAP2, LNPEP). Indeed, one of the strongest ge-netic associations to date with small bowel CD is the loss-of-function polymorphisms in the bacterial sensing gene CARD15/NOD2.[36,37] The dysfunction secondary to

NOD2 mutation has been reported in Paneth cells[38] and monocytes.[39] It seems that dysregulation in the detection of and/or responsiveness to enteric bacteria by innate immune and epithelial cells promotes chronic inflammation in this subgroup of patients. More evidence for their role rests in the efficacy of immune therapy targeted against proinflammatory cytokines produced by innate immune cells. Activated macrophages produce large quantities of TNF-α and IL-12, which are 2 cytokines responsible for the recruitment and activation of pathogenic effector T cells. The efficacy of anti–TNF-α therapy in IBD is well established,[40,41] and promising anti–IL-12/23 studies are ongoing.[42,43]

Another feature in patients with CD is a defective inflammatory response to injury and bacterial products, as evidenced by decreased neutrophil infiltration, lower production of proinflammatory interleukins (IL-8 and IL-1β), and reduced vascular flow as compared with healthy individuals.[44] In addition to defective acute response, there is failure of clearance of bacteria and inflammatory debris, which indicates a disruption in the autophagy pathway. Autophagy (or self-eating) is a process that involves degradation and recycling of intracellular contents and removal of intracellular microbes and is mediated by lysosomes.[45] The GWAS first pointed to the role of autophagy in CD pathogenesis, with many CD-associated genetic loci lying within the category of autophagy homeostatic function (eg, ATG16L1 and IRGM).[46,47] Homozygosity for the ATG16L1 risk allele contributes to Paneth cell dysfunction in mice and humans, but mice do not develop spontaneous intestinal inflammation. Another pathway interconnected with autophagy and that affects intestinal epithelial cells of patients with IBD is unfolded protein response (UPR) from endoplasmic reticulum (ER) stress. Most of the secreted and membrane proteins enter the ER where they fold and assemble with only properly folded proteins exiting the ER via vesicles.[48] When the unfolded proteins accumulate in the ER, it may lead to ER stress and activation of signaling pathways collectively known as UPR that help mitigate the stress.[48] Not only the intestines of patients with IBD have evidence of endoplasmic reticulum (ER) stress[49] but multiple ER stress-related genes like XBP1 have been associated with IBD.[50] Genetic deletion of XBP1 in the intestinal epithelial cells of mice results in the depletion of Paneth cells, inflammatory hyperresponsiveness to TNF-alpha, and spontaneous enteritis.[51]

EVIDENCE FOR BARRIER DYSFUNCTION AND EPITHELIAL INJURY IN THE PATHOGENESIS OF IBD

Numerous studies have shown that disruption of the epithelial barrier may either initiate or perpetuate chronic intestinal inflammation.[46–49] Abnormal intestinal permeability has been established among patients with CD[52,53] and their healthy first-degree relatives[54,55] and may represent a primary abnormality predisposing to excessive antigen uptake, continuous immune stimulation, and eventually mucosal inflammation. Animal models like SAMP1/YitFc have increased intestinal permeability before the development of spontaneous ileitis,[56] and GWAS studies have identified as a CD risk locus MUC19, whose product comprises the intestinal mucous layer.[57] Barrier dysfunction has been directly observed by confocal endomicroscopy in a cohort of patients with IBD, and this dysfunction is predictive of IBD relapse within 12 months of microscopy.[58] The etiologic factors for barrier dysfunction in CD may be environmental or genetic.[59] Diet and nonsteroidal antiinflammatory drugs can affect gut permeability and are variably associated with IBD.[60–63] Furthermore, polymorphic variants in several IBD-associated genes (DLG5, JAK2, HNF4A) seem to primarily affect epithelial permeability and may lead to inappropriate exposure of the mucosal immune system to luminal antigens.[50,64,65] Additionally, epithelial cell death, particularly of

Paneth cells, has been demonstrated to induce terminal ileal inflammation in mice with conditional deletion of caspase-8 in the intestinal epithelium and is associated with CD in humans.[66]

ADAPTIVE INTESTINAL IMMUNITY
T Cells

CD4+ and CD8+ T cells bearing the conventional $\alpha\beta$ TCR are nearly equally represented in the intestinal lamina propria. The intraepithelial space contains unusual T-cell populations that bear the $\gamma\delta$ TCR and CD8+ cells with $\alpha\alpha$ homodimeric expression of TCR. In human and experimental models of IBD, the activated CD4+ TCR $\alpha\beta$ T cells play an essential role in the disease pathogenesis. On maturation in the thymus, naïve T cells (cells that have not yet been exposed to an antigen) circulate in the lymphatic tissues in search of cognate MHC-peptide complex. Naïve T cells constitutively express the selectin CD62L (L-selectin) and the chemokine receptor 7 (CCR7), whereas the endothelial cells of high endothelial venules (HEV) in lymph nodes express vascular addressins like CD34, glycosylation-dependent cell adhesion molecule-1 (GlyCAM-1), and the chemokine ligand 21.[67] The interaction of CD62L and CD34 (among other glycosylated endothelial molecules) promotes a rolling action of the T cell across the endothelial surface. The chemokines present at the luminal surface of HEV activate the surface adhesion molecules like leukocyte function-associated antigen 1 (LFA-1) on T cells. The binding of LFA-1 (on T cells) to the receptors intercellular adhesion molecules (ICAM-1 and ICAM-2) on endothelial cells promotes firm adhesion of T cells and their crossing of the endothelial lining into the lymphoid tissue. Within the underlying lymphoid tissue are DCs loaded with antigen that also secrete chemokines like chemokine (C-C motif) ligand 19 (CCL19, a ligand for CCR7 on T cells) that retain T cells in lymph nodes. Naïve T cells, after entering the lymphoid tissue, scan the surfaces of DCs for a recognizable MHC-peptide complex. If none is found, the cells exit the lymph node, return to the circulation, and reenter other nodes to repeat the process. T cells egress the lymph node (LN) secondary to a concentration gradient of sphingosine-1-phosphate (S1P), which is kept low inside the LN and is at a high concentration in blood and efferent lymphatics. Once a naïve T cell encounters a cognate antigen through its TCR, it gets activated. The complete T-cell activation requires 2 signals: signal 1 is mediated by TCR stimulation, and signal 2 is a costimulatory signal provided by accessory pathways. Costimulation via CD28 (on T cells) and B7.1 or B7.2 (on APC) results in T-cell activation, whereas the costimulation mediated by cytotoxic T-lymphocyte antigen 4 (CTLA-4) (on T cells) by B7.1 or B7.2 results in T cell inhibition. If TCR signaling occurs in the absence of costimulation, it results in anergic T cells (ie, lack of response on reexposure to the same antigen in the future). On activation, CD4+ T cells secrete a particular set of cytokines that determine the type of ensuing immune response and the phenotype of the mature effector T cells. New data continue to enhance our understanding of this complex event, with the most recent data summarized as follows. CD4+ T cells activated in the presence of IL-12 and the absence of IL-4 acquire a T helper 1 (Th1) phenotype, resulting in interferon-γ (IFN-γ)–producing cells effective in the control of intracellular pathogens. CD4+ T cells activated in the presence of IL-4 acquire a Th2 phenotype, generating IL-4–, IL-5–, and IL-13–producing cells effective in the clearance of parasitic infections and allergic responses. Activation in the presence of IL-6, TGF-β, and IL-23 results in cells expressing the Th17 phenotype (ie, IL-17 and IL-6 producing T cells responsible for acute inflammation and recruitment of granulocytes) (**Fig. 2**).[68,69] The activation of T cells and their clonal expansion in lymphoid tissue takes 4 to 5 days; during this process, the T cells

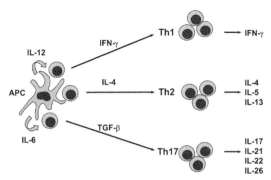

Fig. 2. T-helper (Th) cell differentiation. The naïve T cells differentiate into 3 major types of effector Th cells (Th1, Th2, and Th17). The ultimate functional phenotype of mature effector T cells depends on the type and amount of antigen and the cytokine milieu present at the time of activation. CD was traditionally thought to be the result of aberrant Th1 responses because of increased mucosal levels of interferon γ (IFN-γ), IL-2, and IL-12. However, recent evidence has supported a prominent role for a second Th subset, Th17, as IL-17 and IL-22 are increased in inflamed mucosa of patients with CD. Similarly, UC was thought to be a Th2-mediated disease because of increased mucosal levels of IL-5 and IL-13. However, patients with UC exhibit decreased production of mucosal IL-4 (Th2 cytokine), and natural killer T cells may be responsible for the aberrant production of IL-13. APC, antigen-presenting cell; IL, interleukins; TGF-β, transforming growth factor-β.

downregulate their surface S1P1 receptor to prevent egress from the LN.[70] As T-cell activation wanes and on maturation, the surface S1P1 receptor is upregulated and the effector T cells leave the lymph node returning to the circulation (higher concentration of S1P).[71] On activation, T cells express unique adhesion molecules that direct the T cells to the sites of inflammation[72]; indeed, T cells primed by mucosal DCs are destined to return to the gut through the upregulation of 2 surface molecules, α4β7 integrin and the chemokine receptor CCR9.[28,72] The integrin α4 binds to vascular adhesion molecule 1 (VCAM-1), a molecule expressed on vascular endothelium only at sites of inflammation. The α4β7 integrin recognizes vascular endothelial molecule mucosal addressin adhesion molecule-1, which is upregulated at sites of intestinal inflammation in IBD and, hence, directs migration of effector T cells to the intestinal lamina propria.[73,74] Within the intestinal tissue, recognition of cognate antigen by effector T cells results in the production of proinflammatory cytokines like TNF-α. TNF-α in turn stimulates endothelial cells to upregulate adhesion molecules like E-selectin (recruits monocytes and neutrophils) and VCAM-1 and ICAM-1 (both of which recruit activated T cells). In addition, TNF-α and IFN-γ alter the blood flow, endothelial cell shape, and vascular permeability to enhance the migration of inflammatory cells into the tissue. The inflammatory cascades set in motion by activated T cells lead to significant structural alterations in the inflamed tissue, including ulceration, which eventually triggers the signs and symptoms characteristic of active IBD.

Tregs

In both mice and humans, there is a subpopulation of CD4+ T cells with regulatory potential that restrain not only effector T cells but also innate inflammatory leukocytes.[75] Although there are many different subpopulations of Tregs, the 3 major and not necessarily mutually exclusive subtypes of Tregs are as follows: the naturally occurring CD4+CD25+ cell, the IL-10– and TGF-β–producing Tr1 cell, and the TGF-β–producing Th3 cell derived through oral tolerance.[76] The most-studied Treg cell type is the

CD4+CD25+ T cell expressing the transcription factor forkhead box protein P3 (FOXP3). This cell type has been conclusively shown to suppress mucosal inflammation and murine colitis[77,78]; however, its function in patients with IBD is less well understood, as patients with IBD have more FOXP3+ Tregs at the site of intestinal inflammation[79] and retain potent suppressor activity ex vivo.[80,81] There is evidence that effector T cells obtained from patients with IBD are refractory to suppression by Tregs, but this area requires further study.[82,83]

B Cells

B cells have a membrane-bound immunoglobulin that serves as the B cell receptor for an antigen. A terminally differentiated B cell called plasma cell secretes an immunoglobulin of the same antigen specificity (known as antibody). In GALT, B cells work in collaboration with the epithelium to export secretory IgA (sIgA) and, to some extent, secretory IgM to enhance the mucosal defense from intestinal pathogens. Mucosal B cells exhibit a predominant IgA class switch and, on differentiation to mature plasma cells, produce approximately 3 g of sIgA per day.[84] More than 80% of all human plasma cells are found in the gut, and nearly all of these plasma cells produce IgA.[85] Mucosal plasma cells produce primarily dimeric or polymeric forms of IgA. The joining or J chain of polymeric IgA spontaneously interacts with the polymeric immunoglobulin receptor expressed on the basolateral surface of epithelial cells facilitating exportation of the sIgA to the gastrointestinal lumen.[86] Once in the lumen, the sIgA functions mainly to inhibit the adhesion of viruses and bacteria to the epithelium by agglutinating the bacteria and other antigens, trapping them in the mucous layer, and facilitating their removal from the host. sIgA also promotes M cell–mediated bacterial uptake and target presentation to intestinal DCs and macrophages to provide a positive feedback loop to enhance secretory immunity.[87]

EVIDENCE FOR ADAPTIVE IMMUNE CELLULAR DYSFUNCTION IN THE PATHOGENESIS OF IBD

A multitude of studies strongly support the view that activated CD4+ T cells are a central feature of human IBD. First, T cell–driven animal models of colitis mimic human IBD in both histologic features and responsiveness to similar treatment regimens.[35,88–90] In human IBD, Th17 cells that secrete IL-17 and IL-22 are increased in inflamed patients with CD,[91,92] and an IL-23 receptor variant associated with CD impairs the IL-23–induced Th17 effector function and is a protective genetic variant.[93] In addition, the established and emerging therapies for human IBD are directed toward the destruction of activated effector T cells or the blockade of T cell–derived proinflammatory cytokines.[94] Fourth, clonal populations of T cells (ie, expansion of T cells in response to persistent and specific antigens) have been described in patients with CD in comparison to normal controls.[95] In an animal model of IBD, similar T-cell clones that specifically recognize endogenous gut bacteria have been described.[96] These T-cell clones have pathogenic potential and mediate colitis when transferred into noncolitic recipient mice.[96] Finally, patients with IBD have antibodies directed against particular microbial antigens that point to a pathogenic adaptive immune responses against the intestinal flora.[97]

PUTTING IT ALL TOGETHER: INTEGRATING GUT MICROBES, EPITHELIAL CELLS, LYMPHOCYTES, AND HOST GENETICS IN THE PATHOGENESIS OF IBD

Our knowledge of the human gut microbiota has made rapid strides in the last decade,[98] and the role of the microbiome in both immune system development and function is being increasingly understood.[99] Indeed, the presence of intestinal bacteria is required for the development of inflammation in most animal models of IBD[100,101]; most patients with IBD have antibodies to bacterial antigens. The data from GWAS have yielded important and comprehensive new insights into the pathogenesis of IBD (as an example autophagy pathway) and have implicated the host-microbiota interaction as the driver of disease. **Fig. 3** summarizes the important susceptibility loci identified through GWAS that contribute to the unique and/or combined risk for CD and/or UC.

Similar to the innate immune cells, intestinal epithelial cells constitutively express PRRs like TLR2 and 4 to sense gut bacteria.[102] The interaction between the commensal flora and TLRs enhances the integrity of the intestinal barrier and has been shown to protect against a chemical (dextran sodium sulfate [DSS]) epithelial injury model of colitis.[103,104] The epithelial cells also have NOD1 and NOD2 (intracellular PRRs), with the NOD2 protein shown to have an antibacterial effect in infected epithelial cell lines.[105] Paneth cells in terminal ileum are a very abundant source of NOD2 protein; polymorphisms in NOD2, especially in Paneth cells, have been show to decrease the production of alpha defensins by these cells.[106,107] Paneth cells from NOD2$^{-/-}$ mice have impaired antimicrobial function; but these mice develop

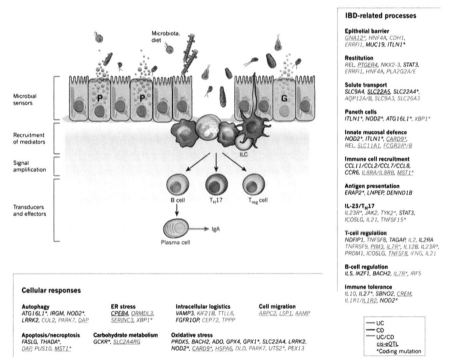

Fig. 3. The illustration shows a model for IBD pathways based on GWAS. Genes that are in linkage disequilibrium with GWAS identified single nucleotide polymorphisms (associated with IBD) were classified according to their function in intestinal inflammation. Text color indicates whether the genes are linked to risk loci associated with CD (*black*), UC (*blue*), or both (*red*). The asterisk denotes corresponding coding mutations; cis-eQTL effects are underlined. G, goblet cell; P, Paneth cell. (*From* Khor B, Gardet A, Xavier RJ. Genetics and pathogenesis of inflammatory bowel disease. Nature 2011;474(7351):309; with permission.)

granulomatous inflammation of the ileum only on inoculation with *Helicobacter hepaticus*, highlighting the role of host genetics and microbial interactions in the development of IBD.[108] Another classic example of gene-environment interaction in IBD is the ATG16L1 allele (T300A) variant, a CD risk-associated allele, which is present in approximately 50% of the Caucasian population but does not cause IBD in a vast majority. The ATG16L1 allele (T300 A in humans and T316A in mice) variant has been shown to affect Paneth cell function in ATG16L1 hypomorph mice (ATG16L1[HM]) that are infected with a murine norovirus (MNV CR6).[109] The ATG16L1[HM] mice derived in an enhanced barrier facility (absence of MNV CR6) do not develop Paneth cell abnormalities. The ATG16L1[HM] mice infected with MNV CR6 only have enhanced susceptibility but do not develop spontaneous intestinal inflammation. A recent study showed that in the presence of cellular stress, caused by starvation or infection with a bacteria like *Yersinia enterocolitica*, resulted in Caspase-3-mediated degradation of the ATG16L1 protein. This degradation of ATG16L1 resulted in impaired autophagy and production of proinflammatory cytokines like TNF-α and IL-1β.[110] The signaling pathways downstream of TLRs, NOD2 lead to dysfunction of autophagy, ER stress response and activation of nuclear factor-κB responsive genes that mediate inflammatory response. An excellent paper provides an in-depth review of these pathways.[111]

The pathogenic and commensal flora interacts with immune cells of the GALT in multiple ways (see **Fig. 1**). First, infected epithelial cells may undergo apoptosis (either spontaneously or killed by effector immune cells); apoptotic fragments containing bacteria may be ingested by resident phagocytic cells (macrophages and DCs) and subsequently presented to host T cells.[112] Second, DCs and macrophages may acquire bacteria directly from the environment and present bacterial antigen on MHC class II to CD4+ T cells. Third, Tregs may contact bacterial antigens directly through their TLRs in the absence of APCs and modify their function.[113] It has been demonstrated that DCs are activated in the mucosa of patients with CD, with upregulation of their PRR in contrast to controls.[26] In the Tbx21$^{-/-}$ X Rag 2$^{-/-}$ ulcerative colitis (TRUC) model, DCs that are deficient in transcription factor T bet secrete large amounts of TNF-α which results in increased epithelial permeability and injury leading to colitis.[114] The colitis is transmitted from the affected mother to not just her progeny but also wild-type mice (genetically intact) progeny cross-fostered from birth, thus, highlighting the role of colitogenic flora in the development of colitis.[114]

It is thought that the reduction in infectious diseases and reduced exposure to microbes in the industrialized world has led to an increase in the incidence of immunologically mediated diseases, such as IBD, type I diabetes, and asthma, over the last few decades.[115] An elegant study has shown that germ-free (GF) mice[116] have increased invariant NKT (iNKT) cells in colonic mucosa as compared with specific pathogen-free mice; this results in more severe oxazolone-induced colitis in GF mice, which is the opposite of murine models that depend on adaptive immunity (reduced disease severity in GF mice).[116] This change in NKT cells is stable throughout life; in fact, colonization with conventional microbiota protects against colitis in neonatal GF mice but not in adult mice.[116] This study highlights the role of early life exposure to microbes as important in developing adult iNKT cell tolerance.

The adaptive immune system first emerged in vertebrates.[99,117] The main characteristics of the adaptive immune system (ie, ability to respond to a wide variety of antigens and to have long-lived memory to those antigens) also facilitated the coevolution of a diverse and more complex microbiota as compared with invertebrates.[99] A more diverse microbiota is advantageous for the vertebrates who extend their metabolic capacity (intestinal microbiota has 100 times the number of human genes) and can harvest energy from a wider selection of foods. The adaptive arm of the immune system allows tailoring of the immune response toward microbiota as either symbiosis or one of host defense. Dysregulation of this crosstalk can lead to autoimmune diseases like IBD. An example of the dynamic interaction of microbiota with adaptive immunity is in the role of Th17 cells in IBD. Patients with CD have been shown to have increased Th17 cells; hence, anti–IL-17 antibody (secukinumab) was tried as a therapeutic strategy. Unexpectedly, secukinumab resulted in the worsening of CD and more adverse events in treated patients, which was attributed to the complex biology of Th17 cells.[118] Segmented filamentous bacteria have been shown to be potent inducers of Th17 cells[119] that are in turn important for protecting the host from bacterial and fungal infections. In fact, the role of Th17 cells in limiting fungal infections like *Candida albicans* and the increased number of mucocutaneous candidiasis noted in the clinical trial in patients treated with anti–IL-17 antibody have been proposed as a reason for the adverse study outcomes.[120]

CD4+ T cell on activation by bacterial antigen recognition interacts with B cells (CD40) through their cell-surface molecule CD40 ligand. This interaction results in the activation of B cells leading to their proliferation and initiation of antibody secretion. Subsequently a cascade of secondary events unfurls that involves production of reactive oxygen metabolites which are directly toxic to cells[121] and proteolytic enzymes like matrix metalloproteinases that digest the extracellular matrix. The necrosis and tissue damage from these secondary events leads to the characteristic morphological features of IBD.

SUMMARY AND FUTURE DIRECTIONS

As discussed earlier, most of the recent advances in IBD, including biologic therapies, have resulted from studies of mucosal immunity in the normal and inflamed intestine.[122] Both murine models of IBD and human studies have shown dysfunction of the epithelial barrier, innate immune cells, and adaptive T cells in the pathogenesis of IBD. Recent advances, including the data from GWAS and microbiome, have started to unravel the complex interaction between host genetics and environmental influences in the pathogenesis of IBD. The insight gained from the study of the aberrant immune system in IBD has led to the identification of molecular targets in the immune system for the design of drugs, some of which are already being used in clinical practice (like TNF-α antibodies and α4 integrin inhibitors), with many others in various phases of development. Unfortunately, most of the clinical trials in IBD have not performed extensive immune phenotyping of patients.

Despite the increased knowledge gained from the aforementioned studies, many aspects of mucosal immunity remain unclear in patients with IBD. As an example, the clinical phenotype may be similar between two patients with IBD; but the underlying aberrations in the immune system, whether it is the presence of susceptibility genes like NOD2, altered microbiota, or a primary defect in innate or adaptive immune system, could be very different. Even in the same patient, the underlying immunopathology may change over time regardless of the initial triggering events. This gap in knowledge can likely be attributed to many reasons, one of which is the limitations of available technology to study the dynamic and complex immune system of patients with IBD. In addition, IBD is identified and characterized based on morphology, an approach that has enhanced our understanding of the natural history of IBD but is also limited by its difficulty to characterize the inherent biologic variability between and within patients with IBD.

Recently, significant progress has been made in high-throughput technologies like genomic sequencing and mass cytometry (cytometry by time-of-flight [CyTOF]) that provide multiparametric data, which can be used to not just define the various immune cells states but also assess how these interact with each other in variety of states.[123,124] The high-throughput technologies coupled with informatics and a systems immunology approach may lead to a new molecular-based definition of complex diseases like IBD.[125–127] These approaches will enhance our understanding of the complex heterogeneity of immune cells and the immunoregulatory pathways and provide a tool to monitor and probe the aberrant immune system of patients with IBD not just at diagnosis but also during the later stages of the disease. A more detailed knowledge of the complexity of immune system in IBD will improve classification of IBD, in developing more representative animal models, and the design of new biologic therapies for a more personalized treatment approach.

REFERENCES

1. Molodecky NA, Soon IS, Rabi DM, et al. Increasing incidence and prevalence of the inflammatory bowel diseases with time, based on systematic review. Gastroenterology 2012;142:46–54.e42 [quiz: e30].
2. Terdiman JP, Gruss CB, Heidelbaugh JJ, et al. American Gastroenterological Association Institute guideline on the use of thiopurines, methotrexate, and anti-TNF-alpha biologic drugs for the induction and maintenance of remission in inflammatory Crohn's disease. Gastroenterology 2013;145:1459–63.
3. Vogelaar L, Spijker AV, van der Woude CJ. The impact of biologics on health-related quality of life in patients with inflammatory bowel disease. Clin Exp Gastroenterol 2009;2:101–9.
4. Bernstein CN, Loftus EV Jr, Ng SC, et al. Hospitalisations and surgery in Crohn's disease. Gut 2012;61:622–9.
5. Abraham C, Cho JH. Inflammatory bowel disease. N Engl J Med 2009;361: 2066–78.
6. Murphy K. Janeway's immunobiology. New York: Garland Science; 2011.
7. Barker N, van Es JH, Kuipers J, et al. Identification of stem cells in small intestine and colon by marker gene Lgr5. Nature 2007;449:1003–7.
8. Fasano A, Shea-Donohue T. Mechanisms of disease: the role of intestinal barrier function in the pathogenesis of gastrointestinal autoimmune diseases. Nat Clin Pract Gastroenterol Hepatol 2005;2:416–22.
9. Tripathi A, Lammers KM, Goldblum S, et al. Identification of human zonulin, a physiological modulator of tight junctions, as prehaptoglobin-2. Proc Natl Acad Sci U S A 2009;106:16799–804.
10. Fagarasan S, Honjo T. Intestinal IgA synthesis: regulation of front-line body defences. Nat Rev Immunol 2003;3:63–72.
11. Ganz T. Defensins: antimicrobial peptides of innate immunity. Nat Rev Immunol 2003;3:710–20.
12. Harwig SS, Tan L, Qu XD, et al. Bactericidal properties of murine intestinal phospholipase A2. J Clin Invest 1995;95:603–10.
13. Newberry RD, Lorenz RG. Organizing a mucosal defense. Immunol Rev 2005; 206:6–21.
14. Owen RL, Bhalla DK. Cytochemical analysis of alkaline phosphatase and esterase activities and of lectin-binding and anionic sites in rat and mouse Peyer's patch M cells. Am J Anat 1983;168:199–212.
15. Pappo J, Owen RL. Absence of secretory component expression by epithelial cells overlying rabbit gut-associated lymphoid tissue. Gastroenterology 1988; 95:1173–7.

16. Ayabe T, Satchell DP, Wilson CL, et al. Secretion of microbicidal alpha-defensins by intestinal Paneth cells in response to bacteria. Nat Immunol 2000;1:113–8.
17. Vaishnava S, Behrendt CL, Ismail AS, et al. Paneth cells directly sense gut commensals and maintain homeostasis at the intestinal host-microbial interface. Proc Natl Acad Sci U S A 2008;105:20858–63.
18. Lee SH, Starkey PM, Gordon S. Quantitative analysis of total macrophage content in adult mouse tissues. Immunochemical studies with monoclonal antibody F4/80. J Exp Med 1985;161:475–89.
19. Smith PD, Ochsenbauer-Jambor C, Smythies LE. Intestinal macrophages: unique effector cells of the innate immune system. Immunol Rev 2005;206: 149–59.
20. Wahl SM, Hunt DA, Wakefield LM, et al. Transforming growth factor type beta induces monocyte chemotaxis and growth factor production. Proc Natl Acad Sci U S A 1987;84:5788–92.
21. Bamias G, Corridoni D, Pizarro TT, et al. New insights into the dichotomous role of innate cytokines in gut homeostasis and inflammation. Cytokine 2012;59: 451–9.
22. Steinbach EC, Plevy SE. The role of macrophages and dendritic cells in the initiation of inflammation in IBD. Inflamm Bowel Dis 2014;20:166–75.
23. Mosser DM, Edwards JP. Exploring the full spectrum of macrophage activation. Nat Rev Immunol 2008;8:958–69.
24. Niess JH, Brand S, Gu X, et al. CX3CR1-mediated dendritic cell access to the intestinal lumen and bacterial clearance. Science 2005;307:254–8.
25. Lelouard H, Fallet M, de Bovis B, et al. Peyer's patch dendritic cells sample antigens by extending dendrites through M cell-specific transcellular pores. Gastroenterology 2012;142:592–601.e3.
26. Hart AL, Al-Hassi HO, Rigby RJ, et al. Characteristics of intestinal dendritic cells in inflammatory bowel diseases. Gastroenterology 2005;129:50–65.
27. Menning A, Loddenkemper C, Westendorf AM, et al. Retinoic acid-induced gut tropism improves the protective capacity of Treg in acute but not in chronic gut inflammation. Eur J Immunol 2010;40:2539–48.
28. Mora JR, Bono MR, Manjunath N, et al. Selective imprinting of gut-homing T cells by Peyer's patch dendritic cells. Nature 2003;424:88–93.
29. Hayday A, Theodoridis E, Ramsburg E, et al. Intraepithelial lymphocytes: exploring the Third Way in immunology. Nat Immunol 2001;2:997–1003.
30. Kanamori Y, Ishimaru K, Nanno M, et al. Identification of novel lymphoid tissues in murine intestinal mucosa where clusters of c-kit+ IL-7R+ Thy1+ lympho-hemopoietic progenitors develop. J Exp Med 1996;184:1449–59.
31. Groh V, Steinle A, Bauer S, et al. Recognition of stress-induced MHC molecules by intestinal epithelial gammadelta T cells. Science 1998;279:1737–40.
32. Thedrez A, Sabourin C, Gertner J, et al. Self/non-self discrimination by human gammadelta T cells: simple solutions for a complex issue? Immunol Rev 2007; 215:123–35.
33. Carding SR, Egan PJ. Gammadelta T cells: functional plasticity and heterogeneity. Nat Rev Immunol 2002;2:336–45.
34. Godfrey DI, MacDonald HR, Kronenberg M, et al. NKT cells: what's in a name? Nat Rev Immunol 2004;4:231–7.
35. Fuss IJ, Heller F, Boirivant M, et al. Nonclassical CD1d-restricted NK T cells that produce IL-13 characterize an atypical Th2 response in ulcerative colitis. J Clin Invest 2004;113:1490–7.

36. Ogura Y, Bonen DK, Inohara N, et al. A frameshift mutation in NOD2 associated with susceptibility to Crohn's disease. Nature 2001;411:603–6.

37. Hugot JP, Chamaillard M, Zouali H, et al. Association of NOD2 leucine-rich repeat variants with susceptibility to Crohn's disease. Nature 2001;411:599–603.

38. Kobayashi KS, Chamaillard M, Ogura Y, et al. Nod2-dependent regulation of innate and adaptive immunity in the intestinal tract. Science 2005;307:731–4.

39. Maeda S, Hsu LC, Liu H, et al. Nod2 mutation in Crohn's disease potentiates NF-kappaB activity and IL-1beta processing. Science 2005;307:734–8.

40. Targan SR, Hanauer SB, van Deventer SJ, et al. A short-term study of chimeric monoclonal antibody cA2 to tumor necrosis factor alpha for Crohn's disease. Crohn's Disease cA2 Study Group. N Engl J Med 1997;337:1029–35.

41. Rutgeerts P, Sandborn WJ, Feagan BG, et al. Infliximab for induction and maintenance therapy for ulcerative colitis. N Engl J Med 2005;353:2462–76.

42. Orenstein R. Anti-interleukin-12 antibody for active Crohn's disease. N Engl J Med 2005;352:627–8.

43. Sandborn WJ, Gasink C, Gao LL, et al. Ustekinumab induction and maintenance therapy in refractory Crohn's disease. N Engl J Med 2012;367:1519–28.

44. Marks DJ, Harbord MW, MacAllister R, et al. Defective acute inflammation in Crohn's disease: a clinical investigation. Lancet 2006;367:668–78.

45. Boya P, Reggiori F, Codogno P. Emerging regulation and functions of autophagy. Nat Cell Biol 2013;15:713–20.

46. Rioux JD, Xavier RJ, Taylor KD, et al. Genome-wide association study identifies new susceptibility loci for Crohn disease and implicates autophagy in disease pathogenesis. Nat Genet 2007;39:596–604.

47. McCarroll SA, Huett A, Kuballa P, et al. Deletion polymorphism upstream of IRGM associated with altered IRGM expression and Crohn's disease. Nat Genet 2008;40:1107–12.

48. Walter P, Ron D. The unfolded protein response: from stress pathway to homeostatic regulation. Science 2011;334:1081–6.

49. Treton X, Pedruzzi E, Cazals-Hatem D, et al. Altered endoplasmic reticulum stress affects translation in inactive colon tissue from patients with ulcerative colitis. Gastroenterology 2011;141:1024–35.

50. Khor B, Gardet A, Xavier RJ. Genetics and pathogenesis of inflammatory bowel disease. Nature 2011;474:307–17.

51. Kaser A, Lee AH, Franke A, et al. XBP1 links ER stress to intestinal inflammation and confers genetic risk for human inflammatory bowel disease. Cell 2008;134:743–56.

52. Jenkins RT, Ramage JK, Jones DB, et al. Small bowel and colonic permeability to 51Cr-EDTA in patients with active inflammatory bowel disease. Clin Invest Med 1988;11:151–5.

53. Wyatt J, Oberhuber G, Pongratz S, et al. Increased gastric and intestinal permeability in patients with Crohn's disease. Am J Gastroenterol 1997;92:1891–6.

54. Hollander D, Vadheim CM, Brettholz E, et al. Increased intestinal permeability in patients with Crohn's disease and their relatives. A possible etiologic factor. Ann Intern Med 1986;105:883–5.

55. Teahon K, Smethurst P, Levi AJ, et al. Intestinal permeability in patients with Crohn's disease and their first degree relatives. Gut 1992;33:320–3.

56. Olson TS, Reuter BK, Scott KG, et al. The primary defect in experimental ileitis originates from a nonhematopoietic source. J Exp Med 2006;203:541–52.

57. Jostins L, Ripke S, Weersma RK, et al. Host-microbe interactions have shaped the genetic architecture of inflammatory bowel disease. Nature 2012;491: 119–24.
58. Kiesslich R, Duckworth CA, Moussata D, et al. Local barrier dysfunction identified by confocal laser endomicroscopy predicts relapse in inflammatory bowel disease. Gut 2012;61(8):1146–53.
59. McGuckin MA, Eri R, Simms LA, et al. Intestinal barrier dysfunction in inflammatory bowel diseases. Inflamm Bowel Dis 2009;15:100–13.
60. Sigthorsson G, Tibble J, Hayllar J, et al. Intestinal permeability and inflammation in patients on NSAIDs. Gut 1998;43:506–11.
61. Ananthakrishnan AN, Higuchi LM, Huang ES, et al. Aspirin, nonsteroidal anti-inflammatory drug use, and risk for Crohn disease and ulcerative colitis: a cohort study. Ann Intern Med 2012;156:350–9.
62. Roberts CL, Keita AV, Duncan SH, et al. Translocation of Crohn's disease Escherichia coli across M-cells: contrasting effects of soluble plant fibres and emulsifiers. Gut 2010;59:1331–9.
63. Ananthakrishnan AN, Khalili H, Konijeti GG, et al. A prospective study of long-term intake of dietary fiber and risk of Crohn's disease and ulcerative colitis. Gastroenterology 2013;145:970–7.
64. Prager M, Buttner J, Haas V, et al. The JAK2 variant rs10758669 in Crohn's disease: altering the intestinal barrier as one mechanism of action. Int J Colorectal Dis 2012;27(5):565–73.
65. Stoll M, Corneliussen B, Costello CM, et al. Genetic variation in DLG5 is associated with inflammatory bowel disease. Nat Genet 2004;36:476–80.
66. Gunther C, Martini E, Wittkopf N, et al. Caspase-8 regulates TNF-alpha-induced epithelial necroptosis and terminal ileitis. Nature 2011;477:335–9.
67. Gunn MD, Tangemann K, Tam C, et al. A chemokine expressed in lymphoid high endothelial venules promotes the adhesion and chemotaxis of naive T lymphocytes. Proc Natl Acad Sci U S A 1998;95:258–63.
68. Weaver CT, Harrington LE, Mangan PR, et al. Th17: an effector CD4 T cell lineage with regulatory T cell ties. Immunity 2006;24:677–88.
69. Iwakura Y, Ishigame H. The IL-23/IL-17 axis in inflammation. J Clin Invest 2006; 116:1218–22.
70. Matloubian M, Lo CG, Cinamon G, et al. Lymphocyte egress from thymus and peripheral lymphoid organs is dependent on S1P receptor 1. Nature 2004; 427:355–60.
71. Shiow LR, Rosen DB, Brdickova N, et al. CD69 acts downstream of interferon-alpha/beta to inhibit S1P1 and lymphocyte egress from lymphoid organs. Nature 2006;440:540–4.
72. Johansson-Lindbom B, Svensson M, Pabst O, et al. Functional specialization of gut CD103+ dendritic cells in the regulation of tissue-selective T cell homing. J Exp Med 2005;202:1063–73.
73. Berlin C, Berg EL, Briskin MJ, et al. Alpha 4 beta 7 integrin mediates lymphocyte binding to the mucosal vascular addressin MAdCAM-1. Cell 1993;74:185–95.
74. Briskin M, Winsor-Hines D, Shyjan A, et al. Human mucosal addressin cell adhesion molecule-1 is preferentially expressed in intestinal tract and associated lymphoid tissue. Am J Pathol 1997;151:97–110.
75. Maloy KJ, Powrie F. Intestinal homeostasis and its breakdown in inflammatory bowel disease. Nature 2011;474:298–306.
76. Shevach EM. From vanilla to 28 flavors: multiple varieties of T regulatory cells. Immunity 2006;25:195–201.

77. Mottet C, Uhlig HH, Powrie F. Cutting edge: cure of colitis by CD4+CD25+ regulatory T cells. J Immunol 2003;170:3939–43.

78. Sakaguchi S, Sakaguchi N, Asano M, et al. Immunologic self-tolerance maintained by activated T cells expressing IL-2 receptor alpha-chains (CD25). Breakdown of a single mechanism of self-tolerance causes various autoimmune diseases. J Immunol 1995;155:1151–64.

79. Maul J, Loddenkemper C, Mundt P, et al. Peripheral and intestinal regulatory CD4+ CD25(high) T cells in inflammatory bowel disease. Gastroenterology 2005;128:1868–78.

80. Saruta M, Yu QT, Fleshner PR, et al. Characterization of FOXP3+CD4+ regulatory T cells in Crohn's disease. Clin Immunol 2007;125:281–90.

81. Yu QT, Saruta M, Avanesyan A, et al. Expression and functional characterization of FOXP3+ CD4+ regulatory T cells in ulcerative colitis. Inflamm Bowel Dis 2007;13:191–9.

82. Fantini MC, Rizzo A, Fina D, et al. Smad7 controls resistance of colitogenic T cells to regulatory T cell-mediated suppression. Gastroenterology 2009;136:1308–16 e1–3.

83. Nguyen DD, Snapper SB. Targeting Smads to restore transforming growth factor-beta signaling and regulatory T-cell function in inflammatory bowel disease. Gastroenterology 2009;136:1161–4.

84. Conley ME, Delacroix DL. Intravascular and mucosal immunoglobulin A: two separate but related systems of immune defense? Ann Intern Med 1987;106:892–9.

85. Brandtzaeg P, Farstad IN, Johansen FE, et al. The B-cell system of human mucosae and exocrine glands. Immunol Rev 1999;171:45–87.

86. Brandtzaeg P, Prydz H. Direct evidence for an integrated function of J chain and secretory component in epithelial transport of immunoglobulins. Nature 1984; 311:71–3.

87. Macpherson AJ, Uhr T. Induction of protective IgA by intestinal dendritic cells carrying commensal bacteria. Science 2004;303:1662–5.

88. Powrie F, Leach MW, Mauze S, et al. Inhibition of Th1 responses prevents inflammatory bowel disease in scid mice reconstituted with CD45RBhi CD4+ T cells. Immunity 1994;1:553–62.

89. Sugawara K, Olson TS, Moskaluk CA, et al. Linkage to peroxisome proliferator-activated receptor-gamma in SAMP1/YitFc mice and in human Crohn's disease. Gastroenterology 2005;128:351–60.

90. Totsuka T, Kanai T, Uraushihara K, et al. Therapeutic effect of anti-OX40L and anti-TNF-alpha MAbs in a murine model of chronic colitis. Am J Physiol Gastrointest Liver Physiol 2003;284:10.

91. Hovhannisyan Z, Treatman J, Littman DR, et al. Characterization of interleukin-17-producing regulatory T cells in inflamed intestinal mucosa from patients with inflammatory bowel diseases. Gastroenterology 2011;140:957–65.

92. Pariente B, Mocan I, Camus M, et al. Activation of the receptor NKG2D leads to production of Th17 cytokines in CD4+ T cells of patients with Crohn's disease. Gastroenterology 2011;141:217–26, 226.e1–2.

93. Di Meglio P, Di Cesare A, Laggner U, et al. The IL23R R381Q gene variant protects against immune-mediated diseases by impairing IL-23-induced Th17 effector response in humans. PLoS One 2011;6:e17160.

94. Danese S. New therapies for inflammatory bowel disease: from the bench to the bedside. Gut 2012;61:918–32.

95. Probert CS, Chott A, Turner JR, et al. Persistent clonal expansions of peripheral blood CD4+ lymphocytes in chronic inflammatory bowel disease. J Immunol 1996;157:3183–91.

96. Cong Y, Brandwein SL, McCabe RP, et al. CD4+ T cells reactive to enteric bacterial antigens in spontaneously colitic C3H/HeJBir mice: increased T helper cell type 1 response and ability to transfer disease. J Exp Med 1998;187:855–64.

97. Lodes MJ, Cong Y, Elson CO, et al. Bacterial flagellin is a dominant antigen in Crohn disease. J Clin Invest 2004;113:1296–306.

98. Dave M, Higgins PD, Middha S, et al. The human gut microbiome: current knowledge, challenges, and future directions. Transl Res 2012;160:246–57.

99. Maynard CL, Elson CO, Hatton RD, et al. Reciprocal interactions of the intestinal microbiota and immune system. Nature 2012;489:231–41.

100. Chassaing B, Darfeuille-Michaud A. The commensal microbiota and enteropathogens in the pathogenesis of inflammatory bowel diseases. Gastroenterology 2011;140:1720–8.

101. Nell S, Suerbaum S, Josenhans C. The impact of the microbiota on the pathogenesis of IBD: lessons from mouse infection models. Nat Rev Microbiol 2010;8:564–77.

102. Sansonetti PJ. War and peace at mucosal surfaces. Nat Rev Immunol 2004;4: 953–64.

103. Cario E, Gerken G, Podolsky DK. Toll-like receptor 2 enhances ZO-1-associated intestinal epithelial barrier integrity via protein kinase C. Gastroenterology 2004; 127:224–38.

104. Rakoff-Nahoum S, Paglino J, Eslami-Varzaneh F, et al. Recognition of commensal microflora by toll-like receptors is required for intestinal homeostasis. Cell 2004;118:229–41.

105. Hisamatsu T, Suzuki M, Reinecker HC, et al. CARD15/NOD2 functions as an antibacterial factor in human intestinal epithelial cells. Gastroenterology 2003; 124:993–1000.

106. Wehkamp J, Harder J, Weichenthal M, et al. NOD2 (CARD15) mutations in Crohn's disease are associated with diminished mucosal alpha-defensin expression. Gut 2004;53:1658–64.

107. Lala S, Ogura Y, Osborne C, et al. Crohn's disease and the NOD2 gene: a role for Paneth cells. Gastroenterology 2003;125:47–57.

108. Biswas A, Liu YJ, Hao L, et al. Induction and rescue of Nod2-dependent Th1-driven granulomatous inflammation of the ileum. Proc Natl Acad Sci U S A 2010;107:14739–44.

109. Cadwell K, Patel KK, Maloney NS, et al. Virus-plus-susceptibility gene interaction determines Crohn's disease gene Atg16L1 phenotypes in intestine. Cell 2010;141:1135–45.

110. Murthy A, Li Y, Peng I, et al. A Crohn's disease variant in Atg16l1 enhances its degradation by caspase 3. Nature 2014;506:456–62.

111. Hamilton MJ, Snapper SB, Blumberg RS. Update on biologic pathways in inflammatory bowel disease and their therapeutic relevance. J Gastroenterol 2012;47(1):1–8.

112. Bevan MJ. Cross-priming. Nat Immunol 2006;7:363–5.

113. Sutmuller RP, Morgan ME, Netea MG, et al. Toll-like receptors on regulatory T cells: expanding immune regulation. Trends Immunol 2006;27:387–93.

114. Garrett WS, Lord GM, Punit S, et al. Communicable ulcerative colitis induced by T-bet deficiency in the innate immune system. Cell 2007;131:33–45.

115. Bach JF. The effect of infections on susceptibility to autoimmune and allergic diseases. N Engl J Med 2002;347:911–20.

116. Olszak T, An D, Zeissig S, et al. Microbial exposure during early life has persistent effects on natural killer T cell function. Science 2012;336:489–93.

117. McFall-Ngai M. Adaptive immunity: care for the community. Nature 2007; 445:153.
118. Hueber W, Sands BE, Lewitzky S, et al. Secukinumab, a human anti-IL-17A monoclonal antibody, for moderate to severe Crohn's disease: unexpected results of a randomised, double-blind placebo-controlled trial. Gut 2012;61: 1693–700.
119. Ivanov II, Atarashi K, Manel N, et al. Induction of intestinal Th17 cells by segmented filamentous bacteria. Cell 2009;139:485–98.
120. Colombel JF, Sendid B, Jouault T, et al. Secukinumab failure in Crohn's disease: the yeast connection? Gut 2013;62:800–1.
121. Pavlick KP, Laroux FS, Fuseler J, et al. Role of reactive metabolites of oxygen and nitrogen in inflammatory bowel disease. Free Radic Biol Med 2002;33: 311–22.
122. Macdonald TT, Monteleone G. Immunity, inflammation, and allergy in the gut. Science 2005;307:1920–5.
123. Newell EW, Sigal N, Bendall SC, et al. Cytometry by time-of-flight shows combinatorial cytokine expression and virus-specific cell niches within a continuum of CD8+ T cell phenotypes. Immunity 2012;36:142–52.
124. Chattopadhyay PK, Gierahn TM, Roederer M, et al. Single-cell technologies for monitoring immune systems. Nat Immunol 2014;15:128–35.
125. Kidd BA, Peters LA, Schadt EE, et al. Unifying immunology with informatics and multiscale biology. Nat Immunol 2014;15:118–27.
126. Virgin HW, Todd JA. Metagenomics and personalized medicine. Cell 2011;147: 44–56.
127. Zitnik M, Janjic V, Larminie C, et al. Discovering disease-disease associations by fusing systems-level molecular data. Sci Rep 2013;3:3202.

Who Should Receive Biologic Therapy for IBD?

The Rationale for the Application of a Personalized Approach

Jennifer Jones, MD, MSc, FRCPC[a],*,
Juan Nicolás Peña-Sánchez, MD, MPH, PhD(c)[b]

KEYWORDS

- IBD • Inflammatory bowel disease • Biologic therapy • Crohn disease
- Ulcerative colitis

KEY POINTS

- The therapeutic approach in inflammatory bowel disease has evolved to target end-organ inflammation to heal intestinal mucosa and avoid structural damage. Objective therapeutic monitoring is required to achieve this goal.
- Earlier intervention with biologic therapy has been shown, indirectly, to be associated with higher clinical response and remission rates.
- A personalized approach to risk stratification with consideration of key clinical factors and inflammatory biomarker concentrations is recommended when deciding whether or not to start a patient on biologic therapy.

BACKGROUND

Inflammatory bowel diseases (IBDs) are a group of incurable, complex, polygenic diseases of the gastrointestinal tract characterized by chronic, relapsing course of intestinal inflammation.[1] IBD is thought to arise from an aberrant mucosal immune response to luminal antigens in the context of predisposing genetic risk factors and environmental exposures. A loss of tolerance to resident microbial flora is considered to be a central event, which triggers a complex cascade of innate and adaptive immune responses leading to intestinal damage.[1] IBD is subclassified into 2 major diagnoses: Crohn disease (CD) and ulcerative colitis (UC).[2] This classification is made on the basis of clinical, endoscopic, and pathologic criteria. Although this classification

[a] Department of Medicine, University of Saskatchewan, 108 Hospital Drive, Saskatoon, Saskatchewan S7N0W8, Canada; [b] Department of Medicine, School of Public Health, University of Saskatchewan, 104 Clinic Place, Saskatoon, Saskatchewan S7N 5E5, Canada
* Corresponding author.
E-mail address: j.jones@usask.ca

Gastroenterol Clin N Am 43 (2014) 425–440
http://dx.doi.org/10.1016/j.gtc.2014.05.004   **gastro.theclinics.com**
0889-8553/14/$ – see front matter © 2014 Elsevier Inc. All rights reserved.

maintains relevance for purposes of clinical decision-making related to medical and surgical management of patients with IBD, it has become apparent that such a crude classification is an oversimplification of this complex disease process with overlapping genetic, and immunopathogenic, processes. These processes result in varied phenotypic expressions of disease. Immune mechanisms in UC and CD have been shown to be somewhat distinct and classified based on the type of T helper cells involved and the cytokines they produce.[1] CD is generally considered to be a Th1 disease (with greater expression of interferon [IFN]-γ and interleukin [IL]-2, as well as the Th1-inducing cytokine IL-12), and UC an atypical disease with expression of both Th1 and Th2 cytokines (IL-5, IL-13, IFN-γ, and no upregulation of IL-4).[3,4] The observed efficacy of anti–tumor necrosis factor-α (TNF-α) therapies in UC further erodes the traditional Th1/Th2 paradigms in IBD. Non-Th1/Th2 pathways also have been identified as being important in the pathogenesis of IBD, including Th17 cells, which produce large quantities of IL-17 (production is upregulated in both CD and UC[1]) and are induced by IL-23.[1]

In the absence of adequate disease control, the chronic inflammatory process of IBD can lead to significant infectious, inflammatory, and structural complications. These complications could result in the need for hospitalizations and surgeries, impaired quality of life, and, in more severe instances, disease-related mortality.[5,6] In the era before biologic therapy was available, a population-based cohort study of patients with CD demonstrated that the rate of hospitalization owing to medical complications, the need for surgery, or both was 194 admissions per 1000 patient-years,[7] and the cumulative surgery rate in the first 10 years after a diagnosis was 40% to 50%.[7] Recent population-based studies estimate colectomy rates in those with UC 20 years after diagnosis of 14.8%.[8] At any time, extraintestinal manifestations can affect up to one-third of patients.[9] In the case of CD, approximately 30% of patients will have a stricturing or penetrating complication at presentation and half of all patients will experience an intestinal complication within 20 years, often leading to the need for surgical intervention.[7,10] Persistent and extensive colonic inflammation in UC or CD and ileal inflammation in CD also increase the risk of developing colorectal and small bowel carcinoma.[4]

THE EVOLUTION OF BIOLOGIC THERAPY FOR IBD

Until fairly recently, the only biologics available for use for the treatment of IBD belonged to the anti–TNF-α class.[11–14] The first anti–TNF-α therapy demonstrated to be efficacious for the treatment of IBD was infliximab (a chimeric monoclonal antibody that specifically binds TNF-α and was initially evaluated in CD).[15] Over time, attempts to humanize the monoclonal antibody to reduce immunogenicity led to the development of second-generation, third-generation, and fourth-generation anti–TNF-α agents (including adalimumab, certolizumab pegol, and golimumab). All of these anti–TNF-α agents have been demonstrated to be efficacious for the induction of clinical response, remission, maintenance of clinical remission, corticosteroid sparing, and mucosal healing in subjects with moderate to severely active IBD, including CD (infliximab, adalimumab, and certolizumab pegol) and UC (infliximab, adalimumab, and golimumab).[16–24] Infliximab also has been shown to be efficacious for the therapy of fistulizing CD, and both infliximab and adalimumab for the prevention of early postoperative endoscopic and histologic recurrence.[25] Post hoc analyses also have suggested that infliximab reduces the 1-year colectomy rate in UC from 17% in the placebo group to 10% in the infliximab-treated group. Despite the proven benefit of these therapies, a significant number of patients with CD (ie, 10% to 40%) will not respond to this class of biologic; this is otherwise referred to as primary treatment failure. Among patients with UC, this number could be as high as 50%.[26] Additionally, only one-third to one-half of patients will have a complete remission, and two-thirds of patients will fail to maintain their response during 12 months of sustained therapy.[26] The inability to maintain response to a biologic is termed secondary treatment failure. Despite these observed limitations in primary and durable response to anti–TNF-α therapies, they remain one of the most well tolerated and effective therapies at our disposal for the therapy of IBD.

The most recent biologic class to demonstrate efficacy and safety in phase 3 clinical trials are the lymphocyte trafficking inhibitors.[3,11] Natalizumab (a humanized immunoglobulin G4 anti–α4-integrin monoclonal antibody that inhibits both α4β7-integrin/MAdCAM-1 interaction and α4β1-integrin/VCAM-1 binding) was the first in this class to be developed.[27] Natalizumab was shown to be effective for induction and maintenance of clinical remission in the Efficacy of Natalizumab as Active Therapy of CD (ENACT-1 and ENACT-2) trials.[27] Its efficacy as a corticosteroid-sparing agent was made evident because all subjects in the ENACT-2 study were able to be withdrawn from corticosteroid therapy. Natalizumab has been demonstrated in randomized controlled clinical trials to be efficacious for the therapy of multiple sclerosis (MS) as well.[28] Despite these early and encouraging results, it was discovered, after natalizumab came to market, that it increased the risk of the development of a serious central nervous system infection called progressive multifocal leukoencephalopathy (PML).[29] PML is a potentially fatal opportunistic infection that arises as a result of reactivation of the clinically latent John Cunningham (JC) polyomavirus. Two patients with MS and 1 patient with CD exposed to natalizumab developed PML within the context of the original clinical trials.[29] These cases, as well as cases reported through postmarketing surveillance after release of the medication, lead the Food and Drug Administration (FDA) to withdraw the medication from the market temporarily. It has since been approved for use in the United States by the FDA for the treatment of MS and CD, with a black box warning about the risk of PML with a mandatory prescribing program and recommended JC virus antibody testing (product monograph).[30] A similar approach for MS has occurred in Canada but not for CD. A second-generation lymphocyte-trafficking inhibitor, vedolizumab, appears to be highly gut selective. Vedolizumab is a α4β7 integrin antagonist that has recently been shown to be efficacious for the induction and maintenance of steroid-free clinical remission in both CD and UC.[12,13] Vedolizumab specifically blocks α4β7 integrin/MAdCAM-1 interactions. In CD, 14.5% of patients randomized to vedolizumab at week 6 attained a CDAI-defined clinical remission (CDAI <150) in comparison with 6.8% of those randomized to placebo. Responders were then re-randomized to receive vedolizumab every 4 weeks or 8 weeks and followed until week 52. Thirty-nine percent and 36.4% of patients receiving vedolizumab every 8 weeks and 4 weeks, respectively, were in clinical remission at week 52, as compared with 21.6% of those assigned to placebo.[27] Similarly, in UC, week 6 clinical response rates were 47.1% and 25.5% in patients receiving vedolizumab induction versus placebo, respectively. At week 52, 41.8% and 44.8% of patients receiving vedolizumab every 8 weeks and 4 weeks, respectively, were in clinical remission (Mayo score $\leq$2 with no endoscopic subscore >1), as compared with 15.9% of those receiving placebo.[13] Although more biologics have been developed, and are being developed, we still grapple with the fairly underwhelming clinical response and remission rates observed in anti–TNF-α induction and maintenance trials and real-world clinical practice.[26] Several factors may contribute to limitations in efficacy observed in clinical trials. It is possible that subject selection was unfavorable in earlier randomized controlled trials (RCTs) of anti–TNF-α therapy from the perspective of disease duration and disease activity. Certainly, mean and median duration of disease was substantially longer than that of clinical trials, such as SONIC, in which the highest rates of steroid-free clinical response and remission for infliximab-treated subjects have been observed to date. Clinical trials of IBD have historically been plagued by high placebo-response rates, partly as a result of the enrollment of patients who lack true inflammatory disease. Instead, alternate disease processes, such as superimposed irritable bowel syndrome, may have resulted in higher clinical disease activity scores.[31] Over the past several years, a movement toward incorporation of objective measures of disease activity, such as colonoscopy or serum/fecal inflammatory biomarkers, has taken place to minimize enrollment of patients who lack active intestinal inflammation.[31]

Consequently, it is hypothesized that the initiation of therapies earlier in disease course, the use of immunosuppressive (IS) and biologic therapies only in individuals with active inflammatory disease, and the optimization of therapies based on the use of objective measures of inflammatory disease activity may enhance the effectiveness of IBD biologic therapy for our patients.

EVOLUTION OF DISEASE MONITORING AND GOALS OF THERAPY

Evidence has accumulated suggesting that patients should be treated with the goal of achieving mucosal healing (MH) rather than simply improvement in clinical symptoms or clinical response with a view to reducing disability and bowel damage.[31–33] This concept of "deep remission" (combined clinical, endoscopic, and biomarker-based remission) is based on the presumption that mucosal healing and inflammatory biomarkers are adequate surrogate markers of end-organ disease. Although there is ample indirect evidence that treating to mucosal healing is associated with reductions in disease relapse as well as improvements in long-term disease-related outcomes, such as the need for hospitalizations and surgeries,[34,35] no direct randomized controlled evidence exists to support this practice. Additionally, no definition of mucosal healing has been validated, and definitions of MH may vary from study to study. To date, only the EXTEND (extend the safety and efficacy of adalimumab through endoscopic healing) trial has attempted to address the concept of "deep remission" as a goal of therapy for IBD.[36] The EXTEND trial showed that subjects achieving deep remission were more likely to have improved disease-specific quality of life, have fewer disease flares, fewer CD-related hospitalizations, greater work productivity, and less activity impairment compared with subjects with mucosal healing alone.[37] Frøslie and colleagues[34] from Norway demonstrated in a population-based inception cohort study that, in UC, MH was associated with a reduced future risk of colectomy, and that, in CD, MH was associated with reduced disease activity after 5 years, as well as reduced future need for corticosteroids. Despite these findings, definitions of disease remission need to be validated in disease modification trials. Not only have treatment definitions evolved to include more rigorous, objective end points of disease control, but therapeutic goals also have evolved to include the evaluation of structural bowel damage and avoidance of IBD-related disability.[32]

The approach to the medical therapy of IBD has evolved rapidly over the past decade as a result of changing treatment goals, as well as new breakthroughs related to the understanding of disease pathogenesis, disease course, and the introduction of more than one class of biologic therapy. Traditional therapeutic paradigms have focused on stepwise, sequential introduction of therapies of differing mechanisms beginning with the least expensive, least systemically active medications and gradually intensifying therapy. This approach has historically been applied across the board to all patients regardless of their clinical and phenotypic features. Improvements in our ability to predict which individuals with IBD are likely to experience an aggressive disease course, along with the development of a larger number of therapeutic options, has led to a paradigm shift in our approach to IBD. Rather than applying a one-size-fits-all approach, we are moving toward a model of personalized medicine based on risk stratification in an effort to modify disease course. A new term has been coined to convey the role of medication therapy for the attainment of this new treatment goal; a term that reflects the philosophy of our rheumatology colleagues. IS and biologic therapies in IBD are now referred to as disease-modifying anti-IBD drugs (DMAIDS).[32] The concept of pursuing a more accelerated step approach to the treatment of individuals at greatest risk for a disabling disease course and intervening with DMAIDs at an earlier time point for these individuals has been embraced by many.

THE CASE FOR EARLIER MEDICATION INTERVENTION IN IBD

The case for earlier intervention with biologic therapy in IBD is supported from observational, subgroup analyses and RCT data in both the adult and pediatric patient populations (**Table 1**).[21,22,35,37–43] RCTs in both adult and pediatric populations, including patients with shorter IBD disease duration (mean 2 years), have demonstrated clinical response and remission rates that are higher than historically observed rates among clinical trial populations with longer disease duration and previous exposure to IS or biologic agents. In the REACH[38] study, pediatric patients with moderate to severely active CD were treated with an open-label 3-dose induction regimen of infliximab, and week 10 responders were re-randomized to infliximab infusion every 8 weeks or 12 weeks. A larger proportion of patients assigned to infliximab every 8 weeks, versus every 12 weeks, were in clinical response or remission. The clinical response rates were 73.1% and 63.5% at 30 and 54 weeks, respectively.[38] The SONIC trial was a randomized controlled double-blind trial in which the efficacy of infliximab monotherapy, azathioprine monotherapy, and the 2 drugs in combination were compared in a population of adult subjects with moderate to severely active CD who were naive to both IS and biologic therapies.[35] The primary end point of corticosteroid-free clinical remission at week 26 was significantly higher in the combination group in comparison with either the infliximab or azathioprine monotherapy group (56.8%, 44.4%, and 30%, respectively).[35] Similar results were observed at week 50. In addition to clinical remission, mucosal healing at week 26 was significantly better in the group receiving combination therapy in comparison with either monotherapy group alone (43.9%, 30.1%, and 16.5%, respectively).[35] Significant differences in the rate of development of serious infections were not observed among the 3 treatment groups.

These remission rates are approximately 20% higher than those observed in the adult population in ACCENT 1, in which the mean disease duration was 7.9 years.[22] The results of subgroup analyses from clinical trials also have suggested that subjects with shorter disease duration appear to have higher disease response and remission rates than those with longer disease duration. In the CHARM study of adalimumab in moderate to severe CD, patients with disease duration of less than 2 years had a 20% increase in remission rates at 26 and 56 weeks compared with patients with disease duration longer than 5 years.[21] Similar observations were made in the PRECISE 2 study of certolizumab pegol in CD.[17] D'Haens[44] conducted an open-label study

Table 1
Evidence in support of the early use of biologic therapies in inflammatory bowel disease

Author, Year	Agent	Study Design	Disease Duration Before Medication	Efficacy Estimate
Löfberg et al,[39] 2012	Adalimumab	Open-label phase IIIb	7.8[a] y	Odds of clinical remission decreases by a factor of 0.96 (0.94–0.98) per unit increase in disease duration (y)
Schreiber et al,[40] 2010	Certolizumab	Post hoc analysis of a randomized, double-blind (Schreiber et al,[17] 2007)	<1 y	Clinical remission (68.4%) and response (89.5%) among those with <1 y vs 57.3% and 44.3% among ≥5 y
Colombel et al,[35] 2010	Infliximab ± azathioprine vs azathioprine	Randomized, double-blind	2.3[a] y	Steroid-free clinical remission Combination: 56.8% Azathioprine: 30% Infliximab: 44.4%
D'Haens et al,[43] 2008	Infliximab/azathioprine	Open-label randomized early combined immunosuppression vs conventional treatment	2[a] y	Clinical remission Absolute difference 19.4% (P = .03)
Hyams et al,[38] 2007	Infliximab	Randomized, open-label Pediatric subjects	1.6[a] y	Clinical response 88.4% and clinical remission 58.9%[b]
Hanauer et al,[22] 2002	Infliximab	Randomized, double-blind	7.9[a] y	Clinical remission and response Median disease duration 7.5 vs nonresponders 9.3

Table does not include results of CHARM subgroup analysis. Although efficacy inversely correlated with disease duration, point estimates were not published.
[a] Median disease duration.
[b] Clinical response (66.7%) and clinical remission (39.1%) observed to be much lower among adults.[22]
Data from Refs.[22,35,38–40,43]

comparing the use of early combined immunosuppression with conventional therapy in newly diagnosed CD. In this study, 133 subjects were assigned to either early combined immunosuppression (infliximab induction at weeks 0, 2, and 6 in combination with azathioprine) or conventional treatment (initial treatment with corticosteroids, followed sequentially by azathioprine and infliximab). The primary outcome measures of this 2-year study were clinical remission without corticosteroids or intestinal resection at weeks 26 and 52. At week 26, 60% of subjects in the combined IS group were in clinical remission compared with 36% in the conventional therapy group (absolute difference 19.3%, 95% confidence interval 2.4–36.3, $P = .0278$).[44] Mucosal healing was significantly higher in the "top-down" group, and complete mucosal healing was associated with a significantly higher steroid-free remission rate in the subsequent 2 years.[44] Rates of serious adverse events were similar between the 2 groups. Within the past 5 years, population-based cohort studies have demonstrated significant reductions in the rates of surgical resections over time. This observed reduction appears to be associated with earlier use of IS therapy in disease course. In a population-based cohort study from Denmark, Jess and colleagues[45] showed that early surgery within 1 year of diagnosis has fallen from 35% (1962–1987) to 12% (2003–2004). Ramadas and colleagues[41] performed a population-based cohort study in which residents of the city of Cardiff with a diagnosis of CD were identified. Surgical resection rates were explored based on year of diagnosis. Patients were divided into three 6-year groups (hexiles): group A, diagnosed between 1986 and 1991; group B, diagnosed between 1992 and 1997; and group C, diagnosed between 1998 and 2003. The median length of follow-up was 92 months (range, 41–261 months) with group A followed for a median of 168 months, group B for 111 months, and group C for 73 months. Rates of first surgery over the course of 5 years differed significantly between the groups (group A, 59%; B, 37%; and C, 25%; $P = .001$).[41] The rates of any surgery within the first 5 years of diagnosis also differed (group A, 60%; B, 42%; C, 35%; $P = .017$). A significant reduction in the rate of long-term corticosteroid use was also observed among the 3 groups (group A, 44%; group B, 31%; and group C, 13%; $P = .001$).[41] Thiopurines were commenced in 38% of patients with a median dose of 100 mg for both azathioprine and 6-mercaptopurine. There was a significant increase in the early use of thiopurines over time (group A, 3%; B, 12%; C, 25%; $P = .001$) as well as in the overall use of thiopurines within 5 years (group A, 11%; group B, 28%; and group C, 45%; $P = .001$).[41] This study was one of the first studies to demonstrate that intervention with IS earlier in the course of IBD is associated with changes in disease course. Triangulation of observations from studies using different study designs and methodology strongly supports the supposition that intervening earlier in the disease course stands to benefit at least some patients with IBD (see **Table 1**). This has led to the development of the "Paris Definition for Early CD," which defines a patient with CD as having early CD if they have had disease for less than 18 months, active disease (as evidence by the Simple Endoscopic Score for Crohn's Disease or Crohn's Disease Endoscopic Index of Severity >4) and radiological evidence of disease activity, clinical symptoms with a CDAI greater than 150, bowel damage (fistula, abscess, stricture), and corticosteroid use (past or current use).[46] If this definition is validated, it will then serve as a way of identifying those individuals who might benefit from earlier, more aggressive intervention with IS or biologic drug therapy; whether classification of patients with UC as having early disease characteristics is valid remains unclear. Until such definitions have been validated, our ability to identify individuals who might benefit the most from biologic therapy is more limited. However, there are clinical features that have been demonstrated to portend a more aggressive disease course.

PREDICTORS OF COMPLEX DISEASE COURSE

To date, research has not been able to demonstrate that serologic or genetic risk factors can reliably predict which individuals are more likely to have an aggressive disease course or progress to complications earlier. Antimicrobial antibodies to anti–*Saccharomyces cerevisiae* (ASCA), *Escherichia coli* outer membrane porin C (Omp-C), bacterial flagellin (anti-CBir1 flagellin), and *Pseudomonas fluorescens* bacterial sequence I2 (anti-I2) have been associated with early-onset CD disease, penetrating and fibrostenosing behavior, need for small-bowel surgery, and higher quantitative titers with more complex disease behavior in pediatric patients with CD.[47–50] However, recent systematic reviews have concluded that there is currently insufficient evidence relating to the accuracy of antibody testing to recommend that they be used to predict disease course or response to therapy.[51] Similarly, the NOD2 gene variants have been shown to be associated with a more complex disease course. Most of the data pertaining to risk stratification by serodiagnostics and genotype have been derived from referral centers, evidence that is subject to selection bias.[48] These results have more recently been confirmed in the IBD CHIP DNA array studies, which have shown that the *NOD2* gene was an independent risk factor need for surgery and most strongly associated with complex disease course.[52] Despite these findings, genetic variants have not been reliable in the prediction course of CD for an individual patient. Clinical risk factors that have been shown to be associated with a more aggressive disease course in CD include ileal disease location, disease located in the upper gastrointestinal tract, smoking, complicated behavior (stricturing, fistulization, or abscess), young age at diagnosis, perianal disease, elevated serum C-reactive protein (CRP),[53] and severe endoscopic lesions or ulcerations.[54] Aggressive UC has recently been defined as disease associated with a high relapse rate, need for surgery, development of colon cancer, and/or the presence of extraintestinal manifestations.[55] Additional clinical risk factors for UC include young age at diagnosis and extensive colitis. Such clinical risk factors can be used to identify patients with IBD in need of earlier intervention with biologic therapy.

CLINICAL PREDICTORS OF RESPONSE TO BIOLOGIC THERAPY

In addition to the identification of those individuals who are more likely to experience an aggressive disease course and require earlier use of biologic therapy, it also is important to identify who is most likely to respond favorably to a biologic agent. Most data relating to this topic have been derived from observational cohort studies, both retrospective and prospective (see **Table 1**).[39,56–66] Common clinical features that have emerged from these studies as being implicated in affecting the likelihood of clinical response to biologic therapy include inflammatory disease burden, disease duration, smoking status, isolated ileitis, isolated colitis, age, previous exposure to biologic agents, and IS use. The same clinical factors have been implicated in both CD and UC.[63–65] In 2003, Arnott and colleagues[59] performed a prospective study of 74 infliximab-treated patients so as to define markers of response at 4 weeks of therapy after a single infusion of infliximab. Stepwise logistic regression identified age, isolated ileitis, and previous surgery as inversely correlated with response, whereas colitis and concomitant IS treatment were positively associated with clinical response (**Table 2**).[59] In their univariate analysis (confirmed by multivariate analysis), smoking and colonic disease emerged as independent predictors for a response to infliximab (odds ratio [OR] 0.24, $P = .035$ and OR 4.87, $P = .035$, respectively).[59] Vermeire and colleagues[61] performed a similar study in which 240 consecutive patients with CD participated in a Belgian infliximab expanded access program, and response to infliximab was evaluated at week 4 or 10. In this study, 1-year relapse rates were significantly different between smokers versus nonsmokers (100.0% vs 39.6%, $P = $ .0026, odds ratio [OR] 3.2), and between patients established on IM versus not (58.0% vs 92.8%, $P = $ .0054, OR 2.6). Multiple studies, including the SONIC trial, have observed that biochemical parameters suggestive of increased inflammatory burden, such as elevated CRP and endoscopic evidence of mucosal inflammation and ulceration, were associated with a better response to infliximab (see **Table 2**).

SAFETY CONSIDERATIONS

In addition to maximizing effectiveness, it is also very important to consider the likelihood of development of adverse effects of therapy when deciding who to treat with a biologic. The increased risk of infectious and malignant events in patients on biologic agents alone or in combination with another IS agent has been well described.[67] Several risk factors for infectious and malignant adverse events in relation to the use of anti-TNF agents have been identified. Cottone and colleagues[68] recently demonstrated age to be an important risk factor for the development of serious adverse events, including severe infections and mortality. This was a prospective study involving 16 Italian referral centers at which patients were initiated on anti-TNF therapy, including either adalimumab (n = 604) or infliximab (n = 2475) between 2000 and 2009. Among patients older than 65 years, more patients suffered severe infections, neoplasms, and death (11%, 3%, and 10%, respectively) in comparison with the control group of those younger than 65 years and treated with biologics (0.5%, 2.0%, and 2.0%, respectively).[68] Only univariate analysis was performed, given the small number of adverse events under study. It is important to note that only 4 of the 10 deaths reported in the older age group were potentially attributable to biologic therapy. The risk of selection bias with inclusion of only the sickest (unwell patients as a result of inclusion of only referral centers) must be noted. Severe infection was determined as the main cause of death for the remaining observed deaths (n = 3).[69] In 2009, Ananthakrishnan and colleagues[70] also showed in a national survey that medically treated elderly patients have a higher mortality in comparison with those who are surgically treated. Advanced age, comorbidities, and *Clostridium difficile* infection were related to higher mortality during hospitalization. The risk of initiation of biologic therapy, with or without concomitant IS therapy, must be weighed against the benefit in any individual patient with risk factors for or with a personal history of tuberculosis, solid tumor malignancies, or hematological malignancies (non-Hodgkin's lymphoma or the fatal hepatosplenic T-cell lymphoma).[71]

SUMMARY AND RECOMMENDATIONS

Evolving goals of IBD care combined with increasing use of more costly biologic agents in an era of increased fiscal constraint in health care spending presents a particularly important challenge to physicians when it comes to prescribing these therapies for patients with IBD. It has become more important than ever to be able to correctly identify those individuals who would be most likely to benefit from the use of biologic therapies and to identify how best to initiate and optimize such therapies. The traditional, nonindividualized, stepwise approach to the treatment of IBD has become substandard for many patients. Such an approach increases the likelihood that structural complications will develop before therapies proven to prevent such complications are introduced. Further, the initiation of therapies for individuals who are less likely to benefit from them results in an inappropriate allocation of health care spending and precious resources, as well as in needless

Table 2
Factors predictive of response to biologic therapy

Author, Year	Biologic Agent	Study Design	Clinical Factors	Adjusted Estimate (95% CI)
CD studies				
Baert et al,[56] 2013	Adalimumab	Retrospective cohort (720 CD)	No prior infliximab (primary response)	1.11 (1.05–1.17)
			Abnormal CRP at start (success of dose escalation)	1.29 (1.04–1.60)
Löfberg et al,[39] 2012	Adalimumab	Open-label phase IIIb trial (945 CD)	CRP levels <5 mg/L	1.46 (1.09–1.97)
			Years with disease	0.96 (0.94–0.98)
			History of surgery	0.59 (0.44–0.79)
			Prior infliximab use	0.68 (0.51–0.91)
			Higher baseline HBI	0.82 (0.78–0.87)
Fefferman et al,[66] 2004	Infliximab	Prospective cohort (200 CD)	Smoking, corticosteroids, IS therapy, gender, age, age of disease onset, disease duration, and disease location	None of the studied factors were significant in the multivariable analysis
Orlando et al,[57] 2005	Infliximab	Retrospective cohort (573 CD)	Single infusion	0.49 (0.28–0.86)
			Previous surgery	0.53 (0.30–0.93)
Lionetti et al,[58] 2003	Infliximab	Retrospective cohort (22 children with CD)	Long disease duration	Higher PCDAI after treatment among late disease, 18.1 vs 5.5 ($P<.05$)[a]

Study	Drug	Study type	Predictor	OR (CI)
Arnott et al,[59] 2003	Infliximab	Prospective cohort (74 CD)	Smoking Colonic disease	0.24 (0.06–0.91) 4.87 (1.12–1.24)
Louis et al,[60] 2002	Infliximab	Prospective cohort (226 CD)	High CRP levels (>5 mg/L) before treatment	OR: 0.26 (0.11–0.63)
Vermeire et al,[61] 2002	Infliximab	Prospective cohort (240 CD)	Age Isolated ileitis Previous surgery Isolated colitis Concomitant IS	0.97 (0.95–0.99) 0.36 (0.18–0.73) 0.43 (0.23–0.79) 1.91 (1.01–3.60) 2.67 (1.43–5.02)
Parsi et al,[62] 2002	Infliximab	Retrospective cohort (100 CD)	Smoking (on response and prolonged response)	0.09 (0.02–0.38) 0.04 (0.01–0.33)
UC studies				
Subramaniam et al,[63] 2014	Infliximab and adalimumab	Retrospective cohort (59 UC)	Acute severe ulcerative colitis	10.64 (3.47–166.7)
García-Bosch et al,[64] 2013	Adalimumab	Retrospective cohort (48 UC)	Prior treatment with infliximab	9.5 (1.64–55.1)
Lee et al,[65] 2013	Infliximab	Retrospective cohort (134 UC)	IM-naïve Hemoglobin ≥11.5 g/dL CRP ≥3 mg/dL	4.89 (1.44–16.66) 4.47 (1.48–13.45) 4.77 (1.43–15.94)

Abbreviations: CD, Crohn disease; CI, confidence interval; CRP, C-reactive protein; HBI, Harvey-Bradshaw Index; IM, immunomodulator; IS, immunosuppressive; OR, odds ratio; PCDAI, Pediatric Crohn's Disease Activity Index; UC, ulcerative colitis.

[a] Unconditional result; adjusted estimated not available.

Data from Refs.[39,56–66]

exposure to therapies that may lead to the development of adverse events. Despite current limitations in our ability to identify those individuals who are most likely to benefit from early initiation of biologic agents, we have identified some clinical predictors of response to biologics that may help to guide clinical practice. It is recommended that the approach to the medical care of each patient be considered on a case-by-case basis, after careful consideration of individual clinical risk factors for complicated IBD course, their likelihood of response to biologic therapy, their likelihood of drug intolerance, risk aversion, personal preferences for drug therapy (if a choice is possible), and risk factors that might place them at higher risk of complications related to drug therapy.

REFERENCES

1. Brown SJ, Mayer L. The immune response in inflammatory bowel disease. Am J Gastroenterol 2007;102(9):2058–69.
2. Abraham C, Cho J. Inflammatory bowel disease. N Engl J Med 2009;361(21): 2066–78.
3. Hamilton MJ, Snapper SB, Blumberg RS. Update on biologic pathways in inflammatory bowel disease and their therapeutic relevance. J Gastroenterol 2012;47(1):1–8.
4. Nielsen OH, Ainsworth MA. Tumor necrosis factor inhibitors for inflammatory bowel disease. N Engl J Med 2013;369(8):754–62.
5. Duricova D, Pedersen N, Elkjaer M, et al. Overall and cause-specific mortality in Crohn's disease: a meta-analysis of population-based studies. Inflamm Bowel Dis 2010;16(2):347–53.
6. Jess T, Winther KV, Munkholm P, et al. Mortality and causes of death in Crohn's disease: follow-up of a population-based cohort in Copenhagen County, Denmark. Gastroenterology 2002;122(7):1808–14.
7. Peyrin-Biroulet L, Loftus EV Jr, Colombel JF, et al. The natural history of adult Crohn's disease in population-based cohorts. Am J Gastroenterol 2010; 105(2):289–97.
8. Targownik LE, Singh H, Nugent Z, et al. The epidemiology of colectomy in ulcerative colitis: results from a population-based cohort. Am J Gastroenterol 2012; 107(8):1228–35.
9. Peyrin-Biroulet L, Loftus EV Jr, Tremaine WJ, et al. Perianal Crohn's disease findings other than fistulas in a population-based cohort. Inflamm Bowel Dis 2012; 18(1):43–8.
10. Thia KT, Sandborn WJ, Harmsen WS, et al. Risk factors associated with progression to intestinal complications of Crohn's disease in a population-based cohort. Gastroenterology 2010;139(4):1147–55.
11. Nakamura K, Honda K, Mizutani T, et al. Novel strategies for the treatment of inflammatory bowel disease: selective inhibition of cytokines and adhesion molecules. World J Gastroenterol 2006;12(29):4628–35.
12. Sandborn WJ, Feagan BG, Rutgeerts P, et al. Vedolizumab as induction and maintenance therapy for Crohn's disease. N Engl J Med 2013;369(8): 711–21.
13. Feagan BG, Rutgeerts P, Sands BE, et al. Vedolizumab as induction and maintenance therapy for ulcerative colitis. N Engl J Med 2013;369(8):699–710.
14. Elliott M, Benson J, Blank M, et al. Ustekinumab: lessons learned from targeting interleukin-12/23p40 in immune-mediated diseases. Ann N Y Acad Sci 2009; 1182:97–110.

15. Targan SR, Hanauer SB, van Deventer SJ, et al. A short-term study of chimeric monoclonal antibody cA2 to tumor necrosis factor alpha for Crohn's disease. Crohn's disease cA2 Study Group. N Engl J Med 1997;337(15):1029–35.
16. Sands BE, Anderson FH, Bernstein CN, et al. Infliximab maintenance therapy for fistulizing Crohn's disease. N Engl J Med 2004;350(9):876–85.
17. Schreiber S, Khaliq-Kareemi M, Lawrance IC, et al. Maintenance therapy with certolizumab pegol for Crohn's disease. N Engl J Med 2007;357(3):239–50.
18. Schreiber S, Rutgeerts P, Fedorak RN, et al. A randomized, placebo-controlled trial of certolizumab pegol (CDP870) for treatment of Crohn's disease. Gastroenterology 2005;129(3):807–18.
19. Sandborn WJ, Feagan BG, Stoinov S, et al. Certolizumab pegol for the treatment of Crohn's disease. N Engl J Med 2007;357(3):228–38.
20. Sandborn WJ, Hanauer SB, Rutgeerts P, et al. Adalimumab for maintenance treatment of Crohn's disease: results of the CLASSIC II trial. Gut 2007;56(9):1232–9.
21. Colombel JF, Sandborn WJ, Rutgeerts P, et al. Adalimumab for maintenance of clinical response and remission in patients with Crohn's disease: the CHARM trial. Gastroenterology 2007;132(1):52–65.
22. Hanauer SB, Feagan BG, Lichtenstein GR, et al. Maintenance infliximab for Crohn's disease: the ACCENT I randomised trial. Lancet 2002;359(9317):1541–9.
23. Sandborn WJ, Feagan BG, Marano C, et al. Subcutaneous golimumab induces clinical response and remission in patients with moderate-to-severe ulcerative colitis. Gastroenterology 2014;146(1):85–95 [quiz: e14–5].
24. Sandborn WJ, Feagan BG, Marano C, et al. Subcutaneous golimumab maintains clinical response in patients with moderate-to-severe ulcerative colitis. Gastroenterology 2014;146(1):96–109.e1.
25. Regueiro M, Schraut W, Baidoo L, et al. Infliximab prevents Crohn's disease recurrence after ileal resection. Gastroenterology 2009;136(2):441–50.e1 [quiz: 716].
26. Peyrin-Biroulet L, Lémann M. Review article: remission rates achievable by current therapies for inflammatory bowel disease. Aliment Pharmacol Ther 2011;33(8):870–9.
27. Sandborn WJ, Colombel JF, Enns R, et al. Natalizumab induction and maintenance therapy for Crohn's disease. N Engl J Med 2005;353(18):1912–25.
28. Miller DH, Khan OA, Sheremata WA, et al. A controlled trial of natalizumab for relapsing multiple sclerosis. N Engl J Med 2003;348(1):15–23.
29. Van Assche G, Van Ranst M, Sciot R, et al. Progressive multifocal leukoencephalopathy after natalizumab therapy for Crohn's disease. N Engl J Med 2005;353(4):362–8.
30. Monograph P. Tysabri (natalizumab) injection, for intravenous use initial U.S. approval: 2004. Cambridge (MA): Biogen Idec Canada Inc.; 2012.
31. Lichtenstein GR, Rutgeerts P. Importance of mucosal healing in ulcerative colitis. Inflamm Bowel Dis 2010;16(2):338–46.
32. Allen PB, Peyrin-Biroulet L. Moving towards disease modification in inflammatory bowel disease therapy. Curr Opin Gastroenterol 2013;29(4):397–404.
33. Peyrin-Biroulet L, Fiorino G, Buisson A, et al. First-line therapy in adult Crohn's disease: who should receive anti-TNF agents? Nat Rev Gastroenterol Hepatol 2013;10(6):345–51.
34. Frøslie KF, Jahnsen J, Moum BA, et al. Mucosal healing in inflammatory bowel disease: results from a Norwegian population-based cohort. Gastroenterology 2007;133(2):412–22.

35. Colombel JF, Sandborn WJ, Reinisch W, et al. Infliximab, azathioprine, or combination therapy for Crohn's disease. N Engl J Med 2010;362(15): 1383–95.

36. Panaccione R, Ghosh S, Middleton S, et al. Combination therapy with infliximab and azathioprine is superior to monotherapy with either agent in ulcerative colitis. Gastroenterology 2014;146(2):392–400.e3.

37. Rutgeerts P, Van Assche G, Sandborn WJ, et al. Adalimumab induces and maintains mucosal healing in patients with Crohn's disease: data from the EXTEND trial. Gastroenterology 2012;142(5):1102–11.e2.

38. Hyams J, Crandall W, Kugathasan S, et al. Induction and maintenance infliximab therapy for the treatment of moderate-to-severe Crohn's disease in children. Gastroenterology 2007;132(3):863–73 [quiz: 1165–6].

39. Löfberg R, Louis EV, Reinisch W, et al. Adalimumab produces clinical remission and reduces extraintestinal manifestations in Crohn's disease: results from CARE. Inflamm Bowel Dis 2012;18(1):1–9.

40. Schreiber S, Colombel JF, Bloomfield R, et al. Increased response and remission rates in short-duration Crohn's disease with subcutaneous certolizumab pegol: an analysis of PRECiSE 2 randomized maintenance trial data. Am J Gastroenterol 2010;105(7):1574–82.

41. Ramadas AV, Gunesh S, Thomas GA, et al. Natural history of Crohn's disease in a population-based cohort from Cardiff (1986-2003): a study of changes in medical treatment and surgical resection rates. Gut 2010;59(9):1200–6.

42. Schnitzler F, Fidder H, Ferrante M, et al. Long-term outcome of treatment with infliximab in 614 patients with Crohn's disease: results from a single-centre cohort. Gut 2009;58(4):492–500.

43. D'Haens G, Baert F, van Assche G, et al. Early combined immunosuppression or conventional management in patients with newly diagnosed Crohn's disease: an open randomised trial. Lancet 2008;371(9613):660–7.

44. D'Haens GR. Top-down therapy for IBD: rationale and requisite evidence. Nat Rev Gastroenterol Hepatol 2010;7(2):86–92.

45. Jess T, Riis L, Vind I, et al. Changes in clinical characteristics, course, and prognosis of inflammatory bowel disease during the last 5 decades: a population-based study from Copenhagen, Denmark. Inflamm Bowel Dis 2007;13(4): 481–9.

46. Peyrin-Biroulet L, Billioud V, D'Haens G, et al. Development of the Paris definition of early Crohn's disease for disease-modification trials: results of an international expert opinion process. Am J Gastroenterol 2012;107(12):1770–6.

47. Ferrante M, Henckaerts L, Joossens M, et al. New serological markers in inflammatory bowel disease are associated with complicated disease behaviour. Gut 2007;56(10):1394–403.

48. Dubinsky MC, Kugathasan S, Mei L, et al. Increased immune reactivity predicts aggressive complicating Crohn's disease in children. Clin Gastroenterol Hepatol 2008;6(10):1105–11.

49. Ryan JD, Silverberg MS, Xu W, et al. Predicting complicated Crohn's disease and surgery: phenotypes, genetics, serology and psychological characteristics of a population-based cohort. Aliment Pharmacol Ther 2013;38(3):274–83.

50. Solberg IC, Cvancarova M, Vatn MH, et al. Risk matrix for prediction of advanced disease in a population-based study of patients with Crohn's disease (the IBSEN Study). Inflamm Bowel Dis 2014;20(1):60–8.

51. Prideaux L, De Cruz P, Ng SC, et al. Serological antibodies in inflammatory bowel disease: a systematic review. Inflamm Bowel Dis 2012;18(7):1340–55.

52. Harris RA, Nagy-Szakal D, Pedersen N, et al. Genome-wide peripheral blood leukocyte DNA methylation microarrays identified a single association with inflammatory bowel diseases. Inflamm Bowel Dis 2012;18(12):2334–41.
53. Vermeire S, Van Assche G, Rutgeerts P. Role of genetics in prediction of disease course and response to therapy. World J Gastroenterol 2010;16(21):2609–15.
54. Allez M, Lemann M. Role of endoscopy in predicting the disease course in inflammatory bowel disease. World J Gastroenterol 2010;16(21):2626–32.
55. D'Haens GR, Panaccione R, Higgins PD, et al. The London Position Statement of the World Congress of Gastroenterology on Biological Therapy for IBD with the European Crohn's and Colitis Organization: when to start, when to stop, which drug to choose, and how to predict response? Am J Gastroenterol 2011; 106(2):199–212 [quiz: 213].
56. Baert F, Glorieus E, Reenaers C, et al. Adalimumab dose escalation and dose de-escalation success rate and predictors in a large national cohort of Crohn's patients. J Crohns Colitis 2013;7(2):154–60.
57. Orlando A, Colombo E, Kohn A, et al. Infliximab in the treatment of Crohn's disease: predictors of response in an Italian multicentric open study. Dig Liver Dis 2005;37(8):577–83.
58. Lionetti P, Bronzini F, Salvestrini C, et al. Response to infliximab is related to disease duration in paediatric Crohn's disease. Aliment Pharmacol Ther 2003; 18(4):425–31.
59. Arnott ID, McNeill G, Satsangi J. An analysis of factors influencing short-term and sustained response to infliximab treatment for Crohn's disease. Aliment Pharmacol Ther 2003;17(12):1451–7.
60. Louis E, Vermeire S, Rutgeerts P, et al. A positive response to infliximab in Crohn disease: association with a higher systemic inflammation before treatment but not with -308 TNF gene polymorphism. Scand J Gastroenterol 2002;37(7): 818–24.
61. Vermeire S, Louis E, Carbonez A, et al. Demographic and clinical parameters influencing the short-term outcome of anti-tumor necrosis factor (infliximab) treatment in Crohn's disease. Am J Gastroenterol 2002;97(9):2357–63.
62. Parsi MA, Achkar JP, Richardson S, et al. Predictors of response to infliximab in patients with Crohn's disease. Gastroenterology 2002;123(3):707–13.
63. Subramaniam K, Richardson A, Dodd J, et al. Early predictors of colectomy and long-term maintenance of remission in ulcerative colitis patients treated using anti-TNF therapy. Intern Med J 2014;44:464–70.
64. García-Bosch O, Gisbert JP, Cañas-Ventura A, et al. Observational study on the efficacy of adalimumab for the treatment of ulcerative colitis and predictors of outcome. J Crohns Colitis 2013;7(9):717–22.
65. Lee KM, Jeen YT, Cho JY, et al. Efficacy, safety, and predictors of response to infliximab therapy for ulcerative colitis: a Korean multicenter retrospective study. J Gastroenterol Hepatol 2013;28(12):1829–33.
66. Fefferman DS, Lodhavia PJ, Alsahli M, et al. Smoking and immunomodulators do not influence the response or duration of response to infliximab in Crohn's disease. Inflamm Bowel Dis 2004;10(4):346–51.
67. Stallmach A, Hagel S, Bruns T. Adverse effects of biologics used for treating IBD. Best Pract Res Clin Gastroenterol 2010;24(2):167–82.
68. Cottone M, Kohn A, Daperno M, et al. Advanced age is an independent risk factor for severe infections and mortality in patients given anti-tumor necrosis factor therapy for inflammatory bowel disease. Clin Gastroenterol Hepatol 2011;9(1): 30–5.

69. Ananthakrishnan AN, McGinley EL, Binion DG. Excess hospitalisation burden associated with *Clostridium difficile* in patients with inflammatory bowel disease. Gut 2008;57(2):205–10.
70. Ananthakrishnan AN, McGinley EL, Binion DG. Inflammatory bowel disease in the elderly is associated with worse outcomes: a national study of hospitalizations. Inflamm Bowel Dis 2009;15(2):182–9.
71. Melmed GY, Spiegel BM, Bressler B, et al. The appropriateness of concomitant immunomodulators with anti-tumor necrosis factor agents for Crohn's disease: one size does not fit all. Clin Gastroenterol Hepatol 2010;8(8):655–9.

Anti–Tumor Necrosis Factor-α Monotherapy Versus Combination Therapy with an Immunomodulator in IBD

CrossMark

Parambir S. Dulai, MBBS[a], Corey A. Siegel, MD, MS[a],
Laurent Peyrin-Biroulet, MD, PhD[b],*

KEYWORDS

- Anti-TNF • Immunomodulator • Monotherapy • Combination therapy

KEY POINTS

- The best available evidence in inflammatory bowel disease demonstrates that the use of infliximab in combination with azathioprine is superior to infliximab monotherapy in both Crohn disease and ulcerative colitis.
- Further direct comparative effectiveness studies are needed to establish the efficacy of combination therapy for anti–tumor necrosis factor (anti-TNF) agents other than infliximab.
- The efficacy of methotrexate as the concomitant immunomodulator agent remains unclear, but the clear impact on immunogenicity and potential reduction in risk for malignancy warrants consideration for use in certain clinical settings.
- In patients at higher risk for serious infection and malignancy, the use of combination therapy should be approached with caution.
- When possible, consideration may be given to transitioning to monotherapy with either an anti-TNF agent or an immunomodulator in patients at low risk for relapse.

INTRODUCTION

Anti–tumor necrosis factor (anti-TNF) therapy is an effective treatment option for inflammatory bowel disease (IBD), and the use of these biologics has risen substantially over the past decade. Despite the increased use and availability of biologics, the

Disclosures: C.A. Siegel serves on the advisory board and as a consultant for Abbvie, Janssen, Takeda and UCB, and has received grant support from AbbVie, Janssen, and UCB. He has delivered CME lectures for Abbvie, Janssen and Merck. Dr C.A. Siegel is supported by Grant number 1R01HS021747-01 from the Agency for Healthcare Research and Quality.
[a] Inflammatory Bowel Disease Center, Dartmouth-Hitchcock Medical Center, One Medical Center Drive, Lebanon, NH 03756, USA; [b] Inserm U954, Department of Hepato-Gastroenterology, Université de Lorraine, Allée du Morvan, Vandoeuvre-lès-Nancy 54511, France
* Corresponding author.
E-mail address: peyrinbiroulet@gmail.com

Gastroenterol Clin N Am 43 (2014) 441–456
http://dx.doi.org/10.1016/j.gtc.2014.05.009
0889-8553/14/$ – see front matter © 2014 Elsevier Inc. All rights reserved.

question of the most effective therapeutic strategy still remains. The most debated of these questions is whether anti-TNF therapy should be used alone or in combination with an immunomodulator. When considering the use of anti-TNF therapy in other inflammatory conditions, such as rheumatoid arthritis (RA), the combination of an anti-TNF agent with an immunomodulator is clearly superior to anti-TNF monotherapy, and the use of combination therapy is now considered standard of care.[1]

In patients with IBD, anti-TNF therapy was initially used as salvage therapy, and combination therapy represented the addition of an anti-TNF in patients failing other therapeutic regimens, including immunomodulators. When the "top-down" approach demonstrated that the use of combination therapy earlier in the disease course was more effective than the traditional "step-up" approach,[2] then combination therapy in patients who were naïve to both drugs was supported. Subsequently, randomized control trials (RCT) demonstrated that the combination of infliximab (IFX) and azathioprine (AZA) was superior to monotherapy with either agent, and this enhanced efficacy correlated with improved pharmacokinetics, similar to that seen in RA.[1,3,4] Concerns arise, however, regarding the long-term efficacy of this approach in IBD, and the safety of combining 2 immunosuppressive drugs for an extended duration of time, especially in young men and the elderly ($\geq$65 years) population with IBD.[5,6] As we have learned more about which patients might be at higher risk for adverse events and for complications of their disease, recent efforts have focused on identifying the patients in whom combination therapy is thought to be most appropriate by taking into account the risk-benefit ratio of each strategy.

In this review, we discuss the currently available evidence regarding the efficacy of anti-TNF therapy in IBD when used as monotherapy versus in combination with an immunomodulator. We will further highlight those populations at greatest risk for adverse events and outline a clinical approach to the use of combination therapy in these patients. Finally, we discuss barriers to initiating therapy and identify tools through which providers may communicate these data to patients at the bedside.

CLINICAL EFFICACY AND PHARMACOKINETICS

The debate surrounding efficacy and the use of anti-TNF therapy in combination with an immunomodulator stems largely from the impact that immunomodulators have on the rate of antidrug antibody formation and subsequent drug concentrations. Episodic use of anti-TNF therapy was initially very common,[7–9] but it quickly became apparent that episodic therapy was associated with impaired anti-TNF pharmacokinetics (specifically the presence of antidrug antibodies and low drug concentrations), which in turn significantly impacted treatment outcomes.[10–13] Although episodic use of anti-TNFs is no longer considered a reasonable treatment approach, it taught us that the use of a concomitant immunomodulator reduced the formation of anti-TNF antibodies and allowed for more consistent drug concentrations, thereby resulting in enhanced treatment efficacy.[14] Evidence for the impact of combination therapy on antibody formation, drug concentrations, and treatment efficacy, when following scheduled anti-TNF treatments, is more inconsistent.

Observational Studies

Several observational studies have attempted to address this question with variable findings (**Table 1**).[15–33] Sokol and colleagues[15] divided IFX treatment periods for a cohort of patients with IBD and subsequently analyzed these data according to whether patients had been treated with IFX monotherapy (n = 319 semesters) or IFX combination therapy (n = 265 semesters). This study demonstrated that the concomitant use of an immunomodulator decreased the risk for an IBD flare (odds ratio [OR] 0.50, 95% confidence interval [CI] 0.32–0.77), and when considering the need for abdominal surgery or switching to adalimumab (ADA), cotreatment with an immunomodulator was again demonstrated to significantly reduce the risk of these events (OR 0.18, 95% CI 0.05–0.63). Given the impact immunomodulator therapy has on pharmacokinetics when using episodic anti-TNF therapy, Ungar and colleagues[17] later assessed the correlation between antidrug antibody formation and clinical response in patients receiving concomitant immunomodulator therapy while undergoing scheduled maintenance therapy. They demonstrated that the use of combination therapy resulted in longer antibody-free survival (P = .003), and survival free of loss of response was significantly longer among patients with no antidrug antibodies (P<.01).

Other observational studies evaluating the correlation between IFX pharmacokinetics and clinical outcomes, however, have found no such correlation among combination therapy, pharmacokinetics, and enhanced efficacy. Maser and colleagues[18] demonstrated that the concurrent use of an immunomodulator did not alter the proportion of patients who achieved complete interval remission (P = .49), a normal C-reactive protein (P = .16), and endoscopic improvement (P = .59). Although this study demonstrated a correlation between IFX concentrations and improved outcomes, it was the use of scheduled maintenance therapy and not concomitant immunomodulator therapy that impacted antibody formation and IFX levels. Seow and colleagues[19] similarly demonstrated that IFX trough levels were associated with increased rates of clinical remission (OR 12.5, 95% CI 4.6–33.9) and endoscopic improvement (OR 7.3, 95% CI 2.9–18.4), but the use of combination therapy had no impact on antidrug antibody formation (P = .88), IFX trough levels (P = .46), clinical remission (OR 1.16, 95% CI 0.47–2.88), or the rate of colectomy (OR 1.13, 95% CI 0.46–2.75). Data regarding the impact of concomitant immunomodulator therapy has similarly been conflicting when considering ADA, certolizumab pegol (CZP), or golimumab, but observational data evaluating the correlation among combination therapy, pharmacokinetics, and clinical efficacy for these anti-TNF agents are limited.

RCTs

Several investigators have suggested that these observational studies more closely represent the real-life experience with these drugs,[34] but the differences in baseline characteristics across studies, variability, and inconsistency in outcome measurements, and method of analysis (subanalyses) significantly limit the conclusions that can be made from these data. RCTs in contrast represent the best-available evidence with regard to treatment efficacy given the rigorous nature of these studies and more consistent measurement of key clinical end points. Subanalyses of anti-TNF RCTs stratified according to baseline immunomodulator use have demonstrated that, despite a clear association between combination therapy and pharmacokinetics, the use of combination therapy appears to have no impact on clinical outcomes (**Table 2**).[35–39]

More recently, a systematic review pooled RCT data for 3 anti-TNF therapies (IFX, ADA, CZP) in Crohn disease (CD) and demonstrated that although there was no overall impact on outcomes (response, remission, fistula closure),[40] the use of combination therapy was more efficacious than monotherapy for 6-month remission rates in IFX-treated patients specifically (OR 1.79, 95% CI 1.06–3.01), but not ADA-treated (OR 0.88, 95% CI 0.58–1.35) or CZP-treated (OR 0.93; 95% CI 0.65–1.34) patients. When attempting to interpret these data, clinicians should be reminded that the ADA and CZP RCTs enrolled a significant proportion of patients who had failed IFX

Table 1
Observational studies assessing impact of combination therapy

	Anti-TNF	Impact of Combination Therapy
Sokol et al,[15] 2010	IFX	Decreased risk of clinical flare, need for abdominal surgery or switching to ADA therapy during follow-up. Flares and complications were less frequently observed when AZA was used as the concomitant immunomodulator as compared with MTX.
Bouguen et al,[16] 2013	IFX	Concomitant immunosuppressive therapy increased the likelihood of fistula closure, and this impact was more pronounced for first fistula closure in patients who were naïve to immunosuppressants. Combination therapy had no impact on fistula or abscess recurrence.
Ungar et al,[17] 2013	IFX	Increased duration of clinical response, but effect was blunted when only patients who were scheduled for maintenance therapy were analyzed.
Maser et al,[18] 2006	IFX	Scheduled maintenance therapy, but not concomitant IM therapy, improved complete interval remission, normalization of CRP, and endoscopic improvement.
Seow et al,[19] 2010	IFX	No impact on antidrug antibody formation, IFX levels, clinical remission, or rate of colectomy.
Baert et al,[20] 2014	IFX	The use of an IM at reinitiation of IFX improved short-term response. Although the overall trough level of IFX was similar between anti-TNF mono and combo groups, within the subgroup having the lowest quartile of trough levels, combo therapy resulted in significantly higher levels. Median ATI was also lower on combo therapy. The presence of ATI was a negative predictor for response, and absence of ATI was a positive predictor for safely restarting IFX therapy.
Bortlik et al,[21] 2013	IFX	Combo therapy resulted in lower ATI levels and higher IFX trough concentrations, and higher trough concentrations (>3 µg/mL) were associated with a decreased risk of treatment failure, but concomitant IM therapy had no direct measurable impact on sustained response to IFX.

Study	Agent	Findings
Baert et al,[22] 2010	IFX	Combo therapy resulted in lower ATI formation and higher IFX concentrations, but it had no overall impact on the duration of response to IFX.
Paul et al,[23] 2013	IFX	No impact on ATI formation, IFX trough concentrations, or clinical remission.
Pariente et al,[24] 2012	IFX	Trend toward lower incidence of ATI formation, but no impact on IFX trough levels or clinical outcomes.
Imaeda et al,[25] 2014	IFX	No impact on IFX trough levels or ATI formation, both of which were predictors of achieving mucosal healing.
Karmiris et al,[26] 2009	ADA	Increased ADA dose, but not concomitant IM therapy, reduced antibody formation, increased trough concentrations, improved initial response to therapy, and improved the likelihood of maintaining a sustained clinical response.
Lofberg et al,[27] 2012	ADA	Increased likelihood of achieving clinical remission after induction therapy (4 wk) and during follow-up (20 wk).
Reenaers et al,[28] 2012	ADA	No overall impact on risk for disease flares or ADA failure, but early use (first 6 mo of ADA) of combination therapy was associated with lower ADA failure rates, and prolonged use (beyond 6 mo) was associated with fewer semesters with flares.
Cohen et al,[29] 2012	ADA	No impact on the need for ADA dose escalation.
Chaparro et al,[30] 2012	ADA	No impact on likelihood of maintaining response to ADA.
Allez et al,[31] 2010	ADA, CZP	When initiating ADA or CZP as the third anti-TNF agent, the use of combo therapy had no impact on the probability of remaining on anti-TNF therapy.
De Silva et al,[32] 2012	Multiple	No impact on clinical response to third anti-TNF agent after failing 2 previous agents.
Bougen et al,[33] 2014	Multiple	No impact on likelihood of achieving mucosal healing when following a treat-to-target approach

Abbreviations: ADA, adalimumab; anti-TNF, anti–tumor necrosis factor; ATI, anti-drug antibody; combo, combination therapy; CRP, C-reactive protein; CZP, certolizumab pegol; IBD, inflammatory bowel disease; IFX, infliximab; IM, immunomodulator (azathioprine, 6-nercaptopurine, methotrexate); mono, monotherapy.

Data from Refs.[15–33]

Table 2
Subgroup analyses of randomized controlled trials stratified for concomitant immunomodulator therapy

	Agent	Clinical Remission (%)		Antidrug Antibody (%)	
		Mono	Combo	Mono	Combo
ACT 1	IFX	36	34	12	3.5
ACT 2	IFX	27	36	15.5	2.5
ACCENT I	IFX	32	37	9.5	5.6
ACCENT II[a]	IFX	38	32	18.1	2.4
PRECISE 2[b]	CZP	64	61	12	2
CLASSIC II	ADA	45	48	3.8	0
PURSUIT[a]	GOL	50	44	3.8	1.1

Abbreviations: ACCENT, A Crohn's Disease Clinical Trial Evaluating Infliximab in a New Long-term Treatment Regimen; ACT, Active Ulcerative Colitis Trials; ADA, adalimumab; Combo, anti–tumor necrosis factor (anti-TNF) therapy in combination with an immunomodulator; CLASSIC, Clinical Assessment of Adalimumab Safety and Efficacy Studied as Induction Therapy in Crohn's Disease; CZP, certolizumab pegol; GOL, golimumab; IFX, infliximab; Mono, anti-TNF monotherapy; PRECISE, Pegylated Antibody Fragment Evaluation in Crohn's Disease: Safety and Efficacy; PURSUIT, Program of Ulcerative Colitis Research Studies Utilizing an Investigational Treatment.
[a] Complete fistula closure used for clinical remission in ACCENT II and clinical response used for clinical remission in PURSUIT.
[b] Week 26 response used in place of clinical remission and data from maintenance group used for antidrug antibody levels.
Data from Refs.[35–39]

therapy, and the use of combination therapy in these studies actually represented the continuation of an immunomodulator in patients switching anti-TNF agents. Furthermore, this meta-analysis excluded patients who were naïve to immunomodulator therapy, and this cohort more closely resembles the classic "step-up" approach to combination therapy, as opposed to the more efficacious "top-down" strategy. As there was no assessment of the impact of combination therapy on pharmacokinetics in this meta-analysis, it is unclear if this benefit for IFX but not ADA and CZP is secondary to a reduction in immunogenicity and improved pharmacokinetics, or variations in study populations and analysis.

An even more recent meta-analysis, pooling data from 6 RCT and 12 observational studies for ADA, demonstrated that the use of ADA in combination with an immunomodulator was superior to ADA monotherapy with regard to induction of remission at 12 weeks (OR 0.78, 95% CI 0.64–0.95), but not for induction of response (OR 0.68, 95% CI 0.37–1.25) or need for ADA dose escalation to achieve a clinical response (OR, 1.24; 95% CI, 0.70–2.20).[41] Similar to the previous meta-analysis by Jones and colleagues,[40] there was again no difference between ADA monotherapy or combination therapy with regard to long-term (52 week) maintenance of response (OR 1.21, 95% CI 0.74–1.99) or remission (OR 1.08, 95% CI 0.87–1.33). Given the variability and inherit limitations of these data with regard to patient populations, previous drug exposure, and outcome assessment, perhaps the most robust assessment of whether combination therapy improves outcomes will come from comparative effectiveness studies directly comparing these 2 strategies in a randomized cohort of patients with IBD.

The Study of Biologic and Immunomodulator Naïve Patients in Crohn's Disease (SONIC) trial randomized patients with moderate-to-severe CD to AZA monotherapy (n = 170), IFX monotherapy (n = 169), or IFX and AZA combination therapy (n = 169), and demonstrated that the combination therapy group had a higher rate of corticosteroid-free remission (*P* = .02) and mucosal healing (*P* = .06) at week 26, with a similar trend being seen at week 50 (**Table 3**).[3] The Combination of Maintenance Methotrexate-Infliximab Trial (COMMIT), which randomized patients with moderate-to-severe CD to IFX monotherapy (n = 63) or IFX and methotrexate (MTX) combination therapy (n = 63), found no significant difference with regard to achieving week 14 steroid-free remission or maintaining this remission out to week 50 (*P* = .63).[42] When considering ulcerative colitis (UC), the UC-SUCCESS trial randomized patients with moderate-to-severe UC to receive AZA monotherapy (n = 76), IFX monotherapy (n = 77), or IFX and AZA combination therapy (n = 78), and, similar to the SONIC trial, demonstrated that the use of IFX in combination with AZA achieved higher rates of steroid-free remission (*P* = .02).[43] Although the overall mucosal healing rate (Mayo endoscopic subscore of 0 or 1) was similar between the 2 groups (*P* = .3), the complete mucosal healing rate (Mayo score of 0) was significantly higher in the combination group (30% vs 12%, *P* = .006).

A confusing part of the story regarding combination therapy is the difference seen when using AZA or MTX. There was clear clinical and pharmacokinetic benefit for IFX in combination with AZA over IFX monotherapy for both CD (SONIC) and UC (UC-SUCCESS). The use of IFX in combination with MTX was not superior to IFX monotherapy in COMMIT, despite the measurable impact MTX had on IFX concentrations and anti-drug antibody formation (see **Table 3**). In fact, the COMMIT IFX monotherapy group achieved an absolute trough IFX concentration (3.75 μg/mL) comparable to that achieved in the SONIC IFX combination therapy group (3.5 μg/mL). There may be 2 explanations for this observation. First, the study population of COMMIT had a milder baseline disease activity as compared with the population enrolled in SONIC. Second, the COMMIT study design used high-dose induction steroid regimens in both groups. Both of these factors (disease activity and steroids) have been shown to impact anti-drug antibody formation and drug concentrations.[44,45] Therefore, the benefit of MTX added to IFX may have been obscured, and the lack of clinical benefit of combination therapy in COMMIT should be interpreted with caution. To corroborate this hypothesis, in the RA literature, the impact of MTX on IFX pharmacokinetics clearly correlates with enhanced clinical efficacy.[46]

Table 3
Direct comparative effectiveness studies assessing anti-TNF monotherapy versus combination therapy with an immunomodulator

| | Clinical Efficacy | | | | Pharmacokinetics | | | |
| | Remission (%) | | Mucosal Healing (%) | | Antidrug Antibody (%) | | IFX Concentrations (μg/mL) | |
	Mono	Combo	Mono	Combo	Mono	Combo	Mono	Combo
SONIC[3]	44	57	30	44	14.6	0.9	1.6	3.5
COMMIT[42]	78	76	n/a	n/a	20.4	4.0	3.8	6.4
UC-SUCCESS[43]	22	40	55	63	19.0	3.0	n/a	n/a

Abbreviations: anti-TNF, anti–tumor necrosis factor; Combo, anti-TNF therapy in combination with an immunomodulator; COMMIT, Combination of Maintenance Methotrexate-Infliximab Trial; IFX, infliximab; Mono, anti-TNF monotherapy; n/a, not assessed; SONIC, Study of Biologic and Immunomodulator Naïve Patients in Crohn's Disease.
Data from Refs.[3,42,43]

There are currently no direct comparative effectiveness studies available to understand the true impact of concomitant immunomodulator therapy with other anti-TNF therapies, and the currently available observational and RCT data are conflicting, but the clear impact on immunogenicity similar to that seen with IFX, and correlation between improved pharmacokinetics and disease activity seen with these agents, suggests that combination therapy is likely beneficial for all anti-TNF agents.

SAFETY OF COMBINATION THERAPY IN SPECIFIC PATIENT POPULATIONS

Although most evidence is largely in support of the use of combination therapy, the heterogeneity in outcomes and variability in patient populations makes a standard approach to this question difficult. Therefore, when considering the risks and benefits of anti-TNF monotherapy versus combination therapy, providers need to identify those populations at greatest risk for harm and make decisions based on an individual patient basis. The 2 adverse events that require the most consideration are the risk of developing a life-threatening infection or cancer.

Elderly Patients

Advanced age is an independent predictor of hospitalization and mortality,[47,48] and patients older than 65 years appear to be at a higher risk for serious infections and infection-related hospitalizations.[47] Although RCTs have found no increased risk for the development of serious infections when comparing anti-TNF monotherapy to combination therapy,[3,35,40,42,43,49] these studies often exclude elderly patients. Observational population-based studies have demonstrated that the risk of serious infection with combination therapy rises with increasing age, and a substantial portion of the overall risk with combination therapy comes from the concomitant use of corticosteroids.[6,47,50–52] When considering the risk of cancer, increasing age has been identified to be an independent predictor of malignancy risk, and pooled analyses of RCTs and observational studies have demonstrated that the use of combination therapy increases the risk for lymphoma above that seen in the general population.[53–55] Therefore, although clinical trial data support the use of a more aggressive "top-down" strategy early in the disease course for most patients, a more conservative approach with anti-TNF monotherapy may be warranted in patients older than 65 years, due to the risk of life-threatening infections and malignancy. Because nearly 20% of elderly patients with IBD become steroid-dependent during their disease course,[56] we still need to treat them with effective steroid-sparing agents. Based on the observation that most if not all of the neoplastic risk is related to thiopurines,[55,57] and this risk subsides with discontinuation of thiopurine therapy,[55,58] a short course of combination therapy with transition to anti-TNF monotherapy may be warranted in this subpopulation to allow for reductions in steroid usage and infection risk.

Young Men

A particularly concerning and often fatal lymphoma, hepatosplenic T-cell lymphoma (HSTCL), has been shown to occur more often in men younger than 35 years who were exposed to long-term ($\geq$2 years) thiopurine therapy.[5] Therefore, careful consideration should be given to the use and duration of combination therapy in these patients. A reasonable approach is to use combination therapy for young male patients with extensive or otherwise high-risk disease (eg, perianal),[16,59] and then withdrawing the thiopurine once remission is achieved. This offers the best chance for disease control while limiting the risk of HSTCL by keeping thiopurine exposure to less than 2 years.

Pregnancy

Another population that warrants special consideration is pregnant patients with IBD. Most IBD medications, with the exception of MTX and thalidomide, have now been demonstrated to be safe for use during gestation.[60] When attempting to understand the role of combination therapy in pregnancy, providers should take into consideration several factors. In patients already on immunomodulator therapy before conception, stopping the thiopurine during pregnancy may precipitate a flare resulting in adverse fetal outcomes.[61] In patients not on an immunomodulator before conception, the initiation of AZA is not recommended for the management of an acute flare because of the risk of bone marrow suppression and pancreatitis.[62] In the prospective Pregnancy in Inflammatory Bowel Disease and Neonatal Outcomes (PIANO) registry, there appeared to be no increased risk of adverse fetal outcomes when using combination therapy; however, when CZP was excluded from this analysis, there was an overall higher rate of infection in the combination therapy group as compared with the anti-TNF monotherapy group.[62,63] This may be secondary to the placental transfer of IFX and ADA (not CZP) and, therefore, in patients who are naïve to biologic therapy starting anti-TNF therapy during pregnancy, consideration should be given to the use of CZP, which has minimal placental transfer.[62,64] In all cases, the most risk to the fetus comes from disease activity, and efforts should focus on disease control and optimization based on these considerations. Anti-TNF monotherapy may be preferable for maintenance of disease control or management of acute flares in patients not already on an immunomodulator. In patients already on an immunomodulator, therapy should be continued throughout pregnancy, and anti-TNF therapy should be added if needed for flares.

Azathioprine Versus MTX

In nonpregnant patients with IBD, consideration may be given to using MTX in place of AZA as the concomitant immunomodulator. This is of particular importance when considering the association between thiopurines and Epstein-Barr virus–associated lymphomas, and the risk of HSTCL in young men.[5,65–67] Providers should be reminded, however, that although MTX and AZA are similar in their ability to improve anti-TNF pharmacokinetics (antidrug antibody and drug concentrations),[14] we do not have supportive data to confirm that adding MTX to an anti-TNF agent is clinically beneficial.[15,42] Furthermore, we must recognize that there is a lack of safety data in patients with IBD when using MTX as the concomitant immunomodulator agent, and the true oncogenic potential of MTX in this population is unknown. In RA, the comparative risk of cancer with MTX is higher than that seen with anti-TNF therapy, suggesting that some increased risk may be present when using this agent in IBD as well.[68]

Duration of Combination Therapy

The greatest hesitation to the use of an immunomodulator resides in the increased risk for malignancy with these agents, particularly when using these agents for an extended duration, as the risk of lymphoma rises exponentially with thiopurine use beyond 2 years.[5,58] It has now been demonstrated that the risk of malignancy in patients discontinuing immunomodulators appears to be similar to that seen in patients without previous exposure,[58] and therefore consideration may be given to stopping immunomodulator therapy in patients at a low risk for relapse after achieving clinical remission while on combination therapy (**Box 1**).[69] This approach is likely most appropriate in young men with limited disease, given the measurable risk of HSTCL with

---

Box 1
Factors associated with an attenuated response to therapy or disease relapse after stopping an immunomodulator or anti-TNF agent

Immunomodulators

- Male gender
- Extensive disease
- Elevated inflammatory markers (CRP, platelet count, white blood count)
- Evidence of mucosal activity on endoscopy
- Short duration in remission before stopping
- Short duration of steroid-free remission

Anti-TNF agents

- Long duration of disease before anti-TNF therapy
- Endoscopic or biologic (CRP) disease activity
- Short duration of remission or combination therapy use
- Impaired pharmacokinetics with initial use (antidrug antibodies or low drug concentrations)

Abbreviations: Anti-TNF, anti-tumor necrosis factor; CRP, C-reactive protein.

---

extended-duration thiopurines.[59] These patients should, however, be carefully monitored for disease relapse, as this strategy has been associated with dropping anti-TNF drug concentrations and antidrug antibody formation.[70] We can take a similar approach in the elderly based on the increased risk for both opportunistic and nonopportunistic infections.[50] For elderly patients who were induced into remission with combination therapy, withdrawing the thiopurine after documenting good disease control (eg, mucosal healing) and optimizing anti-TNF is very reasonable. Although we are starting to gather data that anti-TNF withdrawal may be acceptable in certain treatment scenarios, we need further prospective data to support this treatment algorithm.[20,71,72]

SHARED DECISION MAKING: HELPING PATIENTS DECIDE THE OPTIMAL APPROACH ON AN INDIVIDUALIZED BASIS

Based on these data, we have outlined an approach for providers to consider when counseling patients regarding the use of combination therapy in clinical practice (**Fig. 1**). Although the use of anti-TNF therapy in combination with an immunomodulator has several clear clinical benefits, this decision remains a preference-sensitive decision in IBD given the risks associated with the choice.[73] When helping patients decide on the most appropriate strategy at an individual level, providers have several tools to rely on. One type of decision aid that has gained popularity is an Option Grid, which is a 1-page summary table outlining head-to-head comparisons of key outcomes with different treatment strategies. These Option Grids help providers more easily explain treatment options to patients and enhance patient involvement in collaborative decision making.[74] Two Option Grids are currently available for use when considering anti-TNF monotherapy versus combination therapy in adult and pediatric patients with CD (http://www.optiongrid.org/).[75] Although these decision aids can be helpful, they do not incorporate specific patient characteristics into the decision-making process.

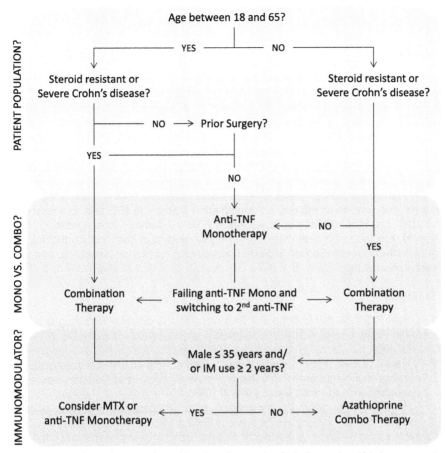

Fig. 1. Approach to the use of combination therapy in clinical practice. This is a suggested approach for the use of anti-TNF therapy in combination with an immunomodulator. Ultimately, providers should make these decisions with patients on an individual basis after carefully weighing the risks and benefits of each strategy. Anti-TNF agents are IFX, ADA, certolizumab pegol, golimumab. Combo, combination therapy; IM, immunomodulator (azathioprine, 6-mercaptopurine, methotrexate); Mono, monotherapy.

The Building Research in IBD Globally (BRIDGe) group recently applied a RAND panel methodology across various clinical scenarios and created an online tool (www.BRIDGeIBD.com) for use that allows for consideration of various patient and disease characteristics when deciding on the appropriateness of combination therapy.[59] Providers are able to input clinical variables and then output a rating of appropriate, inappropriate, or uncertain with regard to use of combination therapy versus anti-TNF monotherapy in CD. Another shared decision-making tool currently under investigation is a Web-based program linking a video Decision Aid about the benefits and risks of CD therapy to a personalized decision-making tool that presents a prediction of disease severity based on patient demographics, disease characteristics, genetic variables, and serologic markers. Providers are able to input these data in the program, which then graphically depicts a patient's individual risk for disease-related complications. This Web-based patient communication tool has now been validated in both adult and pediatric patients with CD, and the impact of this tool on provider and patient decisions is currently under investigation.[76,77]

SUMMARY

In conclusion, the use of AZA in combination with IFX is clearly superior to IFX monotherapy in both CD and UC. Further direct comparative effectiveness studies are needed to establish the efficacy of combination therapy for other anti-TNF agents, but the clear impact on pharmacokinetics suggests that combination therapy is likely beneficial for all anti-TNF agents. The use of combination therapy in high-risk populations (young men, elderly, patients who are pregnant) should be approached with caution given the risk of serious infection and malignancy with this approach. When attempting to make these decisions on an individualized basis, providers have several tools to rely on as patients and providers decide together on the most appropriate strategy. The long-term efficacy of combination therapy in IBD and its impact on the natural history of disease course (disability, bowel damage, hospitalizations, and surgeries) has yet to be determined, and the risk-benefit of combination therapy will require further investigation to guide decision making for chronic, disabling, and progressive conditions.

REFERENCES

1. Emery P, Sebba A, Huizinga TW. Biologic and oral disease-modifying antirheumatic drug monotherapy in rheumatoid arthritis. Ann Rheum Dis 2013;72: 1897–904.
2. D'Haens G, Baert F, van Assche G, et al. Early combined immunosuppression or conventional management in patients with newly diagnosed Crohn's disease: an open randomised trial. Lancet 2008;371:660–7.
3. Colombel JF, Sandborn WJ, Reinisch W, et al. Infliximab, azathioprine, or combination therapy for Crohn's disease. N Engl J Med 2010;362:1383–95.
4. Panaccione R, Ghosh S, Middleton S, et al. Combination therapy with infliximab and azathioprine is superior to monotherapy with either agent in ulcerative colitis. Gastroenterology 2014;146:392–400.e3.
5. Kotlyar DS, Osterman MT, Diamond RH, et al. A systematic review of factors that contribute to hepatosplenic T-cell lymphoma in patients with inflammatory bowel disease. Clin Gastroenterol Hepatol 2011;9:36–41.e1.
6. Stallmach A, Hagel S, Gharbi A, et al. Medical and surgical therapy of inflammatory bowel disease in the elderly—prospects and complications. J Crohns Colitis 2011;5:177–88.
7. Hanauer SB, Feagan BG, Lichtenstein GR, et al. Maintenance infliximab for Crohn's disease: the ACCENT I randomised trial. Lancet 2002;359:1541–9.
8. Sands BE, Anderson FH, Bernstein CN, et al. Infliximab maintenance therapy for fistulizing Crohn's disease. N Engl J Med 2004;350:876–85.
9. Rutgeerts P, Feagan BG, Lichtenstein GR, et al. Comparison of scheduled and episodic treatment strategies of infliximab in Crohn's disease. Gastroenterology 2004;126:402–13.
10. Nanda KS, Cheifetz AS, Moss AC. Impact of antibodies to infliximab on clinical outcomes and serum infliximab levels in patients with inflammatory bowel disease (IBD): a meta-analysis. Am J Gastroenterol 2013;108:40–7.
11. Colombel JF, Sandborn WJ, Allez M, et al. Association between plasma concentrations of certolizumab pegol and endoscopic outcomes of patients with Crohn's disease. Clin Gastroenterol Hepatol 2014;12:423–31.e1.

12. Schreiber S, Rutgeerts P, Fedorak RN, et al. A randomized, placebo-controlled trial of certolizumab pegol (CDP870) for treatment of Crohn's disease. Gastroenterology 2005;129:807–18.
13. Hanauer SB, Wagner CL, Bala M, et al. Incidence and importance of antibody responses to infliximab after maintenance or episodic treatment in Crohn's disease. Clin Gastroenterol Hepatol 2004;2:542–53.
14. Vermeire S, Noman M, Van Assche G, et al. Effectiveness of concomitant immunosuppressive therapy in suppressing the formation of antibodies to infliximab in Crohn's disease. Gut 2007;56:1226–31.
15. Sokol H, Seksik P, Carrat F, et al. Usefulness of co-treatment with immunomodulators in patients with inflammatory bowel disease treated with scheduled infliximab maintenance therapy. Gut 2010;59:1363–8.
16. Bouguen G, Siproudhis L, Gizard E, et al. Long-term outcome of perianal fistulizing Crohn's disease treated with infliximab. Clin Gastroenterol Hepatol 2013; 11:975–81.e1–4.
17. Ungar B, Chowers Y, Yavzori M, et al. The temporal evolution of antidrug antibodies in patients with inflammatory bowel disease treated with infliximab. Gut 2013. [Epub ahead of print].
18. Maser EA, Villela R, Silverberg MS, et al. Association of trough serum infliximab to clinical outcome after scheduled maintenance treatment for Crohn's disease. Clin Gastroenterol Hepatol 2006;4:1248–54.
19. Seow CH, Newman A, Irwin SP, et al. Trough serum infliximab: a predictive factor of clinical outcome for infliximab treatment in acute ulcerative colitis. Gut 2010; 59:49–54.
20. Baert F, Drobne D, Gils A, et al. Early trough levels and antibodies to infliximab predict safety and success of re-initiation of infliximab therapy. Clin Gastroenterol Hepatol 2014. [Epub ahead of print].
21. Bortlik M, Duricova D, Malickova K, et al. Infliximab trough levels may predict sustained response to infliximab in patients with Crohn's disease. J Crohns Colitis 2013;7:736–43.
22. Baert F, Moortgat L, Van Assche G, et al. Mucosal healing predicts sustained clinical remission in patients with early-stage Crohn's disease. Gastroenterology 2010;138:463–8 [quiz: e10–1].
23. Paul S, Del Tedesco E, Marotte H, et al. Therapeutic drug monitoring of infliximab and mucosal healing in inflammatory bowel disease: a prospective study. Inflamm Bowel Dis 2013;19:2568–76.
24. Pariente B, Pineton de Chambrun G, Krzysiek R, et al. Trough levels and antibodies to infliximab may not predict response to intensification of infliximab therapy in patients with inflammatory bowel disease. Inflamm Bowel Dis 2012;18:1199–206.
25. Imaeda H, Bamba S, Takahashi K, et al. Relationship between serum infliximab trough levels and endoscopic activities in patients with Crohn's disease under scheduled maintenance treatment. J Gastroenterol 2014;49:674–82.
26. Karmiris K, Paintaud G, Noman M, et al. Influence of trough serum levels and immunogenicity on long-term outcome of adalimumab therapy in Crohn's disease. Gastroenterology 2009;137:1628–40.
27. Lofberg R, Louis EV, Reinisch W, et al. Adalimumab produces clinical remission and reduces extraintestinal manifestations in Crohn's disease: results from CARE. Inflamm Bowel Dis 2012;18:1–9.
28. Reenaers C, Louis E, Belaiche J, et al. Does co-treatment with immunosuppressors improve outcome in patients with Crohn's disease treated with adalimumab? Aliment Pharmacol Ther 2012;36:1040–8.

29. Cohen RD, Lewis JR, Turner H, et al. Predictors of adalimumab dose escalation in patients with Crohn's disease at a tertiary referral center. Inflamm Bowel Dis 2012; 18:10–6.

30. Chaparro M, Panes J, Garcia V, et al. Long-term durability of response to adalimumab in Crohn's disease. Inflamm Bowel Dis 2012;18:685–90.

31. Allez M, Vermeire S, Mozziconacci N, et al. The efficacy and safety of a third anti-TNF monoclonal antibody in Crohn's disease after failure of two other anti-TNF antibodies. Aliment Pharmacol Ther 2010;31:92–101.

32. de Silva PS, Nguyen DD, Sauk J, et al. Long-term outcome of a third anti-TNF monoclonal antibody after the failure of two prior anti-TNFs in inflammatory bowel disease. Aliment Pharmacol Ther 2012;36:459–66.

33. Bouguen G, Levesque BG, Pola S, et al. Endoscopic assessment and treating to target increase the likelihood of mucosal healing in patients with Crohn's disease. Clin Gastroenterol Hepatol 2014;12:978–85.

34. Ha C, Ullman TA, Siegel CA, et al. Patients enrolled in randomized controlled trials do not represent the inflammatory bowel disease patient population. Clin Gastroenterol Hepatol 2012;10:1002–7 [quiz: e78].

35. Lichtenstein GR, Diamond RH, Wagner CL, et al. Clinical trial: benefits and risks of immunomodulators and maintenance infliximab for IBD-subgroup analyses across four randomized trials. Aliment Pharmacol Ther 2009;30:210–26.

36. Sandborn WJ, Hanauer SB, Rutgeerts P, et al. Adalimumab for maintenance treatment of Crohn's disease: results of the CLASSIC II trial. Gut 2007;56:1232–9.

37. Sandborn WJ, Feagan BG, Stoinov S, et al. Certolizumab pegol for the treatment of Crohn's disease. N Engl J Med 2007;357:228–38.

38. Sandborn WJ, Feagan BG, Marano C, et al. Subcutaneous golimumab maintains clinical response in patients with moderate-to-severe ulcerative colitis. Gastroenterology 2014;146:96–109.e1.

39. Sandborn WJ, Feagan BG, Marano C, et al. Subcutaneous golimumab induces clinical response and remission in patients with moderate-to-severe ulcerative colitis. Gastroenterology 2014;146:85–95 [quiz: e14–5].

40. Jones J, Kaplan GG, Peyrin-Biroulet L, et al. Impact of concomitant immunomodulator treatment on efficacy and safety of anti-TNF therapy in Crohn's disease: a meta-analysis of placebo controlled trials with individual patient-level data. Gastroenterology 2013;144:S-179.

41. Kopylov U, Al-Taweel T, Yaghoobi M, et al. Adalimumab monotherapy versus combination therapy with adalimumab and immunomodulators for Crohn's disease: a meta-analysis. Gastroenterology 2014;146:S-201.

42. Feagan BG, McDonald JW, Panaccione R, et al. Methotrexate in combination with infliximab is no more effective than infliximab alone in patients with Crohn's disease. Gastroenterology 2014;146:681–8.e1.

43. Panaccione R, Ghosh S, Middleton S, et al. Infliximab, azathioprine, or infliximab and azathioprine for treatment of moderate to severe ulcerative colitis: the UC success trial. Gastroenterology 2011;140:A-202.

44. Billioud V, Sandborn WJ, Peyrin-Biroulet L. Loss of response and need for adalimumab dose intensification in Crohn's disease: a systematic review. Am J Gastroenterol 2011;106:674–84.

45. Farrell RJ, Alsahli M, Jeen YT, et al. Intravenous hydrocortisone premedication reduces antibodies to infliximab in Crohn's disease: a randomized controlled trial. Gastroenterology 2003;124:917–24.

46. Maini RN, Breedveld FC, Kalden JR, et al. Therapeutic efficacy of multiple intravenous infusions of anti-tumor necrosis factor alpha monoclonal antibody

combined with low-dose weekly methotrexate in rheumatoid arthritis. Arthritis Rheum 1998;41:1552–63.

47. Ananthakrishnan AN, McGinley EL. Infection-related hospitalizations are associated with increased mortality in patients with inflammatory bowel diseases. J Crohns Colitis 2013;7:107–12.

48. Lichtenstein GR, Feagan BG, Cohen RD, et al. Serious infection and mortality in patients with Crohn's disease: more than 5 years of follow-up in the TREAT registry. Am J Gastroenterol 2012;107:1409–22.

49. Lichtenstein GR, Rutgeerts P, Sandborn WJ, et al. A pooled analysis of infections, malignancy, and mortality in infliximab- and immunomodulator-treated adult patients with inflammatory bowel disease. Am J Gastroenterol 2012;107: 1051–63.

50. Toruner M, Loftus EV Jr, Harmsen WS, et al. Risk factors for opportunistic infections in patients with inflammatory bowel disease. Gastroenterology 2008;134:929–36.

51. Marehbian J, Arrighi HM, Hass S, et al. Adverse events associated with common therapy regimens for moderate-to-severe Crohn's disease. Am J Gastroenterol 2009;104:2524–33.

52. Deepak P, Stobaugh DJ, Ehrenpreis ED. Infectious complications of TNF-alpha inhibitor monotherapy versus combination therapy with immunomodulators in inflammatory bowel disease: analysis of the Food and Drug Administration Adverse Event Reporting System. J Gastrointestin Liver Dis 2013;22:269–76.

53. Siegel CA, Marden SM, Persing SM, et al. Risk of lymphoma associated with combination anti-tumor necrosis factor and immunomodulator therapy for the treatment of Crohn's disease: a meta-analysis. Clin Gastroenterol Hepatol 2009;7: 874–81.

54. Lichtenstein GR, Feagan BG, Cohen RD, et al. Drug therapies and the risk of malignancy in Crohn's disease: results from the TREAT registry. Am J Gastroenterol 2014;109:212–23.

55. Beaugerie L, Brousse N, Bouvier AM, et al. Lymphoproliferative disorders in patients receiving thiopurines for inflammatory bowel disease: a prospective observational cohort study. Lancet 2009;374:1617–25.

56. Charpentier C, Salleron J, Savoye G, et al. Natural history of elderly-onset inflammatory bowel disease: a population-based cohort study. Gut 2014;63:423–32.

57. Osterman MT, Sandborn WJ, Colombel JF, et al. Increased risk of malignancy with adalimumab combination therapy, compared with monotherapy, for Crohn's disease. Gastroenterology 2014;146:941–9.

58. Khan N, Abbas AM, Lichtenstein GR, et al. Risk of lymphoma in patients with ulcerative colitis treated with thiopurines: a nationwide retrospective cohort study. Gastroenterology 2013;145:1007–15.e3.

59. Melmed GY, Spiegel BM, Bressler B, et al. The appropriateness of concomitant immunomodulators with anti-tumor necrosis factor agents for Crohn's disease: one size does not fit all. Clin Gastroenterol Hepatol 2010;8:655–9.

60. Habal FM, Huang VW. Review article: a decision-making algorithm for the management of pregnancy in the inflammatory bowel disease patient. Aliment Pharmacol Ther 2012;35:501–15.

61. Mahadevan U, Kane S. American gastroenterological association institute technical review on the use of gastrointestinal medications in pregnancy. Gastroenterology 2006;131:283–311.

62. Ng SW, Mahadevan U. Management of inflammatory bowel disease in pregnancy. Expert Rev Clin Immunol 2013;9:161–73 [quiz: 174].

63. Mahadevan U, Martin CF, Sandler RS, et al. 865 PIANO: a 1000 patient prospective registry of pregnancy outcomes in women with IBD exposed to immunomodulators and biologic therapy. Gastroenterology 2012;142:S-149.

64. Mahadevan U, Wolf DC, Dubinsky M, et al. Placental transfer of anti-tumor necrosis factor agents in pregnant patients with inflammatory bowel disease. Clin Gastroenterol Hepatol 2013;11:286–92 [quiz: e24].

65. Sokol H, Beaugerie L, Maynadie M, et al. Excess primary intestinal lymphoproliferative disorders in patients with inflammatory bowel disease. Inflamm Bowel Dis 2012;18:2063–71.

66. Dayharsh GA, Loftus EV Jr, Sandborn WJ, et al. Epstein-Barr virus-positive lymphoma in patients with inflammatory bowel disease treated with azathioprine or 6-mercaptopurine. Gastroenterology 2002;122:72–7.

67. Magro F, Santos-Antunes J, Albuquerque A, et al. Epstein-Barr virus in inflammatory bowel disease—correlation with different therapeutic regimens. Inflamm Bowel Dis 2013;19:1710–6.

68. Solomon DH, Kremer JM, Fisher M, et al. Comparative cancer risk associated with methotrexate, other non-biologic and biologic disease-modifying anti-rheumatic drugs. Semin Arthritis Rheum 2014;43:489–97.

69. Clarke K, Regueiro M. Stopping immunomodulators and biologics in inflammatory bowel disease patients in remission. Inflamm Bowel Dis 2012;18:174–9.

70. Van Assche G, Magdelaine-Beuzelin C, D'Haens G, et al. Withdrawal of immunosuppression in Crohn's disease treated with scheduled infliximab maintenance: a randomized trial. Gastroenterology 2008;134:1861–8.

71. Louis E, Mary JY, Vernier-Massouille G, et al. Maintenance of remission among patients with Crohn's disease on antimetabolite therapy after infliximab therapy is stopped. Gastroenterology 2012;142:63–70.e5 [quiz: e31].

72. Brandse JF, Peters CP, Gecse KB, et al. Effects of infliximab retreatment after consecutive discontinuation of infliximab and adalimumab in refractory Crohn's disease. Inflamm Bowel Dis 2014;20:251–8.

73. Siegel CA. Shared decision making in inflammatory bowel disease: helping patients understand the tradeoffs between treatment options. Gut 2012;61:459–65.

74. Elwyn G, Lloyd A, Joseph-Williams N, et al. Option Grids: shared decision making made easier. Patient Educ Couns 2013;90:207–12.

75. Dulai PS, Siegel CA, Dubinsky MC. Balancing and communicating the risks and benefits of biologics in pediatric inflammatory bowel disease. Inflamm Bowel Dis 2013;19:2927–36.

76. Siegel CA, Siegel LS, Hyams JS, et al. Real-time tool to display the predicted disease course and treatment response for children with Crohn's disease. Inflamm Bowel Dis 2011;17:30–8.

77. Siegel CA, Horton H, Siegel LS, et al. A validated web-based patient communication tool to display individualized Crohn's disease predicted outcomes based on clinical, serological and genetic variables. Gastroenterology 2014;146:S-433–4.

Update on Anti-Tumor Necrosis Factor Agents in Crohn Disease

Siddharth Singh, MD, Darrell S. Pardi, MD, MS*

KEYWORDS

- Anti-tumor necrosis factor • Infliximab • Adalimumab • Certolizumab pegol
- Crohn disease

KEY POINTS

- Anti-TNF therapy is effective in induction and maintenance of remission as well as mucosal healing in adults and children with Crohn disease.
- Anti-TNF therapy also decreases the risk of hospitalization and surgery in patients with Crohn disease, improves quality of life, and decreases postoperative recurrence after surgical remission.
- Approximately one-third of patients do not respond to induction therapy with anti-TNF therapy (primary nonresponders).
- Approximately 13% to 20% of initial responders may lose response to anti-TNF therapy annually; these patients may be managed with dose escalation or switching within or outside the anti-TNF class of medications.

INTRODUCTION

Tumor necrosis factor-α (TNF) is a key pro-inflammatory cytokine in Crohn disease (CD).[1] Produced mainly by activated macrophages and T lymphocytes, TNF induces many other pro-inflammatory cytokines, including interleukin-1 and interleukin-6, enhances leukocyte migration by inducing expression of adhesion molecules by endothelial cells and leukocytes, activates leukocytes, induces acute phase reactants and metalloproteinases, and inhibits apoptosis of inflammatory cells. Anti-TNF agents, by binding to membrane-bound and soluble TNF, induce destruction of immune cells by antibody-dependent cellular toxicity, induce T-cell apoptosis by binding to membrane-bound TNF, and neutralize the effects of soluble TNF.[2] Currently, anti-TNF agents are the mainstay of treatment for the induction and maintenance of remission in patients with moderate to severe CD.

Inflammatory Bowel Disease Clinic, Division of Gastroenterology and Hepatology, Department of Internal Medicine, Mayo Clinic, 200 First Street South West, Rochester, MN 55905, USA
* Corresponding author.
E-mail address: Pardi.Darrell@mayo.edu

Gastroenterol Clin N Am 43 (2014) 457–478
http://dx.doi.org/10.1016/j.gtc.2014.05.008
0889-8553/14/$ – see front matter © 2014 Elsevier Inc. All rights reserved.
gastro.theclinics.com

Three anti-TNF agents have been approved by the US Food and Drug Administration for the management of CD: infliximab (IFX), adalimumab (ADA), and certolizumab pegol (CZP).[2] IFX is a chimeric monoclonal immunoglobulin G1 (IgG1) antibody against TNF composed of 75% human and 25% murine sequences. It is administered intravenously, over 1 to 3 hours, with standard weight-based dosing of 5 mg/kg body weight at weeks 0, 2, and 6 for induction, followed by 5 mg/kg every 8 weeks for maintenance of remission. ADA is a fully human, monoclonal IgG1 antibody against TNF. It is administered subcutaneously with standard dosing of 160 mg and 80 mg at weeks 0 and 2 for induction, followed by 40 mg every 2 weeks for maintenance of remission. CZP contains the Fab fragment of a humanized anti-TNF monoclonal antibody, and to increase plasma half-life, the Fab fragment is covalently attached to a polyethylene glycol moiety, far removed from the antigen-binding site, to prevent interference. Like ADA, it is administered subcutaneously, with standard dosing of 400 mg at weeks 0, 2, and 4 for induction, followed by 400 mg every 4 weeks for maintenance of remission. In this review, the efficacy, predictors of response, primary and secondary nonresponse to anti-TNF therapy, as well as the use of anti-TNF therapy in special situations are discussed. Evidence on optimal use of anti-TNF therapy (step-up vs top-down therapy; withdrawal of anti-TNF therapy), combination immunosuppressive therapy, and therapeutic drug monitoring is discussed elsewhere in this issue.

EFFICACY OF ANTI-TNF THERAPY

The goals of therapy in CD are to induce and maintain corticosteroid-free remission, achieve mucosal healing, improve quality of life, reduce the need for surgery and hospitalization, as well as reduce long-term risk of small intestinal and colorectal adenocarcinoma.[3] Anti-TNF therapy is effective in achieving these goals in moderate to severe luminal CD, especially in steroid-dependent patients, patients intolerant to or with progressive disease despite immunomodulator therapy, and for penetrating CD.[3] It also appears to be an effective maintenance therapy in patients at high risk of CD recurrence after surgically induced remission. Currently, a minority of patients are treated with anti-TNF agents based on nationwide administrative database studies,[4,5] although, with increasing understanding of disease behavior and the potential for disease modification by anti-TNFs, their use is likely to increase.

Clinical Remission

Tables 1 and **2** summarize the key randomized controlled trials (RCTs) of induction and maintenance of remission with anti-TNF therapy in luminal CD. Overall, in RCTs of patients with moderate to severe luminal CD, clinical remission rates at weeks 4 to 12 were 33% to 72% for IFX,[6–8] 21% to 43% for ADA (36%–43% in anti-TNF-naïve patients, 21%–26% in anti-TNF-exposed patients),[9–11] and 22% to 32% for CZP (32%–40% in anti-TNF-naïve patients, 24% in anti-TNF-exposed patients).[12–14] On meta-analysis, remission of CD was achieved in 456/1598 anti-TNF-treated patients (28.5%) at 4 to 12 weeks, compared with 223/1158 placebo-treated patients (19.3%); rates of clinical response were higher.[15] These rates correspond to a 13% lower risk of failure to achieve remission (95% confidence interval [CI], 6%–20%) and 8 patients would need to be treated with IFX to achieve clinical remission in one more patient after induction therapy compared with placebo (number needed to treat [NNT], 8; 95% CI, 6–17). At 10 to 12 weeks, induction therapy with IFX achieved remission in 45.3% of patients (compared with 25.3% of patients treated

Table 1
Key RCT on the efficacy of anti-TNF therapy for induction of remission in luminal CD

Study, Year of Publication	Location, Time Period	Participants	Intervention (and Comparator)	Outcomes of Interest	Key Results
INFLIXIMAB					
Targan et al,[8] 1997	North America and Europe, 18 sites; 1995–1996	Luminal, moderate-severe CD (CDAI 220–450); 16% ileal, 54% ileocolonic, 30% colonic; 108 patients	IFX 5 mg/kg, 10 mg/kg, or 20 mg/kg at week 0; placebo	Remission: CDAI <150, week 4 and 12; Response: 70-point decrease in CDAI, week 4 and 12	1. Remission: IFX (all doses) vs placebo: 33% vs 4% (week 4), 24% vs 8% (week 12); 2. Response: IFX (all doses) vs placebo: 65% vs 16% (week 4), 41% vs 12% (week 12)
Lemann et al,[7] 2006	France, 22 sites; 2000–2002	Luminal moderate-severe CD, all patients with steroid-dependent CD; 20% ileal, 51% ileocolonic, 29% colonic; 115 patients	IFX 5 mg/kg or 10 mg/kg at weeks 0, 2, and 6; placebo (all patients received azathioprine or 6-mercaptopurine)	Remission: CDAI <150 (steroid-free), week 12 and 24	1. Steroid-free remission: IFX (all doses) vs placebo: 72% vs 36% (week 12), 53% vs 26% (week 24)
Colombel et al (SONIC),[6] 2010	Multinational, 92 sites; 2005–2008	Luminal, moderate-severe CD (CDAI 220–450), all patients were immunomodulator-naïve; 36% ileal, 42% ileocolonic, 22% colonic; 508 patients	IFX 5 mg/kg at weeks 0, 2, and 6, and then every 8 wk; azathioprine 2.5 mg/kg/d; IFX + azathioprine (combination)	Remission: CDAI <150 (steroid-free), week 10; Response: 100-point decrease in CDAI, week 10; Mucosal healing: absence of mucosal ulceration at week 26 in patients who had confirmed mucosal ulceration at baseline	1. Steroid-free remission: IFX vs AZA (vs combination): 37% vs 24% (vs 47%); 2. Response: IFX vs AZA (vs combination): 56% vs 39% (vs 69%); 3. Mucosal healing: IFX vs AZA (vs combination): 30% vs 16% (vs 44%)

(continued on next page)

Table 1
(continued)

Study, Year of Publication	Location, Time Period	Participants	Intervention (and Comparator)	Outcomes of Interest	Key Results
ADALIMUMAB					
Hanauer et al (CLASSIC-I),[9] 2006	Multinational, 55 sites; 2002–2003	Luminal, moderate-severe CD (CDAI 220–450); 62% ileal, 9% ileocolonic, 25% colonic; 299 patients	ADA 40/20 mg, 80/40 mg, or 160/80 mg at weeks 0 and 2; placebo (excluded patients with previous anti-TNF therapy)	Remission: CDAI <150, week 4 Response: 100-point decrease in CDAI, week 4	1. Remission: ADA 160/80 vs placebo: 36% vs 12% 2. Response: ADA 160/80 vs placebo: 50% vs 25%
Sandborn et al (GAIN),[10] 2007	North America and Europe, 52 sites; 2005–2006	Luminal, moderate-severe CD (CDAI 220–450), with prior intolerance to IFX or loss of response; 325 patients	ADA 160/80 mg at weeks 0 and 2; placebo	Remission: CDAI <150, week 4 Response: 100-point decrease in CDAI, week 4	1. Remission: ADA vs placebo: 21% vs 7% 2. Response: ADA vs placebo: 38% vs 25%
Watanabe et al,[11] 2012	Japan, 2007	Luminal, moderate-severe CD (CDAI 220–450); 113 patients	ADA 80/40 mg, or 160/80 mg at weeks 0 and 2; placebo	Remission: CDAI <150, week 4 Response: 100-point decrease in CDAI, week 4; analysis stratified by previous anti-TNF exposure	In anti-TNF exposed patients: 1. Remission: ADA 160/80 vs placebo: 26% vs 8% 2. Response: ADA 160/80 vs placebo: 42% vs 15% In anti-TNF naïve patients: 3. Remission: ADA 160/80 vs placebo: 43% vs 20% 4. Response: ADA 160/80 vs placebo: 50% vs 20%

CERTOLIZUMAB PEGOL

Study	Setting	Population	Treatment	Outcome definitions	Results
Schreiber et al,[14] 2005	Multinational, 58 centers; 2001–2002	Luminal, moderate-severe CD (CDAI 220–450); 291 patients	CZP 100 mg, 200 mg, or 400 mg at weeks 0, 4, and 8; placebo	Remission: CDAI <150, week 12; Response: 100-point decrease in CDAI, week 12	1. Remission: CZP (all doses) vs placebo: 24% vs 23%; 2. Response: CZP (all doses) vs placebo: 39% vs 36%
Sandborn et al (PRECISE 1),[13] 2007	Multinational, 171 centers; 2003–2005	Luminal, moderate-severe CD (CDAI 220–450); 28% ileal, 48% ileocolonic, 24% colonic; 659 patients	Certolizumab 400 mg at weeks 0, 2, and 4; placebo	Remission: CDAI <150, week 6; Response: 100-point decrease in CDAI, week 6; analysis stratified by previous anti-TNF exposure	1. Remission: CZP vs placebo: 22% vs 17%; 2. Response: CZP vs placebo: 35% vs 27% In anti-TNF exposed patients: 3. Response: CZP vs placebo: 24% vs 20% In anti-TNF naïve patients: 4. Response: CZP vs placebo: 40% vs 29%
Sandborn et al,[84] 2011	Multinational, 120 sites; 2008–2009	Luminal, moderate-severe CD (CDAI 220–450); 27% ileal, 41% ileocolonic, 29% colonic; 421 patients	Certolizumab 400 mg at weeks 0, 2, and 4; placebo (excluded patients with previous anti-TNF therapy)	Remission: CDAI <150, week 6; Response: 100-point decrease in CDAI, week 6	1. Remission: CZP vs placebo: 32% vs 25%; 2. Response: CZP vs placebo: 40% vs 34%

Abbreviation: CDAI, Crohn disease activity index.
Data from Refs.[6–14,84]

Table 2
Key RCT on the efficacy of anti-TNF therapy for maintenance of remission in patients with luminal CD

Study, Year of Publication	Location, Time Period	Participants	Intervention (and Comparator)	Outcomes of Interest	Key Results
INFLIXIMAB					
Rutgeerts et al,[31] 2004	North America and Europe, 17 sites;	Luminal, moderate-severe CD (CDAI 220–450); 14% ileal, 55% ileocolonic, 31% colonic; 73 patients	Initial response to placebo or single-dose IFX (5, 10, or 20 mg/kg) (CR-70) (nonresponders given IFX 10 mg/kg at week 12), then responders randomized to IFX 10 mg/kg at 8-weekly intervals thereafter; placebo	Relapse: CDAI ≥150, or need for surgery, or escalation of medical therapy, week 44 Maintenance of remission: CDAI <150, week 44	1. Relapse: IFX vs placebo: 51% vs 81% 2. Remission: IFX vs placebo: 49% vs 19%
Hanauer et al (ACCENT-I),[16] 2002	Multinational, 55 sites	Luminal, moderate-severe CD (CDAI 220–400); 22% ileal, 55% ileocolonic, 22% colonic; 335 patients	Initial response to open-label single-dose IFX (5 mg/kg), then responders (CR-70), randomized to IFX 5 mg/kg at week 2 and 6, then 5 mg/kg or 10 mg/kg at 8-weekly intervals thereafter; placebo	Relapse: CDAI ≥150, or need for surgery, or escalation of medical therapy, week 30 Maintenance of remission: CDAI <150, week 30	1. Relapse: IFX vs placebo: 58% vs 79% 2. Remission: IFX vs placebo: 42% vs 21%
ADALIMUMAB					
Colombel et al (CHARM),[18] 2007	Multinational, 92 sites; 2003–2005	Luminal and penetrating, moderate-severe CD (CDAI 220–450); 499 patients	Initial open-label ADA 80/40, then randomized (stratified by responder status) at week 4 to ADA 40 mg weekly or 40 mg every other week thereafter; placebo	Relapse: CDAI ≥150, week 56 Maintenance of remission in week 4-responders: CDAI <150, week 56 in patients with 70-point decrease in CDAI at week 4	1. Relapse: ADA vs placebo: 62% vs 88% 2. Remission, in week 4 responders: ADA vs placebo: 38% vs 12%

Sandborn et al (CLASSIC-II),[19] 2007	North America and Europe, 53 sites; 2002–2005	Luminal, moderate-severe CD (CDAI 220–450), enrolled in CLASSIC-I trial: included only patients in remission 4 and 8 wk after 2 induction doses of ADA; 55 patients	Initial ADA or placebo as part of CLASSIC-I, then patients with remission (CDAI <150 at week 4 and after 40 mg open-label at week 8) randomized to ADA 40 mg weekly or 40 mg every other week, thereafter; placebo	Relapse: CDAI $\geq$150, week 56 Maintenance of remission: CDAI <150, week 56	1. Relapse: ADA vs placebo: 19% vs 56% 2. Remission: ADA vs placebo: 81% vs 44%
CERTOLIZUMAB PEGOL					
Schreiber et al (PRECISE 2),[20] 2007	Multinational, 147; 2004–2005	Luminal and penetrating, moderate-severe CD (CDAI 220–450); 428 patients	Initial open-label CZP 400 mg at weeks 0, 2, 4, then patients with response (CR100) at week 6, randomized to CZP 400 mg every 4 wk; placebo	Relapse: CDAI $\geq$150, week 26 Maintenance of remission: CDAI <150, week 26	1. Relapse: CZP vs placebo: 52% vs 72% 2. Remission: CZP vs placebo: 29% vs 48%

Abbreviation: CDAI, Crohn disease activity index.
Data from Refs.[16,18–20,31]

with placebo); this corresponds to a 32% lower risk of failure to achieve remission (95% CI, 10%–48%) and NNT of 4 (95% CI, 3–7). Likewise, induction therapy with ADA achieved remission in 24.2% of patients (compared with 9.1% of patients treated with placebo); this corresponds to a 15% lower risk of failure to achieve remission (95% CI, 9%–21%) and an NNT of 7 (95% CI, 5–12.5). On the other hand, on meta-analysis of 4 RCTs of CZP induction therapy, remission was achieved in 24.7% of CZP-treated patients and 21% of placebo-treated patients. Induction therapy with CZP was not superior to placebo in achieving remission (relative risk [RR], 0.95; 95% CI, 0.90–1.01). However, it should be noted that there were differences in trial design, especially for CZP, which may account for some of the differences in the observed efficacy of these agents.

In RCTs evaluating maintenance of remission after open-label induction, clinical remission rates at weeks 30 to 56 were 42% to 49% for IFX,[16,17] 38% to 81% for ADA,[11,18,19] and 48% for CZP in luminal CD.[20] On pooling data from 5 RCTs of maintenance therapy with anti-TNF, 44.1% of initial responders to induction therapy, who continued on anti-TNF therapy, were able to maintain remission 26 to 60 weeks later; in contrast, only 21.6% of patients treated with placebo were able to maintain remission.[15] The RR of relapse with anti-TNF compared with placebo was 0.71 (95% CI, 0.65–0.76), with the corresponding NNT to prevent one CD patient from relapsing of 4 (95% CI, 3–5). For IFX, ADA, and CZP, the RR of relapse after achieving remission, compared with placebo was 0.72 (95% CI, 0.63–0.83), 0.54 (95% CI, 0.27–1.07), and 0.73 (0.63–0.85), respectively. Steroid-free remission was reported in 12% to 16% of patients at weeks 48 to 52 for IFX and 23% to 29% for ADA.[21]

Similar results have been observed for clinical response (defined as decrease in Crohn Disease Activity Index score by 70 points) to anti-TNF therapy.[22] Patients treated with anti-TNF agents were 64% more likely to achieve clinical response at week 4 after induction therapy than placebo (RR, 1.64; 95% CI, 1.37–1.95); likewise, among patients with initial response to induction therapy, maintenance therapy with anti-TNF agents was twice as likely to maintain clinical response than placebo (RR, 2.06; 95% CI, 1.32–3.23).

Table 3 summarizes the RCTs of fistula healing with anti-TNF therapy. Of note, only IFX has been specifically studied with fistula healing as the primary endpoint in an RCT in patients with penetrating CD[23,24]; RCTs of other agents have reported fistula healing as a secondary endpoint in a subset of patients with penetrating disease. In these RCTs, complete fistula closure rates at weeks 18 to 56 were 36% to 46% for IFX,[23,24] 33% for ADA,[18] and 30% to 54% for CZP[13,20]; fistula closure was observed in only 8% to 12% of ADA-treated patients in short-term 4-week induction trials.[9,10] On meta-analysis, the RR of failing to achieve fistula healing with anti-TNF therapy was 0.80 (95% CI, 0.65–0.98) when short-term trials were excluded.[15] Partial fistula healing rates (at least 50% reduction in the number of draining fistulae) are expectedly higher, with 62% of IFX-treated patients achieving partial response, as compared with 26% of placebo-treated patients.[23]

Long-term follow-up of patients enrolled in these RCTs demonstrate continued benefit with extended use of anti-TNF agents. In a follow-up of the CHARM and ADHERE trials, of the 329 patients with an initial 4-week response to ADA, more than 30% maintained clinical remission extending to 4 years.[25] In a subset of patients who were in remission at week 54, more than half maintained remission at the end of 4 years of follow-up. In a prospective cohort study of 469 patients with CD treated with IFX, 61% of those with response to induction therapy had sustained benefit at end of 4.5 years of follow-up; the estimated 5-year sustained benefit was 56%.[26]

Mucosal Healing

Mucosal healing has been associated with clinical response, durable steroid-free remission, reduced need for surgery and hospitalization, and reduced risk of colitis-associated colorectal cancer.[27,28] In a Norwegian population-based cohort study of patients with CD, mucosal healing 1 year after diagnosis was associated with decreased need for corticosteroids and a trend toward lower risk of intestinal resection over the next 7 years, as compared with patients with continued endoscopic disease activity.[29] In the endoscopic substudy of the "top-down/step-up" study of newly diagnosed, treatment-naïve patients with CD, patients with complete mucosal healing 2 years after treatment initiation were 4.3 times more likely to maintain steroid-free remission 3 and 4 years after treatment initiation.[30]

Anti-TNF agents are currently the most effective agents in achieving mucosal healing. In the ACCENT I trial, scheduled IFX induction at weeks 0, 2, and 6 led to mucosal healing in 29% of patients, as compared with 3% patients given only a single dose of IFX at week 10; subsequent scheduled IFX maintenance every 8 weeks led to mucosal healing in 44% of patients at week 54, as compared with 18% patients who received episodic IFX.[16,31] In the SONIC trial, IFX monotherapy achieved mucosal healing in 30% of patients, as compared with only 16% of azathioprine-treated patients at week 26; combination therapy with IFX and azathioprine was superior to either of these strategies with 44% of patients achieving mucosal healing.[6] In the EXTEND trial, patients who received scheduled ADA were more likely than placebo-treated patients to achieve mucosal healing at both weeks 12 (27% vs 13%) and 52 (24% vs 0%), respectively.[32] Similar results were observed with CZP: rates of complete endoscopic remission and mucosal healing at week 10 and 54 compared with placebo were 10% and 4%, and 14% and 8%, respectively.[33] Differences in the definition of endoscopic remission and mucosal healing partly account for the differences observed in rates of mucosal healing for different anti-TNF agents.

Although retrospective studies and post-hoc analysis of RCTs have demonstrated better outcomes associated with achievement of mucosal healing, prospective data on the ability of mucosal healing to modify natural history of CD are lacking. Moreover, the definition of mucosal healing has been variable across studies, and it is not clarified in the literature how mucosal healing should ideally be defined in CD (ie, whether it should be based on biochemical, endoscopic, radiographic, or histologic parameters, or a combination of these). Although the understanding of mucosal healing continues to evolve, it is premature to recommend universal treatment to achieve mucosal healing.

Quality of Life in CD

Multiple RCTs have demonstrated improvement in health-related quality of life in patients who respond to anti-TNF therapy. In the CHARM trial of maintenance therapy with ADA in patients with moderate to severe CD, patients who continued ADA for maintenance reported significantly less depression, fewer fatigue symptoms, greater improvements in the inflammatory bowel disease (IBD) questionnaire, greater Short Form Health Survey-36 physical component summary scores, and less abdominal pain from weeks 12 to 56, compared with patients who were assigned to placebo after ADA induction therapy.[34] In the open-label, multicenter CARE trial of ADA in patients with moderate to severe CD, 60% of IFX-naïve patients achieved clinically important improvements on the short IBD questionnaire, and 51% had improved work productivity.[35] Overall, at week 20, 64% of IFX-naïve patients

Table 3
Key RCT on the efficacy of anti-TNF therapy for treatment of enterocutaneous and perianal fistulae in patients with penetrating CD

Study, Year of Publication	Location, Time Period	Participants	Intervention (and Comparator)	Outcomes of Interest	Key Results
INFLIXIMAB					
Present et al,[23] 1999	US and Europe, 12 sites; 1996	Penetrating CD, single or multiple draining enterocutaneous or perianal fistulae; 94 patients	IFX 5 mg/kg or 10 mg/kg at weeks 0, 2, and 6; placebo	Fistula remission: absence of any draining fistula at 2 consecutive visits, week 18 Fistula improvement: reduction of number of draining fistulae by ≥50% (fistula response) at 2 consecutive visits, week 18	1. Fistula remission: IFX (all doses) vs placebo: 46% vs 13% 2. Fistula improvement: IFX (all doses) vs placebo: 62% vs 26%
Sands et al (ACCENT-II),[24] 2004	Multinational, 45 sites; 2000–2001	Penetrating CD, single or multiple draining enterocutaneous or perianal fistulae	Initial response to open-label IFX (5 mg/kg, at weeks 0, 2, and 6), then responders (fistula improvement) randomized at week 14 to IFX 40 mg every 8 wk thereafter; placebo	Fistula remission: absence of any draining fistula, week 54	1. Fistula remission: IFX vs placebo: 36% vs 19%
ADALIMUMAB					
Hanauer et al (CLASSIC-I),[9] 2006	Multinational, 55 sites; 2002–2003	Enterocutaneous or perianal fistulae at baseline; 32 patients	ADA 40/20 mg, 80/40 mg, or 160/80 mg at weeks 0 and 2; placebo (excluded patients with previous anti-TNF therapy)	Fistula remission: absence of any draining fistula at 2 consecutive visits, week 4 Fistula improvement: reduction of number of draining fistulae by ≥50% (fistula response) at 2 consecutive visits, week 4	1. Fistula remission: ADA (all doses) vs placebo: 12% vs 17% 2. Fistula improvement: ADA (all doses) vs placebo: 23% vs 33%

Study	Location/sites; years	Population	Treatment	Definitions	Results
Sandborn et al (GAIN),[10] 2007	North America and Europe, 52 sites; 2005–2006	Luminal and penetrating, moderate-severe CD, with enterocutaneous or perianal fistulae at baseline in CD patients with prior intolerance to IFX or loss of response (excluded primary nonresponders to IFX); 45 patients	ADA 160/80 mg at weeks 0 and 2; placebo	Fistula remission: absence of any draining fistula at 2 consecutive visits, week 4. Fistula improvement: reduction of number of draining fistulae by ≥50% (fistula response) at 2 consecutive visits, week 4	1. Fistula remission: ADA vs placebo: 8% vs 5%. 2. Fistula improvement: ADA vs placebo: 20% vs 15%
Colombel et al (CHARM),[18] 2007	Multinational, 92 sites; 2003–2005	Luminal and penetrating, moderate-severe CD, with enterocutaneous or perianal fistulae at baseline; 117 patients	Initial response to open-label ADA 80/40, then randomized at week 4 to ADA 40 mg weekly or 40 mg every other week thereafter; placebo	Fistula remission: absence of any draining fistula at 2 consecutive visits, weeks 26 and 56	1. Fistula remission: ADA (all doses) vs placebo: 30% vs 13% (week 26), 33% vs 13% (week 56)

CERTOLIZUMAB PEGOL

Study	Location/sites; years	Population	Treatment	Definitions	Results
Sandborn et al (PRECISE 1),[13] 2007	Multinational, 171 centers; 2003–2005	Luminal and penetrating, moderate-severe CD, with enterocutaneous or perianal fistulae at baseline; 107 patients	Certolizumab 400 mg at weeks 0, 2, and 4, then 400 mg at 4-weekly intervals thereafter; placebo	Fistula remission: absence of any draining fistula at 2 consecutive visits, week 26	1. Fistula remission: CZP vs placebo: 30% vs 31%
Schreiber et al (PRECISE 2),[20] 2007	Multinational, 147 centers; 2004–2005	Luminal and penetrating, moderate-severe CD, with enterocutaneous or perianal fistulae at baseline; 58 patients	Initial response to open-label certolizumab (400 mg at weeks 0, 2, 4), then responders (CR-100) randomized to certolizumab 400 mg at week 8, then 400 mg at 4-weekly intervals thereafter; placebo	Fistula remission: absence of any draining fistulae on gentle compression at any 2 consecutive visits after baseline, week 26	1. Fistula remission: CZP vs placebo: 54% vs 43%

Abbreviation: CDAI, Crohn disease activity index.
Data from Refs.[9,10,13,18,20,23,24]

achieved clinically important improvement in total activity impairment with ADA therapy. Based on these findings, the investigators concluded that ADA therapy resulted in a per-patient indirect cost savings of €2577, owing to reductions in CD-related work loss and productivity impairment, with work productivity improving as early as 4 weeks after initiation. Similar improvements in work productivity, daily activities, and health-related quality of life were observed in patients with active CD treated with CZP.[36]

Hospitalization and Surgery in CD

Anti-TNF therapy has been associated with decreased risk of hospitalization and surgery in patients with CD, in both RCTs and observational studies. In the ACCENT I trial in patients with moderate to severe CD, patients treated with scheduled IFX were significantly less likely to require hospitalization or surgery, as compared with patients treated with episodic IFX.[31] Likewise, in the ACCENT II study of patients with fistulizing CD, those who initially responded to IFX therapy and then received IFX maintenance had significantly fewer mean hospitalization days (0.5 vs 2.5 days, $P<.05$), mean number (per 100 patients) of hospitalizations (11 vs 31, $P<.05$), all surgeries and procedures (65 vs 126, $P<.05$), inpatient surgeries and procedures (7 vs 41, $P<.01$), and major surgeries (2 vs 11, $P<.05$), compared with those who received placebo maintenance.[37] In a meta-analysis of 3 RCTs, IFX use was associated with a 52% lower risk of hospitalization (odds ratio [OR], 0.48; 95% CI, 0.34–0.67) and 69% lower risk of surgery at 1 year (OR, 0.31 95% CI, 0.15–0.64), as compared with placebo[38]; likewise, on meta-analysis of 9 observational studies, patients treated with IFX had a 72% lower risk of hospitalization (OR, 0.28; 95% CI, 0.18–0.46), and 68% lower risk of surgery (OR, 0.32; 95% CI, 0.21–0.49), as compared with patients not on IFX. In a single-center, retrospective cohort study, initiation of IFX was associated with decreased risk of surgery (11% vs 24%, $P<.001$) and hospitalization (55% vs 31%, $P<.001$), and a shorter duration of hospital stay (6.3 d/y vs 11.3 d/y, $P<.001$) compared with the pre-IFX period.[39]

Similar benefits have also been observed with ADA. In the CHARM trial in responders to initial open-label ADA, patients who received maintenance ADA were less likely to have all-cause or CD-related hospitalization, as compared with patients randomized to placebo.[40] The rate of all-cause hospitalization at 12 months in ADA-treated and placebo-treated patients was 12.6% and 25.2%, respectively. Long-term efficacy data on the risk of hospitalization and surgery are not available for CZP currently, but are expected to be similar.

COMPARATIVE EFFECTIVENESS OF ANTI-TNF AGENTS

Despite multiple trials demonstrating the superiority of anti-TNF agents over placebo, there are no comparative-effectiveness clinical trials comparing one agent to another. Clinical trials have suggested that a 4-week induction of remission rates may be slightly lower with ADA and CZP, as compared with IFX, although it is not valid to directly compare results across clinical trials. In an open-label, single-center SWITCH trial of patients with CD with sustained clinical response on maintenance IFX, elective switching from IFX to ADA was associated with intolerance or loss of efficacy in 47% of patients switched to ADA, compared with 16% of patients continued on IFX.[41] In an observational comparative-effectiveness cohort study comparing outcomes in first-time users of anti-TNF agents among Medicare beneficiaries, Osterman and colleagues[42] found no significant difference among IFX-treated or ADA-treated patients with CD, although numerically the risk of surgery was lower in IFX-treated patients (5.5

vs 6.9 surgeries per 100 person-years; adjusted hazard ratio [HR], 0.79; 95% CI, 0.60–1.05). Given the Medicare population, most patients in this study were older than 65 years of age, and hence, were not representative of the average patient with CD; interestingly, in a subset of patients younger than 65 years, it appeared that IFX use was associated with lower risk of surgery as compared with ADA (adjusted OR, 0.66; 95% CI, 0.47–0.93).

In a Bayesian network meta-analysis of 17 RCTs on the efficacy of anti-TNF therapy in first-time users with moderate to severe CD, induction therapy with IFX was 4.2 times more likely to achieve clinical remission than CZP (OR, 4.2; 95% CI, 1.4–14.3) but was comparable to ADA (OR, 2.0; 95% CI, 0.5–9.1) (Singh S, personal observation, 2014). IFX, ADA and CZP were comparable to each other in maintaining remission among responders to induction therapy. As noted above, there were differences in trial design, especially for CZP, which may account for some of the differences in the observed efficacy of these agents. Hence, in the absence of any direct comparison, the quality of evidence is low and warrants further evaluation through prospective studies.

PREDICTORS OF RESPONSE TO ANTI-TNF THERAPY

Several clinical and biologic factors have been identified that may predict response to anti-TNF therapy in CD.[43–45] The most consistent and predictive factor is a shorter duration of disease. In the CHARM trial with ADA, remission rates approached 60% in patients who had CD for less than 2 years compared with 40% ($P<.05$) in those with a longer duration of disease.[18] Presence of an inflammatory and not fibrostenotic CD phenotype, isolated colonic disease, less severe disease, nonsmoking status, and young age may also be associated with better response to anti-TNF therapy.[43,45–49] In patients with penetrating CD, the presence of a rectovaginal fistula may be associated with poor response to IFX.[50]

Among biologic factors, an elevated CRP, and a return to normal after initiation of therapy, predicts a good response to anti-TNF therapy. In a Belgian cohort of IFX-treated patients, baseline CRP greater than 5 mg/L before the start of IFX was associated with higher response (76%) compared with patients with normal CRP (46%; OR of nonresponse to anti-TNF in patients with high CRP, compared with patients with normal CRP, 0.26; 95% CI, 0.11–0.63)[51]; similar results have also been observed with ADA,[13,14] but not with CZP.[52] Serologic markers may also predict response to anti-TNF therapy: increased perinuclear anti-neutrophil cytoplasmic antibodies (pANCA) levels may be associated with decreased response to IFX in patients with CD, particularly in the absence of associated ASCA antibodies, although these findings are not consistent.[53,54] Pharmacogenomic studies have suggested genetic markers that may be potential predictors of response to anti-TNF therapies. Genetic variants in the TNF and TNF receptor pathways or NOD2 mutations have not shown a consistent relationship with IFX response.[44] Consistent with the observation that IFX acts through induction of apoptosis of activated T cells, a Belgian cohort of 287 patients found that the presence of 3 single nucleotide polymorphisms in apoptosis-related genes influenced short-term response to IFX in luminal and penetrating CD and developed an "apoptotic pharmacogenetic index," which correlates with IFX response and remission.[55,56]

Composite models based on genotype, phenotype, and serologic biomarkers have been proposed that may identify patients who would be anti-TNF responsive, with good discriminatory value.[57] However, these findings are preliminary and warrant further validation in a prospective cohort of patients.

Primary Nonresponse to Anti-TNF Therapy

Primary nonresponse refers to lack of clinical improvement with induction therapy with anti-TNF, typically assessed 8 to 12 weeks after initiation of therapy. Approximately one-third of patients are classified as primary nonresponders.[45] Lack of response may be due to an alternative pro-inflammatory pathway beyond TNF-mediated inflammation, a differential role of TNF in certain stages of disease, individual differences in bioavailability and pharmacokinetics, inadequate concentrations of a biologic secondary to immunogenicity (innate neutralizing or nonneutralizing antibodies, or unmeasured or unknown antibody), or other factors that increase drug clearance, including high consumption in severe disease. Other, as yet unidentified, factors may play a role, such as genetic or serologic backgrounds of individual patients or absence of inflammation accounting for clinical symptoms.[43,45]

The best treatment strategy for patients with primary nonresponse to anti-TNF agents is unclear. Clinical trials of ADA and CZP typically excluded patients who were primary nonresponders to IFX or another anti-TNF agent. Only a few uncontrolled studies have evaluated the efficacy of secondary anti-TNF therapy in primary nonresponders with CD, with suboptimal results. In a cohort of 118 patients treated with ADA at Mayo Clinic, 9 patients were primary nonresponders to IFX. Of these 9 patients, only 1 patient had complete clinical response (11.1%), compared with 47.8% of patients with loss of response to IFX who achieved complete clinical response on switching to ADA therapy.[58] In the open-label, multicenter CHOICE trial of 673 patients with penetrating CD with previous failure of IFX (17% primary nonresponders), ADA achieved complete fistula healing in 30.8% of primary nonresponders and 40.0% of patients with loss of response to IFX.[59] In contrast, in another open-label, multicenter European trial of ADA therapy in patients with luminal CD (the CARE study), similar rates of response were observed in IFX primary nonresponders and those who discontinued IFX because of secondary loss of response or adverse events; clinical remission was achieved in 29% of IFX primary nonresponders by week 4, and 37% by week 20, and 38% and 43% by weeks 4 and 20, respectively, in patients who discontinued IFX because of other reasons.[60]

The availability of alternative biologic agents, such as an IL-12/23 antagonist (ustekinumab) and leukocyte trafficking blockers (natalizumab, vedolizumab), has increased options available to physicians and patients in the management of patients with primary nonresponse to anti-TNF.[61-63] Surgical resection may be an option for patients with limited disease extent.

Loss of Response to Anti-TNF Therapy

Loss of response, or secondary failure, refers to recurrence of disease activity during maintenance therapy after achieving an appropriate induction response. Multiple factors contribute to loss of response: subtherapeutic drug levels, either secondary to immunogenicity or other factors that increase drug clearance (such as high consumption in severe disease), shift in the dominant mechanism of inflammation to a non-TNF-mediated pathway (loss of the pharmacodynamic effect), or development of symptoms unrelated to active inflammation (for example, concomitant bacterial overgrowth, bile salt-induced diarrhea, irritable bowel syndrome, gastrointestinal infections such as *Clostridium difficile*, or the development of fibrostenotic disease).[43,45]

In a systematic review of 16 studies of IFX on 2236 patients with CD followed for 6284 person-years, the annual risk for loss of IFX response was estimated to be 13%.[64] The mean time to loss of response or need for dose intensification varied from 9.5 months to 18 months. Likewise, on systematic review of 11 studies of

ADA, the annual risk of loss of response was 20%, and a significant proportion of patients required ADA dose intensification annually.[65] It is important to note that the incidence of loss of response is not linear: two-thirds of patients who lose response to anti-TNF do so within the first 12 months of therapy, and the remaining third do so at a much slower rate. Typically, the rate of loss of response within 12 months of anti-TNF therapy in CD patients ranges between 23% and 46% for both IFX and ADA.[66]

Predictors of loss of response to anti-TNF therapy include a combination of demographic (male gender, current/former smoker status, family history of IBD), disease-specific (isolated colonic disease, presence of extra-intestinal manifestations, longer disease duration, greater baseline disease activity), previous therapy-related (previous primary nonresponse to anti-TNF agent and anti-TNF-exposed status), and other drug-related characteristics (concomitant corticosteroid use, no deep remission, use of suboptimal doses, and low trough anti-TNF level).[65,66]

Strategies for management of loss of response are discussed in detail elsewhere in this issue. Dose intensification may be an effective strategy for management of loss of response, especially in patients with subtherapeutic drug levels. In the ACCENT I trial, 88% of patients who had initially responded to IFX but lost response during maintenance therapy regained response by increasing the dose to 10 mg/kg.[17] In a pooled analysis of 9 studies, ADA dose escalation led to regain of response in 71%, with remission in 40% of patients.[65] Switching to another anti-TNF is another effective strategy. The efficacy of a second anti-TNF agent in patients with loss of response to the first anti-TNF agent has been specifically studied in 2 RCTs. In the GAIN trial, 325 patients with moderate to severe CD with loss of response or intolerance to IFX were randomized to receive induction ADA therapy or placebo.[19] At week 4, 21% of ADA-treated patients achieved remission as compared with only 7% of placebo-treated patients. Similarly, in the WELCOME trial, 539 CD patients with loss of response or intolerance to IFX received open-label CZP and subsequently responders were randomized to maintenance CZP every 2 or 4 weeks. Overall, 62% of the participants achieved clinical response, with 39% achieving remission at week 6.[12] At week 26, 30% of patients remained in remission with maintenance CZP.

In patients who have lost response to 2 anti-TNF agents, treatment with a third anti-TNF can also be considered. In a single-center retrospective cohort study of 63 patients with IBD (57 with CD) with loss of response to 2 anti-TNF agents, the probability of remaining on the third anti-TNF, 1 and 2 years after commencement, was 55% and 37%, respectively.[67] Primary nonresponse to the first anti-TNF agent (HR, 6.4; 95% CI, 2.5–16.1) and persistent disease activity 3 months after initiation of the third anti-TNF agent (HR, 3.2; 95% CI, 1.3–7.8) were predictive of poor response to the third anti-TNF agent.

ANTI-TNF USE IN SPECIAL SITUATIONS
Postoperative Prophylaxis

In a small, single-center, placebo-controlled RCT, Regueiro and colleagues[68] observed that patients randomized to IFX within 4 weeks after surgery were significantly less likely to develop endoscopic recurrence 12 months after therapy (9.1%), as compared with placebo (84.6%); none of the patients who received IFX developed clinical recurrence. In a subsequent 5-year, open-label prospective follow-up of this cohort, patients who continued on IFX had a 13.5 times lower risk of endoscopic recurrence than patients who chose not to use IFX.[69] This initial study on efficacy of IFX for postoperative prophylaxis is being followed up with a large, multicenter RCT.

In a comparative-efficacy RCT, Savarino and colleagues[70] observed that patients randomized to ADA after surgical remission of CD were significantly less likely to develop endoscopic (6.3%) and clinical (12.5%) recurrence than patients who received azathioprine (64.7%, 64.7%) or 5-aminosalicylates (83.3%, 50.0%) 2 years after randomization. Hence, for patients at highest risk of recurrence after surgical resection of CD (young adults, with a history of penetrating CD, prior intestinal resection, perianal disease, and active smoking), anti-TNF therapy started within 4 weeks of surgery may be the preferred strategy. Follow-up endoscopic evaluation 9 to 12 months after initiation of postoperative prophylaxis is useful to ensure appropriate response.

Pediatric CD

The safety and efficacy of anti-TNF therapy in patients who had failed conventional therapy with corticosteroids and immunomodulators have also been established in pediatric CD, although there are no placebo-controlled RCTs. In the multicenter, open-label REACH study of 112 children, mean age 13.3 years, Hyams and colleagues[71] observed that 10-week clinical remission and response rate after induction therapy with IFX were 58.9% and 88.4%, respectively. Among patients who responded to induction IFX therapy, 55.8% and 63.5% were in clinical remission and response at week 54. In addition, IFX therapy was associated with improvement in quality of life, decreased corticosteroid requirement as well as increase in height. Likewise, in another multicenter, open-label, IMAgINE 1 trial, Hyams and colleagues[72] observed that of 188 patients who received open-label induction therapy with ADA, 82.4% had a clinical response at week 4% and 27.7% achieved clinical remission. Of the patients who had an initial response, 33.5% were in clinical remission at week 26. The superiority of anti-TNF therapy over immunomodulators in early, inflammatory CD was observed in a prospective cohort study. In analyzing data from the RISK study, Walters and colleagues[73] observed that early treatment with anti-TNF (within 3 months of CD diagnosis) was superior to immunomodulator monotherapy in achieving remission (85.3% vs 60.4%) and improved overall clinical and growth outcomes at 1 year. In a retrospective, multicenter RESEAT cohort of 100 pediatric CD patients who had previously been treated with IFX, Rosh and colleagues[74] observed clinical response rates with ADA of 70% and 71% at 6 and 12 months, respectively, and 33% and 42% steroid-free clinical remission rates, respectively. Hence, anti-TNF agents are effective in inducing and maintaining clinical remission, mucosal healing, improving quality of life, and growth in pediatric CD; they also appear to be safe.[75] However, it is unclear whether top-down therapy with early use of aggressive anti-TNF with or without concomitant immunomodulators is superior to step-up therapy in children with CD.

CD in the Elderly

There is an increasing incidence of CD in the elderly, who generally have a milder course with predominant colonic involvement. Anti-TNF medications are used in only 2% to 9% of elderly patients with IBD.[76] In a population-based cohort of elderly patients, the cumulative probability of receiving anti-TNF agents at 5 and 10 years was 5% and 9%, respectively.[77] In a study of 54 elderly patients with CD, the rate of complete and partial response to anti-TNF therapy was 61%, as compared with 83% with younger patients; 70% of elderly patients had discontinued anti-TNF therapy after a mean follow-up of 2 years.[78] There is a higher rate of adverse events with use of biologic therapy in the elderly than in younger patients. In the authors' experience of 58 elderly IBD patients treated with anti-TNF, 22% developed a serious infection, as compared with 8% of younger patients, even after adjusting for disease extent, severity, and comorbidities.[79] In an Italian cohort of 95 elderly patients with IBD (58 with CD) treated with anti-TNF agents, 11% developed serious infection and 10% died; the corresponding proportions in elderly IBD patients not treated with anti-TNF agents were 2.6% and 1%, respectively.[80] Hence, although anti-TNF agents are effective for treatment of CD in elderly patients, there is a higher incidence of adverse events, particularly of infections, which requires careful monitoring.

Extra-intestinal Manifestations

Anti-TNF agents are effective in the management of ankylosing spondylitis, regardless of the presence of coexistent IBD.[81] In a controlled study of 24 patients with active or quiescent CD and spondyloarthropathy, patients treated with scheduled IFX had rapid and significant improvement in gastrointestinal as well as articular and periarticular manifestations of spondyloarthropathy and peripheral arthritis.[82] IFX is also effective for the treatment of pyoderma gangrenosum. In a multicenter, placebo-controlled trial of 30 patients with pyoderma gangrenosum (19 with associated IBD), a single dose of IFX 5 mg/kg was associated with a reduction in size, depth, and degree of undermining of skin lesions in 46% of patients, as compared with only 6% of placebo-treated patients. Following open-label IFX infusions, by week 6, 69% of patients had clinical improvement. Likewise, the safety and efficacy of anti-TNF therapy have been demonstrated in patients with IBD-associated immune-mediated ocular diseases such as uveitis.[83]

SUMMARY

Anti-TNF therapy is the cornerstone of management of moderate to severe luminal and penetrating CD, effective in inducing and maintaining clinical remission, inducing mucosal healing, improving quality of life, and decreasing risk of surgery and hospitalization. Future research in comparative effectiveness of the different anti-TNF agents is warranted. In addition, a better understanding of predictors of clinical response, primary nonresponse, and secondary failure is required to enable greater optimization of anti-TNF therapy.

REFERENCES

1. Abraham C, Cho JH. Inflammatory bowel disease. N Engl J Med 2009;361(21): 2066–78.
2. Nielsen OH, Ainsworth MA. Tumor necrosis factor inhibitors for inflammatory bowel disease. N Engl J Med 2013;369(8):754–62.
3. Lichtenstein GR, Hanauer SB, Sandborn WJ, et al. Management of Crohn's disease in adults. Am J Gastroenterol 2009;104(2):465–83.
4. Herrinton LJ, Liu L, Fireman B, et al. Time trends in therapies and outcomes for adult inflammatory bowel disease, Northern California, 1998-2005. Gastroenterology 2009;137(2):502–11.
5. Long MD, Martin C, Sandler RS, et al. Increased risk of pneumonia among patients with inflammatory bowel disease. Am J Gastroenterol 2013;108(2): 240–8.
6. Colombel JF, Sandborn WJ, Reinisch W, et al. Infliximab, azathioprine, or combination therapy for Crohn's disease. N Engl J Med 2010;362(15):1383–95.
7. Lemann M, Mary JY, Duclos B, et al. Infliximab plus azathioprine for steroid-dependent Crohn's disease patients: a randomized placebo-controlled trial. Gastroenterology 2006;130(4):1054–61.

8. Targan SR, Hanauer SB, van Deventer SJ, et al. A short-term study of chimeric monoclonal antibody cA2 to tumor necrosis factor alpha for Crohn's disease. Crohn's Disease cA2 Study Group. N Engl J Med 1997;337(15):1029–35.

9. Hanauer SB, Sandborn WJ, Rutgeerts P, et al. Human anti-tumor necrosis factor monoclonal antibody (adalimumab) in Crohn's disease: the CLASSIC-I trial. Gastroenterology 2006;130(2):323–33.

10. Sandborn WJ, Rutgeerts P, Enns R, et al. Adalimumab induction therapy for Crohn disease previously treated with infliximab: a randomized trial. Ann Intern Med 2007;146(12):829–38.

11. Watanabe M, Hibi T, Lomax KG, et al. Adalimumab for the induction and maintenance of clinical remission in Japanese patients with Crohn's disease. J Crohns Colitis 2012;6(2):160–73.

12. Sandborn WJ, Abreu MT, D'Haens G, et al. Certolizumab pegol in patients with moderate to severe Crohn's disease and secondary failure to infliximab. Clin Gastroenterol Hepatol 2010;8(8):688–95.

13. Sandborn WJ, Feagan BG, Stoinov S, et al. Certolizumab pegol for the treatment of Crohn's disease. N Engl J Med 2007;357(3):228–38.

14. Schreiber S, Rutgeerts P, Fedorak RN, et al. A randomized, placebo-controlled trial of certolizumab pegol (CDP870) for treatment of Crohn's disease. Gastroenterology 2005;129(3):807–18.

15. Ford AC, Sandborn WJ, Khan KJ, et al. Efficacy of biological therapies in inflammatory bowel disease: systematic review and meta-analysis. Am J Gastroenterol 2011;106(4):644–59.

16. Hanauer SB, Feagan BG, Lichtenstein GR, et al. Maintenance infliximab for Crohn's disease: the ACCENT I randomised trial. Lancet 2002;359(9317): 1541–9.

17. Rutgeerts P, D'Haens G, Targan S, et al. Efficacy and safety of retreatment with anti-tumor necrosis factor antibody (infliximab) to maintain remission in Crohn's disease. Gastroenterology 1999;117(4):761–9.

18. Colombel JF, Sandborn WJ, Rutgeerts P, et al. Adalimumab for maintenance of clinical response and remission in patients with Crohn's disease: the CHARM trial. Gastroenterology 2007;132(1):52–65.

19. Sandborn WJ, Hanauer SB, Rutgeerts P, et al. Adalimumab for maintenance treatment of Crohn's disease: results of the CLASSIC II trial. Gut 2007;56(9): 1232–9.

20. Schreiber S, Khaliq-Kareemi M, Lawrance IC, et al. Maintenance therapy with certolizumab pegol for Crohn's disease. N Engl J Med 2007;357(3):239–50 [Erratum appears in N Engl J Med 2007;357(13):1357].

21. Peyrin-Biroulet L, Deltenre P, Suray N, et al. Efficacy and safety of tumor necrosis factor antagonists in Crohn's disease: meta-analysis of placebo-controlled trials. Clin Gastroenterol Hepatol 2008;6(6):644–53.

22. Kawalec P, Mikrut A, Wisniewska N, et al. Tumor necrosis factor-alpha antibodies (infliximab, adalimumab and certolizumab) in Crohn's disease: systematic review and meta-analysis. Arch Med Sci 2013;9(5):765–79.

23. Present DH, Rutgeerts P, Targan S, et al. Infliximab for the treatment of fistulas in patients with Crohn's disease. N Engl J Med 1999;340(18):1398–405.

24. Sands BE, Anderson FH, Bernstein CN, et al. Infliximab maintenance therapy for penetrating Crohn's disease. N Engl J Med 2004;350(9):876–85.

25. Panaccione R, Colombel JF, Sandborn WJ, et al. Adalimumab maintains remission of Crohn's disease after up to 4 years of treatment: data from CHARM and ADHERE. Aliment Pharmacol Ther 2013;38(10):1236–47.

26. Eshuis EJ, Peters CP, van Bodegraven AA, et al. Ten years of infliximab for Crohn's disease: outcome in 469 patients from 2 tertiary referral centers. Inflamm Bowel Dis 2013;19(8):1622–30.

27. Neurath MF, Travis SP. Mucosal healing in inflammatory bowel diseases: a systematic review. Gut 2012;61(11):1619–35.

28. Peyrin-Biroulet L, Ferrante M, Magro F, et al. Results from the 2nd Scientific Workshop of the ECCO. I: impact of mucosal healing on the course of inflammatory bowel disease. J Crohns Colitis 2011;5(5):477–83.

29. Froslie KF, Jahnsen J, Moum BA, et al. Mucosal healing in inflammatory bowel disease: results from a Norwegian population-based cohort. Gastroenterology 2007;133(2):412–22.

30. Baert F, Caprilli R, Angelucci E. Medical therapy for Crohn's disease: top-down or step-up? Dig Dis 2007;25(3):260–6.

31. Rutgeerts P, Feagan BG, Lichtenstein GR, et al. Comparison of scheduled and episodic treatment strategies of infliximab in Crohn's disease. Gastroenterology 2004;126(2):402–13.

32. Rutgeerts P, Van Assche G, Sandborn WJ, et al. Adalimumab induces and maintains mucosal healing in patients with Crohn's disease: data from the EXTEND trial. Gastroenterology 2012;142(5):1102–11.

33. Hebuterne X, Lemann M, Bouhnik Y, et al. Endoscopic improvement of mucosal lesions in patients with moderate to severe ileocolonic Crohn's disease following treatment with certolizumab pegol. Gut 2013;62(2):201–8.

34. Loftus EV, Feagan BG, Colombel JF, et al. Effects of adalimumab maintenance therapy on health-related quality of life of patients with Crohn's disease: patient-reported outcomes of the CHARM trial. Am J Gastroenterol 2008;103(12):3132–41.

35. Louis E, Lofberg R, Reinisch W, et al. Adalimumab improves patient-reported outcomes and reduces indirect costs in patients with moderate to severe Crohn's disease: results from the CARE trial. J Crohns Colitis 2013;7(1):34–43.

36. Feagan BG, Sandborn WJ, Wolf DC, et al. Randomised clinical trial: improvement in health outcomes with certolizumab pegol in patients with active Crohn's disease with prior loss of response to infliximab. Aliment Pharmacol Ther 2011;33(5):541–50.

37. Lichtenstein GR, Yan S, Bala M, et al. Infliximab maintenance treatment reduces hospitalizations, surgeries, and procedures in penetrating Crohn's disease. Gastroenterology 2005;128(4):862–9.

38. Costa J, Magro F, Caldeira D, et al. Infliximab reduces hospitalizations and surgery interventions in patients with inflammatory bowel disease: a systematic review and meta-analysis. Inflamm Bowel Dis 2013;19(10):2098–110.

39. Taxonera C, Rodrigo L, Casellas F, et al. Infliximab maintenance therapy is associated with decreases in direct resource use in patients with luminal or penetrating Crohn's disease. J Clin Gastroenterol 2009;43(10):950–6.

40. Feagan BG, Panaccione R, Sandborn WJ, et al. Effects of adalimumab therapy on incidence of hospitalization and surgery in Crohn's disease: results from the CHARM study. Gastroenterology 2008;135(5):1493–9.

41. Van Assche G, Vermeire S, Ballet V, et al. Switch to adalimumab in patients with Crohn's disease controlled by maintenance infliximab: prospective randomised SWITCH trial. Gut 2012;61(2):229–34.

42. Osterman MT, Haynes K, Delzell E, et al. Comparative effectiveness of infliximab and adalimumab for Crohn's disease. Clin Gastroenterol Hepatol 2013. http://dx.doi.org/10.1016/j.cgh.2013.06.010.

43. D'Haens GR, Panaccione R, Higgins PD, et al. The London Position Statement of the World Congress of Gastroenterology on Biological Therapy for IBD with the European Crohn's and Colitis Organization: when to start, when to stop, which drug to choose, and how to predict response? Am J Gastroenterol 2011; 106(2):199–212.

44. Gerich ME, McGovern DP. Towards personalized care in IBD. Nat Rev Gastroenterol Hepatol 2013. http://dx.doi.org/10.1038/nrgastro.2013.242.

45. Yanai H, Hanauer SB. Assessing response and loss of response to biological therapies in IBD. Am J Gastroenterol 2011;106(4):685–98.

46. Arnott ID, McNeill G, Satsangi J. An analysis of factors influencing short-term and sustained response to infliximab treatment for Crohn's disease. Aliment Pharmacol Ther 2003;17(12):1451–7.

47. Lichtenstein GR, Olson A, Travers S, et al. Factors associated with the development of intestinal strictures or obstructions in patients with Crohn's disease. Am J Gastroenterol 2006;101(5):1030–8.

48. Parsi MA, Achkar JP, Richardson S, et al. Predictors of response to infliximab in patients with Crohn's disease. Gastroenterology 2002;123(3):707–13.

49. Vermeire S, Louis E, Carbonez A, et al. Demographic and clinical parameters influencing the short-term outcome of anti-tumor necrosis factor (infliximab) treatment in Crohn's disease. Am J Gastroenterol 2002;97(9):2357–63.

50. Topstad DR, Panaccione R, Heine JA, et al. Combined seton placement, infliximab infusion, and maintenance immunosuppressives improve healing rate in penetrating anorectal Crohn's disease: a single center experience. Dis Colon Rectum 2003;46(5):577–83.

51. Louis E, Vermeire S, Rutgeerts P, et al. A positive response to infliximab in Crohn disease: association with a higher systemic inflammation before treatment but not with -308 TNF gene polymorphism. Scand J Gastroenterol 2002;37(7): 818–24.

52. Shao LM, Chen MY, Cai JT. Meta-analysis: the efficacy and safety of certolizumab pegol in Crohn's disease. Aliment Pharmacol Ther 2009;29(6): 605–14.

53. Esters N, Vermeire S, Joossens S, et al. Serological markers for prediction of response to anti-tumor necrosis factor treatment in Crohn's disease. Am J Gastroenterol 2002;97(6):1458–62.

54. Taylor KD, Plevy SE, Yang H, et al. ANCA pattern and LTA haplotype relationship to clinical responses to anti-TNF antibody treatment in Crohn's disease. Gastroenterology 2001;120(6):1347–55.

55. Hlavaty T, Ferrante M, Henckaerts L, et al. Predictive model for the outcome of infliximab therapy in Crohn's disease based on apoptotic pharmacogenetic index and clinical predictors. Inflamm Bowel Dis 2007;13(4):372–9.

56. Hlavaty T, Pierik M, Henckaerts L, et al. Polymorphisms in apoptosis genes predict response to infliximab therapy in luminal and penetrating Crohn's disease. Aliment Pharmacol Ther 2005;22(7):613–26.

57. Dubinsky MC, Mei L, Friedman M, et al. Genome wide association (GWA) predictors of anti-TNFalpha therapeutic responsiveness in pediatric inflammatory bowel disease. Inflamm Bowel Dis 2010;16(8):1357–66.

58. Swoger JM, Loftus EV, Tremaine WJ, et al. Adalimumab for Crohn's disease in clinical practice at Mayo Clinic: the first 118 patients. Inflamm Bowel Dis 2010;16(11):1912–21.

59. Lichtiger S, Binion DG, Wolf DC, et al. The CHOICE trial: adalimumab demonstrates safety, fistula healing, improved quality of life and increased work

productivity in patients with Crohn's disease who failed prior infliximab therapy. Aliment Pharmacol Ther 2010;32(10):1228–39.

60. Lofberg R, Louis EV, Reinisch W, et al. Adalimumab produces clinical remission and reduces extraintestinal manifestations in Crohn's disease: results from CARE. Inflamm Bowel Dis 2012;18(1):1–9.

61. Sandborn WJ, Colombel JF, Enns R, et al. Natalizumab induction and maintenance therapy for Crohn's disease. N Engl J Med 2005;353(18):1912–25.

62. Sandborn WJ, Feagan BG, Rutgeerts P, et al. Vedolizumab as induction and maintenance therapy for Crohn's disease. N Engl J Med 2013;369(8):711–21.

63. Sandborn WJ, Gasink C, Gao LL, et al. Ustekinumab induction and maintenance therapy in refractory Crohn's disease. N Engl J Med 2012;367(16):1519–28.

64. Gisbert JP, Panes J. Loss of response and requirement of infliximab dose intensification in Crohn's disease: a review. Am J Gastroenterol 2009;104(3):760–7.

65. Billioud V, Sandborn WJ, Peyrin-Biroulet L. Loss of response and need for adalimumab dose intensification in Crohn's disease: a systematic review. Am J Gastroenterol 2011;106(4):674–84.

66. Ben-Horin S, Chowers Y. Review article: loss of response to anti-TNF treatments in Crohn's disease. Aliment Pharmacol Ther 2011;33(9):987–95.

67. de Silva PS, Nguyen DD, Sauk J, et al. Long-term outcome of a third anti-TNF monoclonal antibody after the failure of two prior anti-TNFs in inflammatory bowel disease. Aliment Pharmacol Ther 2012;36(5):459–66.

68. Regueiro M, Schraut W, Baidoo L, et al. Infliximab prevents Crohn's disease recurrence after ileal resection. Gastroenterology 2009;136(2):441–50.

69. Regueiro M, Kip KE, Baidoo L, et al. Postoperative therapy with infliximab prevents long-term Crohn's disease recurrence. Clin Gastroenterol Hepatol 2014. http://dx.doi.org/10.1016/j.cgh.2013.12.035.

70. Savarino E, Bodini G, Dulbecco P, et al. Adalimumab is more effective than azathioprine and mesalamine at preventing postoperative recurrence of Crohn's disease: a randomized controlled trial. Am J Gastroenterol 2013;108(11):1731–42.

71. Hyams J, Crandall W, Kugathasan S, et al. Induction and maintenance infliximab therapy for the treatment of moderate-to-severe Crohn's disease in children. Gastroenterology 2007;132(3):863–73.

72. Hyams JS, Griffiths A, Markowitz J, et al. Safety and efficacy of adalimumab for moderate to severe Crohn's disease in children. Gastroenterology 2012;143(2):365–74.

73. Walters TD, Kim MO, Denson LA, et al. Increased effectiveness of early therapy with anti-tumor necrosis factor-alpha vs an immunomodulator in children with Crohn's disease. Gastroenterology 2014;146(2):383–91.

74. Rosh JR, Lerer T, Markowitz J, et al. Retrospective evaluation of the safety and effect of adalimumab therapy (RESEAT) in pediatric Crohn's disease. Am J Gastroenterol 2009;104(12):3042–9.

75. Dulai PS, Thompson KD, Blunt HB, et al. Risks of serious infection or lymphoma with anti-tumor necrosis factor therapy for pediatric inflammatory bowel disease: a systematic review. Clin Gastroenterol Hepatol 2014. http://dx.doi.org/10.1016/j.cgh.2014.01.021.

76. Katz S, Surawicz C, Pardi DS. Management of the elderly patients with inflammatory bowel disease: practical considerations. Inflamm Bowel Dis 2013;19(10):2257–72.

77. Charpentier C, Salleron J, Savoye G, et al. Natural history of elderly-onset inflammatory bowel disease: a population-based cohort study. Gut 2014;63(3):423–32.

78. Desai A, Zator ZA, de Silva P, et al. Older age is associated with higher rate of discontinuation of anti-TNF therapy in patients with inflammatory bowel disease. Inflamm Bowel Dis 2013;19(2):309–15.

79. Bhushan A, Pardi DS, Loftus EV, et al. Association of age with adverse events from biologic therapy in patients with inflammatory bowel disease. Gastroenterology 2010;138:S413.

80. Cottone M, Kohn A, Daperno M, et al. Advanced age is an independent risk factor for severe infections and mortality in patients given anti-tumor necrosis factor therapy for inflammatory bowel disease. Clin Gastroenterol Hepatol 2011;9(1): 30–5.

81. Spadaro A, Lubrano E, Marchesoni A, et al. Remission in ankylosing spondylitis treated with anti-TNF-alpha drugs: a national multicentre study. Rheumatology (Oxford) 2013;52(10):1914–9.

82. Generini S, Giacomelli R, Fedi R, et al. Infliximab in spondyloarthropathy associated with Crohn's disease: an open study on the efficacy of inducing and maintaining remission of musculoskeletal and gut manifestations. Ann Rheum Dis 2004;63(12):1664–9.

83. Barrie A, Regueiro M. Biologic therapy in the management of extraintestinal manifestations of inflammatory bowel disease. Inflamm Bowel Dis 2007; 13(11):1424–9.

84. Sandborn WJ, Schreiber S, Feagan BG, et al. Certolizumab pegol for active Crohn's disease: a placebo-controlled, randomized trial. Clin Gastroenterol Hepatol 2011;9(8):670–8.

An Update on Anti-TNF Agents in Ulcerative Colitis

Mark A. Samaan, MBBS[a], Preet Bagi, MD[b], Niels Vande Casteele, PharmD, PhD[b], Geert R. D'Haens, MD, PhD[a], Barrett G. Levesque, MS, MD[b,*]

KEYWORDS

- Ulcerative colitis • UC • Anti-TNF • Infliximab • Adalimumab • Golimumab

KEY POINTS

- Large randomized controlled trials have demonstrated the efficacy of multiple anti-tumor necrosis factor (TNF) agents in delivering mucosal healing, reducing clinical disease activity, and improving long-term outcomes in patients with moderate-to-severe ulcerative colitis.
- A head-to-head trial has shown that infliximab may be as effective as cyclosporin when used as rescue therapy in severe colitis.
- Combining infliximab with an immunomodulator is more effective than infliximab alone in inducing a response in moderate-to-severe ulcerative colitis.
- Therapeutic drug monitoring and dose optimization of anti-TNF agents can maximize their efficacy.

INTRODUCTION

The advent of biologic therapies has led to significant changes in treatment strategies for ulcerative colitis (UC). Before biologic therapies, options for treatment primarily consisted of the stepwise use of mesalamine, corticosteroids, and immunomodulators for disease of increasing severity. Mesalamine was used to achieve and maintain remission in mild-to-moderate cases with the addition of corticosteroids for those failing to respond or with severe disease.[1,2] Patients with colitis refractory to intravenous (IV) corticosteroids received cyclosporin[3] or underwent colectomy. Over the past decade, multiple clinical trials have shown the efficacy of anti-tumor necrosis factor-α (anti-TNF) therapies for these patients with moderate-to-severe UC.[4–6] Therefore, anti-TNF agents are key tools in current treatment algorithms for both chronically active and acute severe UC.[7]

The effectiveness of biologic agents has also changed treatment goals in UC, which is evident in the evolution of endpoints used for clinical trials and targets used in

[a] Department of Gastroenterology, Academic Medical Centre, Meibergdreef 9, Amsterdam 1105 AZ, The Netherlands; [b] Division of Gastroenterology, University of California, San Diego, 9500 Gilman Drive, La Jolla, CA 92093-0956, 92103, USA
* Corresponding author.
E-mail address: bglevesque@ucsd.edu

Gastroenterol Clin N Am 43 (2014) 479–494
http://dx.doi.org/10.1016/j.gtc.2014.05.006
0889-8553/14/$ – see front matter © 2014 Elsevier Inc. All rights reserved.

gastro.theclinics.com

clinical practice.[8] Conventional and established goals of treatment focused predominantly on achieving symptomatic remission. The cessation of corticosteroid use and achieving mucosal healing (MH) were secondary goals.[9] However, in the era of anti-TNF agents with the ability to heal colonic mucosa when other drugs have failed, MH and steroid-free clinical remission have gained prominence as therapeutic targets.

In this update, data are reviewed from randomized controlled trials (RCTs) and comparative effectiveness research and the impact of anti-TNF agents on long-term disease outcomes and their safety data is assessed. In addition, ongoing research is discussed on the pharmacokinetics and pharmacodynamics of TNF-antagonists in UC. Also considered is what may lie ahead as it is aimed to maximize the benefit this group of drugs can deliver.

INFLIXIMAB

Infliximab (Remicade) is a chimeric IgG_1 monoclonal antibody that binds with high affinity and specificity to soluble TNF-α. This process prevents the proinflammatory cytokine binding to cell receptors and propagating the inflammatory cascade.[10] Infliximab also mediates inflammatory processes by binding to membrane-bound TNF-α on inflammatory cells, thereby inducing apoptosis.[11] Infliximab is administered as an IV infusion with weight-based dosing and a regimen that includes an induction phase followed by maintenance treatment.

The first randomized, placebo-controlled study of infliximab for UC was published in 2001. Described as a pilot study, it included just 11 patients with severely active, steroid-refractory UC (defined as a Truelove and Witts[12] score >10 and Blackstone[13] endoscopic grade of 3 or 4). Although the trial was not sufficient to draw meaningful conclusions, it provided an initial signal of the drug's efficacy with response seen in 4 of the 8 patients treated, compared with none in the placebo group.[14] This study was followed by several uncontrolled trials[15,16] before a larger randomized, double-blind, placebo-controlled trial using only a single dose of 4 to 5 mg/kg of infliximab was carried out in Sweden.[17] That study included 45 patients with moderate, severe, or fulminant colitis (based on the Seo[18] or fulminant colitis index[19]) who were refractory to conventional therapies. Their results demonstrated the value of infliximab as a rescue therapy with 7 of 24 (29%) treated patients requiring colectomy at 3 months compared with 14 of 21 (67%) given placebo ($P = .017$). The first RCT to implement an induction regimen of 5 mg/kg at 0, 2, and 6 weeks demonstrated the superiority of infliximab when compared with IV methylprednisolone.[20]

Clinical Efficacy: Moderate-to-Severe Disease and Maintenance Therapy

Infliximab has also been evaluated for use in patients with ongoing moderate to severely active UC, despite conventional therapy. In 2005, infliximab became the first anti-TNF agent approved by the US Food and Drug Administration (FDA) for use in moderate-to-severe UC. A year later, this approval was extended to include maintenance, as well as induction therapy, and European approval was also granted. This evidence was generated in 2 large, randomized, placebo-controlled, double-blind trials[4]: Active Ulcerative Colitis Trials 1 and 2 (ACT 1 and ACT 2). The 2 trials ran concurrently for 3 years at multiple sites over 4 continents. Each trial included 364 patients and studied the effect of infliximab given at doses of 5 or 10 mg/kg at weeks 0, 2, and 6 followed by maintenance treatment scheduled at 8 weekly intervals. Both studies included patients with moderate-to-severe disease activity (defined as a Mayo[21] score >6, with an endoscopic subscore of ≥2) and their inclusion criteria regarding concomitant medications differed only slightly. Both included patients taking corticosteroids and/or thiopurines as well as those who were no longer taking them but had previously failed or had contraindications (or intolerance) to these medications in the past. In addition to these groups, ACT 2 also included 5-aminosalicylate drugs using the same criteria. Therefore, patients did not necessarily need to be receiving corticosteroids at baseline (61% and 51% were in ACT 1 and 2, respectively). Although the 2 studies had identical induction regimens, the duration of treatment and follow-up period differed. Patients were given maintenance treatment until week 46 in ACT 1 and followed until 56 weeks. In ACT 2, the corresponding time points were week 22 and 30. Clinical response at week 8 was the primary endpoint of the ACT trials. The authors defined this as a decrease from baseline in the total Mayo score of at least 3 points and at least 30%, with an accompanying decrease in the subscore for rectal bleeding of at least 1 point or an absolute subscore for rectal bleeding of 0 or 1. Both trials showed that patients treated with infliximab (at either dose) were significantly more likely to have a clinical response at week 8 and 30. The 2 dosing regimens delivered similar efficacy, and response rates at these time points in treated patients were greater than 60% at week 8 and greater than 47% at week 30. Placebo response rates were less than 38% and 30% at the corresponding time points. With its extended follow-up period, ACT 1 showed this response to be durable at week 54 with 45.5% and 44.3% of treated patients (5 mg/kg and 10 mg/kg, respectively) responding compared with 19.8% on placebo. Clinical remission rates followed a similar pattern to clinical response and the effect of infliximab was again significant. In ACT 1, remission rates at 54 weeks were 34.7%, 34.4%, and 16.5% of patients treated with infliximab 5 mg/kg, 10 mg/kg, or placebo, respectively ($P = .01$).

Corticosteroid-Free Remission

Remission in the absence of corticosteroid treatment has become an important endpoint for clinical trials in UC. Of the 61% of patients in ACT 1 on steroids at baseline, the proportion in clinical remission following corticosteroid cessation at week 30 was significantly higher with infliximab 5 mg/kg than with placebo (24.3% vs 10.1%, respectively; $P = .03$). The durability of this effect was evident at week 54 when the corresponding corticosteroid-free remission rates were 25.7% versus 8.9%, respectively ($P = .006$). Furthermore, at baseline, the median dose was 20 mg/d in all groups. By week 54, this had fallen to 5 mg/d in the group given infliximab 5 mg/kg, whereas it remained at 20 mg/d in the placebo group.

Mucosal Healing

MH is an outcome measure with important implications for remission rates, future steroid use, and risk of colectomy in UC. Evidence is growing that complete mucosal reconstitution or significant improvement of endoscopic appearance can have multiple clinical benefits.[22,23] MH was defined in the trials as a Mayo endoscopic subscore of 0 or 1 following treatment. Analysis of data from ACT 1 using this definition showed that at all time points, 5 mg/kg infliximab was significantly superior to placebo in this regard. At week 8, 62% achieved MH on this dose compared with 33.9% on placebo. This difference was maintained at weeks 30 (50.4% vs 24.8%, respectively) and 54 (45.5% vs 18.2%, respectively) with all comparisons reaching statistical significance ($P<.001$).

As debate is on-going[23] regarding whether Mayo grade 1 (abnormal vascular pattern and some friability but no erosions, ulcerations, or active bleeding) should be included in the group achieving MH, subgroup analysis including only those with grade 0 (completely normal mucosa) has subsequently been carried out.[24] Using this more stringent definition, MH was achieved in 22.3% of infliximab patients and 12.4% of placebo patients at week 8, and 32.2% and 15.7%, respectively, at week 54.

Hospitalizations, Colectomy, and Long-Term Efficacy

Hospitalization and colectomy rates from the ACT trials were studied in a post-hoc analysis, which included 630 (87%) of the original 728 patients.[25] When assessed at week 54, the cumulative incidence of colectomy was 10% in the infliximab-treated group compared with 17% in the placebo group (P = .02). Infliximab therefore delivers an absolute risk reduction of 7% for colectomy in patients with moderate-to-severe UC. In their post-hoc analysis, the authors also showed that infliximab halved the rate of hospital admissions compared with placebo. Through week 54, there were 40 hospitalizations per 100 patient-years (PY) in the placebo group and 20 per 100 PY with infliximab (P = .003).

To assess the long-term efficacy, effect on quality of life (QoL), and safety of infliximab, a 3-year open-label extension to the ACT trials was carried out.[26] Any patient participating in the original trials who could benefit from ongoing treatment, as deemed by the investigator (without specific criteria), was eligible for inclusion. Ongoing infliximab, given at 8 weekly intervals, was shown to deliver maintained clinical benefit and health-related QoL while reducing corticosteroid use.

Combination Therapy Versus Monotherapy

Panaccione and colleagues[27] conducted the UC SUCCESS trial to compare the efficacy of infliximab monotherapy with the combination of infliximab and azathioprine. To compare these 2 approaches, they recruited 239 biologic-naïve patients with moderate-to-severe UC (Mayo score $\geq$6). Ninety percent were azathioprine-naïve and 10% had stopped azathioprine more than 3 months before trial entry. The original trial design had planned the enrollment of 600 patients to the first phase (described here) to allow 200 to subsequently enter a longer-term observational study in the second phase. However, enrollment was terminated prematurely by the sponsor, because of higher than expected serious infusion reactions with an intermittent infliximab regimen in an unrelated study of patients with psoriasis.[28] Patients were randomized to 1 of 3 treatment arms: azathioprine and placebo; infliximab and placebo; infliximab and azathioprine. A standard induction regimen of 5 mg/kg infliximab and/or 2.5 mg/kg azathioprine was administered to the relevant groups and endpoints were judged at week 16. The primary endpoint investigated was steroid-free remission (defined as total Mayo score $\leq$2 with no subscore >1). In this regard, combination therapy performed significantly better than either infliximab (40% vs 22%, P = .017) or azathioprine (40% vs 24%, P = .032) alone. Patients on combination therapy were significantly more likely to achieve MH (endoscopic Mayo of 0 or 1) than those on azathioprine monotherapy. MH rates were 63% with combination therapy compared with 55% with infliximab monotherapy (P = .295) and 37% with azathioprine monotherapy (P = .001).

Safety

The TREAT (Crohn Therapy, Resource, Evaluation, and Assessment Tool) registry was designed specifically to investigate the long-term safety of anti-TNF therapy in patients with Crohn disease (CD).[29] More than 5 years of data from this ongoing, prospective, observational study was published in 2012 and, although the study only includes patients with CD, results are certainly relevant to anti-TNF-treated patients with UC. Based on analysis of more than 6000 patients, the authors demonstrated no increase in mortality or neoplasia between patients receiving infliximab and those receiving other treatments only. Analysis of this data also confirmed the increased risk of serious infections that had been previously seen (hazard ratio 1.98; 95% confidence interval [CI] 1.11, 1.84; $P = .006$). It should be noted, however, that increased risk was not relative to cumulative infliximab dose because neither the number of infusions nor the dose escalation to 10 mg/kg significantly impacted it.

Of significant concern in the treatment of fulminant colitis with infliximab is its possible effect on postoperative complication rates among nonresponder who require colectomy. This group of patients are often already at increased risk of infectious complications owing to the use of immunomodulators and corticosteroids. A literature review[30] and meta-analysis[31] of trials have been conducted to examine this issue. Although the studies included[17,32–36] are all retrospective, use different endpoints, and report mixed results, limited conclusions can be drawn. It seems that if the use of preoperative infliximab increases the risk of postoperative complications (infectious or otherwise) at all, the effect is minimal.

Clinical Efficacy: Rescue Therapy

Before infliximab, therapeutic options for patients with severe or fulminant colitis unresponsive to IV corticosteroids were only cyclosporin or colectomy. Given the risks for toxicity with cyclosporin,[37] the benefit of infliximab in clinical trials of moderate-to-severe UC suggested a potential alternative for patients hospitalized with severe UC. However, until recently the 2 agents had not been compared in a head-to-head trial to assess their relative efficacy. This comparison was recently carried out in a study involving 27 centers in France and Belgium as part of a parallel, open-label, RCT.[38] Patients experiencing a severe flare (defined as a Lichtiger[39] score >10) with an insufficient response to IV corticosteroids received either cyclosporin (2 mg/kg/d for 1 week, followed by oral drug until day 98) or infliximab (5 mg/kg at 0, 2, and 6 weeks). All 115 patients included were naïve to the trial agents and those with a satisfactory response to either drug commenced azathioprine at day 7. The primary outcome was "treatment failure," and the authors defined this as the absence of a clinical response at day 7, a relapse between day 7 and day 98, absence of steroid-free remission at day 98, a severe adverse event leading to treatment interruption, colectomy, or death. Failure of therapy was seen in 60% (35) of those receiving cyclosporin and 54% (31) given infliximab (absolute risk difference 6%, 95% CI −7 to 19; odds ratio 1.3, 95% CI 0.6–2.7). Roughly 85% of patients in both groups had a clinical response at day 7 measured by the Lichtiger score (a secondary endpoint). The proportion of severe adverse events was also similar among the 2 arms with 9 (16%) and 14 (25%) suffering these in the cyclosporin and infliximab groups, respectively. No deaths and few serious infections were reported. Overall, the authors concluded that treatment choice should be guided by physician and center experience. When considered in the context of the monitoring cyclosporin blood levels, the significant potential toxicity of cyclosporin, and the emerging evidence regarding the pharmacodynamics of infliximab, infliximab may soon become the rescue therapy of choice for many practitioners.[40] The overriding practical issue in relation to cyclosporin is that its use is restricted to centers that can regularly monitor concentrations and have sufficient clinical experience in the use of drugs not routinely used in outpatient practices. Evidence has also emerged demonstrating that patients with severe, steroid-refractory colitis may fail to respond to infliximab because of accelerated clearance of the drug.[41] Dose optimization with higher or more frequent doses may therefore improve response rates, an aspect that was not studied in the head-to-head comparison. This theory is supported by post-hoc analysis from the ACT 1 and 2 demonstrating that higher infliximab trough concentrations were associated with greater likelihood of response, remission, and MH than were low or absent trough concentrations.[42]

It is also important to consider the patient who has a severe flair despite thiopurine maintenance therapy in whom there is no subsequent maintenance option if rescue cyclosporin is chosen and succeeds. Infliximab, therefore, has a significant advantage in this group. Further data regarding the efficacy and cost-effectiveness of each agent will be available when the UK-wide CONSTRUCT trial (COmparison of iNfliximab and cyclosporin in STeroid Resistant Ulcerative Colitis: a Trial) is completed in August 2014.

ADALIMUMAB

After FDA approval of infliximab for induction and maintenance of UC, the next anti-TNF agent to achieve FDA approval for the treatment of UC was adalimumab (Humira). Adalimumab is a TNF-α targeted fully human monoclonal antibody. It is administered via the subcutaneous route and is FDA approved as therapy for moderate-to-severe CD as well. In addition, adalimumab is currently in use for the therapy for psoriasis, psoriatic arthritis, rheumatoid arthritis, and ankylosing spondylitis. Initially, case reports and many small open-label studies showed efficacy in UC.[43–46] Recently, a multicenter RCT, ULTRA1, was conducted to examine the efficacy of adalimumab in induction of clinical remission in moderate-to-severe UC.[5] This phase III, randomized, double-blind, placebo-controlled study was conducted across 94 European and North American centers. Enrolled subjects were required to have a full Mayo score ranging from 6 to 12, with an endoscopic subscore of 2 to 3. Subjects were required to be anti-TNF naïve. Prior failure of oral corticosteroid and/or immunomodulator therapy with azathioprine or 6-mercaptopurine was required for study enrollment. Subjects were randomized to either placebo or induction with subcutaneous adalimumab 160/80 mg or 80/40 mg. This dosing selection was based on adalimumab dosing in the CHARM and CLASSIC-I CD trials and regulatory agency guidance.[47,48] The 160/80 mg group received subcutaneous adalimumab 160 mg at week 0, 80 mg at week 2, followed by 40 mg at weeks 4 and 6. The 80/40 mg group received 80 mg at week 0 followed by 40 mg at weeks 2, 4, and 6.

The study's primary endpoint was the proportion of subjects in clinical remission by week 8, defined as a composite Mayo score less than or equal to 2 with no individual subscore of 1 or more. At the study's end, the adalimumab 160/80 mg group achieved clinical remission in 18.5% of subjects, which was double the placebo rate of 9.2% ($P = .031$). The adalimumab 80/40 mg group reached a clinical remission rate that was similar to placebo at 10% ($P = .833$). Furthermore, secondary endpoints revealed that the adalimumab 160/80 mg group did achieve greater rates of MH, clinical response, and improvement to less than or equal to 1 in all components of the Mayo score in comparison to placebo. Subanalyses revealed that subjects with a greater composite Mayo score on study entry, CRP more than or equal to 10 mg/L at baseline, and higher study entry weight achieved lower rates of remission than those with a lower Mayo score. The safety profile of adalimumab appeared to be comparable to that of placebo. Overall, the results of ULTRA1 conclude that adalimumab 160/80 mg is effective for induction of remission in moderate-to-severe UC subjects who are failing corticosteroids and/or thiopurines. The optimal dose regimen in UC may, however, not have been reached because the dose-response curve suggests that efficacy may be improved with doses more than the current standard dosing regimen.

Following ULTRA1, the ULTRA2 study was conducted as a phase III, randomized, double-blind, placebo-controlled trial to examine the efficacy of adalimumab in long-term maintenance of remission in moderate-to-severe UC.[49] Before enrollment, subjects were required to have 3 months of active moderate-to-severe UC defined as a composite Mayo score of 6 to 12 and an endoscopic subscore of 2 or more. Subjects had moderate-to-severe UC despite corticosteroid or azathioprine/6-mercaptopurine. Concomitant 5-ASA therapy was allowed but not a requirement, and prior use of infliximab was permitted after a more than or equal to 8-week washout period. In total, 40% of subjects had prior anti-TNF exposure. Randomization to placebo or subcutaneous adalimumab 160 mg at week 0, 80 mg at week 2, and then 40 mg every other week was done in a 1:1 fashion. After week 12, subjects who showed poor response were able to enter the open-label phase using adalimumab 40 mg every other week. In addition, subjects were permitted to dose escalate to adalimumab 40 mg every week in the case of inadequate response to every other week dosing.

The study followed subjects for a total of 52 weeks with assessments of primary and secondary endpoints at weeks 8, 32, and 52. The primary endpoint of clinical remission was defined as a composite Mayo score less than or equal to 2 with no individual subscore greater than 1. By week 8, 16.5% of subjects who received adalimumab were in clinical remission, whereas the placebo remission rate was 9.3% ($P = .019$). By week 52, remission rates were 17.3% and 8.5% in the adalimumab and placebo group, respectively ($P = .004$). Secondary endpoints included clinical response and MH. Clinical response was defined as a decrease in Mayo score of more than or equal to 3 from baseline and a decrease in Mayo score more than or equal to 30% from baseline and decrease in rectal bleeding subscore more than or equal to 1 or an absolute score of 0 or 1. By week 8, the adalimumab group achieved clinical response in 50.4% of subjects compared with 34.6% in the placebo group ($P<.001$). By week 52, the adalimumab group revealed response in 30.2% compared with 18.3% placebo response ($P = .002$). MH was achieved by reaching an endoscopic subscore of 0 or 1. At week 8, 41.1% of subjects achieved MH compared with 31.7% on placebo ($P = .032$). In comparison, by week 52, the adalimumab group achieved MH in 25% compared with 15.4% in the placebo group ($P = .009$). Further subanalyses revealed that subjects who were anti-TNF naïve had a greater chance of achieving clinical remission at weeks 8 and 52 compared with the anti-TNF exposed group. Safety results were also comparable between the treatment and placebo groups.

An additional study analyzing the safety of adalimumab using a benefit-to-risk balance assessed the likelihood of achieving efficacy without serious adverse events in the intention-to-treat group.[50] This analysis showed a favorable adverse event profile and overall positive benefit/risk balance when remission or response was achieved at weeks 8 and 52 in adalimumab-treated subjects. One notable difference between the ULTRA2 trial and the infliximab trials (ACT 1 and 2) is that the infliximab studies did not allow for rescue therapy. Another variation is that a significant portion of the ULTRA2 subjects had been exposed to anti-TNF, whereas all the infliximab study subjects were anti-TNF naïve at enrollment. These variations may explain in part the lower remission rates seen with adalimumab versus infliximab.

In summary, the ULTRA2 study results confirm findings from ULTRA1. Combined, these studies show that adalimumab 160 mg at week 0, 80 mg at week 2, followed by 40 mg every other week is effective in induction and maintenance of remission in moderate-to-severe UC.

To study the long-term safety of adalimumab, the PYRAMID registry was initiated in 2007.[51] In common with the TREAT registry for infliximab, only patients with CD are included, but once again the results are also certainly of relevance to those on long-term adalimumab treatment of UC. Although not due for completion until 2015 with a planned 6-year study duration for each patient, an interim safety analysis was carried out at year 3. This study demonstrated very low rates of opportunistic infection (0.1 per 100 PY) as well as malignancy (0.6 per 100 PY) and lymphoma (<0.1 per 100 PY) with no new safety signals. At that point, more than 8000 PY had been studied with a median exposure to adalimumab of 19 months, suggesting that long-term treatment can be considered safe.

GOLIMUMAB

In 2013, the FDA expanded the armamentarium for treatment of moderate-to-severe UC with the approval of golimumab (Simponi), a fully human monoclonal antibody to TNF-α administered subcutaneously. Golimumab is also approved for the treatment of rheumatoid arthritis, psoriatic arthritis, and ankylosing spondylitis. PURSUIT-SC was a randomized, double-blind, placebo-controlled integrated phase 2 and 3 study to assess the safety as well as efficacy of golimumab in inducing remission in moderate-to-severe UC subjects.[6] Subjects were required to have had failed or inadequately responded to standard therapy including oral 5-aminosalyciates, thiopurines, or oral corticosteroids. Prior anti-TNF therapy was an exclusion criterion. A composite Mayo score of 6 to 12 with an endoscopic subscore of 2 or more was required for study entry. The initial phase 2 portion of the study was conducted to determine the dose-response relationship of subcutaneous golimumab, and this information was applied to the phase 3 efficacy portion. Enrolled subjects were randomized to either placebo or 1 of 3 induction regimens 2 weeks apart (100/50 mg, 200/100 mg, or 400/200 mg). After safety, pharamacokinetic, and efficacy analyses, the 200/100 mg and 400/200 mg doses were selected for continuation in the phase 3 study portion. For the phase 3 portion, subjects were assessed at week 6 for primary and secondary endpoints. The study's primary endpoint was week 6 clinical response measured by a decline in the baseline composite Mayo score by 30% or more and 3 points or more (with a bleeding subscore of 0 or 1 or decrease ≥ 1). Clinical remission was a secondary endpoint and was defined by the authors as a composite Mayo score less than or equal to 2 and no subscore greater than 1. In addition, week 6, MH was also assessed and defined as an endoscopy subscore of 0 or 1. QoL assessment was made as well using the Inflammatory Bowel Disease Questionnaire (IBDQ). By the end of phase 3, the study demonstrated favorable findings for primary and all secondary endpoints. A larger proportion of subjects in the 400/200 mg golimumab group had achieved clinical response, clinical remission, or MH or had greater IBDQ scores when compared with placebo. Clinical response was greatest in the 400/200 mg (54.9%) and 200/100 mg (51%) groups compared with placebo (30.3%), indicating that the study was able to meet its primary endpoint. Improvement in MH was noted at week 2 and was greater by week 6 in the 400/200 mg and 200/100 mg groups compared with placebo. Furthermore, mean C-reactive protein concentrations declined to a greater extent in the 400/200 mg and 200/100 mg groups compared with placebo. Adverse events were similar in the treatment and placebo groups with the most notable being headache and nasopharyngitis. There was no noted dose-dependent accumulation of adverse events. In summary, induction with 400/200 mg and 200/100 mg of golimumab at weeks 0 and 2 resulted in statistically significant induction of remission by week 6 in subjects suffering from moderate-to-severe UC.

Additional analysis of serum golimumab concentration using a validated assay revealed that serum concentrations were dose-proportional and those with higher serum concentrations had greater rates of clinical response and remission and greater improvement in median composite Mayo scores.

All subjects from the PURSUIT-SC study were eligible for enrollment in the PURSUIT-Maintenance study in which subjects received 54 weeks of golimumab

50 mg or 100 mg every 4 weeks as maintenance.[52] This study's primary endpoint of maintenance of clinical response by week 54 was achieved at rates of 49.7% and 47% in the 100 mg and 50 mg groups, respectively, compared with 31.2% placebo response. Secondary endpoints of clinical remission, MH, and corticosteroid-free remission by week 54 were greater in the 100 mg and 50 mg golimumab groups compared with placebo.

It is too early for any safety registry data for golimumab in inflammatory bowel disease (IBD) to mirror the results from infliximab (TREAT[29]) and adalimumab (PYRAMID[51]) registries. However, safety analyses were made as part of the PURSUIT trials. Overall, the safety signals were reassuring and consistent with experience gained from use in rheumatoid arthritis but should prompt a note of caution.[53] Four cases of tuberculosis were seen, all in golimumab-treated patients (who were also receiving corticosteroids) living in endemic regions, with one resulting death. This finding should serve to underscore the importance of robust pretreatment screening for tuberculosis in clinical practice.

ALTERING PRACTICE? TREATING TO TARGET, MUCOSAL, AND HISTOLOGIC HEALING

Progress related to the advent of anti-TNF agents has seen MH become an established endpoint for clinical trials. In conjunction with this, interest in alternative, nonclinical endpoints has also grown. Histologic healing is one such alternative and offers significant promise. As is the case with ongoing endoscopic activity, studies have shown that clinical remission in the presence of ongoing histologic inflammation is less durable than if histologic healing is achieved.[54,55] Also, mirroring the situation in MH, a validated definition for histologic healing remains elusive. Nonetheless, it is likely to feature to some degree as an endpoint in future clinical trials,[56] possibly alongside MH as a part of a composite endpoint.

To investigate the feasibility of using these endpoints as targets in a predefined treatment algorithm for UC, Bouguen and colleagues[8] performed a retrospective cohort study of 60 patients undergoing serial endoscopies. Multivariate analysis demonstrated that anti-TNF use at baseline (along with disease duration <2 years and family history of IBD) predicted MH (hazard ratio 4.47; 95% CI 1.58–11.96). Although anti-TNF treatment during the course of the study (median follow-up 76 weeks) was not associated with higher rates of MH, use of the treatment algorithm approach was. This approach was based on adapting therapy to the target of MH, meaning optimizing biologic therapy by increasing the dose, adjusting to target serum infliximab concentrations, switching biologics, and adding immunosuppressive agents as needed to reach MH. Using this approach allowed 60% of those with endoscopic disease at baseline to achieve MH (with a stringent definition of Mayo 0) at week 76. A similar pattern was seen on a microscopic level, whereby adjustments in medical therapy in response to ongoing histologic activity resulted in higher rates of histologic healing. Preliminary experience regarding treat-to-target algorithms has also been gained from those used in the management of rheumatoid arthritis. The structure of a corresponding proposal for specific recommendations in IBD can be made based on these (**Fig. 1**).[57] However, long-term studies with similar algorithms are necessary, and it appears that this type of target-driven approach could optimize the benefit gained from anti-TNF agents.

THERAPEUTIC DRUG MONITORING

In the setting of anti-TNF treatment optimization as suggested in the algorithm by Bouguen and colleagues,[57] therapeutic drug monitoring (TDM) could be an objective

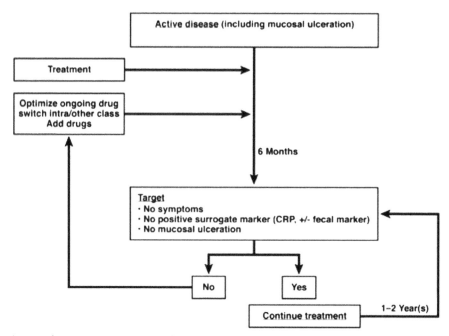

Fig. 1. Schematic representation for a treat-to-target based strategy for UC. On the basis of preliminary experience from RA, proposal algorithm for UC includes careful selection of patients to active treatment, use of MH as the optimal target, and a time frame to assess treatment efficacy.

tool to guide treatment decisions. Prospective studies using TDM are currently, however, lacking.

Concentration-Effect Relationship

The correlation between anti-TNF trough concentrations, anti-drug antibodies, and clinical outcomes, such as clinical response, remission, and MH, has been investigated. In a retrospective study including 115 UC patients treated with 3-dose induction followed by scheduled maintenance infliximab, the authors found that detectable as opposed to undetectable infliximab trough concentrations were associated with clinical remission (69% vs 15%; $P<.001$), endoscopic improvement (76% vs 28%; $P<.001$), and endoscopic remission (27% vs 8%; $P = .021$).[58] Moreover, an undetectable infliximab trough concentration predicted an increased risk for colectomy (odds ratio 9.3; 95% CI 2.9 to 29.9; $P<.001$). This dichotomous cutoff of presence or absence of detectable infliximab trough concentration was later refined in a follow-up study including 134 patients with steroid refractory active UC treated with 3-dose induction followed by scheduled maintenance therapy.[59] An infliximab trough concentration greater than 2 μg/mL, without or with Antibodies Toward Infliximab, was associated with a higher rate of clinical steroid-free remission (69% vs 16%; $P<.001$) that was sustained over the follow-up period of a median of 19.9 months. These results were recently corroborated in a post-hoc analysis of the ACT 1 and 2 trials whereby the proportion of patients achieving clinical response, remission, and MH at week 8, 30, and 54 increased with increasing quartiles of infliximab concentration.[42] Interestingly, the same concentration-effect relationship (although it was dose-proportional) was observed in the PURSUIT trial as the change from baseline Mayo score and rates of clinical response and clinical remission at week 6 increased with increasing quartiles of serum golimumab concentration.[6] In the subsequent maintenance trial with golimumab, a combined analysis of patients randomized to golimumab 50-mg and 100-mg groups showed that greater proportions of patients in the higher serum golimumab concentration quartiles achieved clinical response through week 54 or clinical remission at both weeks 30 and 54 when compared with those in the lower serum concentration quartiles.[52] MH has emerged as an important target and it is therefore of interest to investigate the correlation between MH and anti-TNF trough concentrations. In a cross-sectional study in 40 IBD patients treated with adalimumab therapy, the outcome of endoscopic evaluation was correlated to the adalimumab trough concentration.[60] The authors found that an absence of MH was associated with an adalimumab trough concentration less than 4.9 mg/mL (likelihood ratio, 4.3; sensitivity, 66%; specificity, 85%). Although the authors did not find these results to vary with type of IBD, the number of CD and UC patients did become small in subgroup analysis (22 and 18 patients, respectively). Nevertheless, these concentration-effect relationships indicate that when the predefined target is not met, a TDM approach with measurement of serum anti-TNF drug concentrations could be used to optimize anti-TNF treatment further.

TDM-guided Treatment

In a simulated model, Velayos and colleagues[61] showed that a testing-based strategy is more cost-effective than the empiric dose-escalation strategy to address secondary loss of response. In a recent Scandinavian RCT of 69 CD patients with secondary loss of response, the TDM strategy was shown to reduce treatment costs with up to 34% at similar efficacy rates (a response rate of 58% vs 53% for the testing-based and empiric approach, respectively).[62] A similar approach can be applied to further optimize treatment in patients who have insufficient response to the drug (**Table 1**). When response to the current anti-TNF is inadequate and the patient has adequate anti-TNF trough concentrations, switching to an out-of-class drug may be the preferred strategy. In this case, patients might not respond to the drug because of pharmacodynamic problems (a non-TNF-driven disease). In the case of a low anti-TNF trough concentration, dose optimization should be considered if antidrug antibodies are absent. If antidrug antibodies are sustained, the preferred strategy is to switch to another anti-TNF drug. These therapeutic monitoring strategies must be confirmed in UC in prospective clinical trials.

Table 1
TDM algorithm used to optimize anti-TNF therapy in patients failing to improve with standard dosing

		Serum Anti-TNF Trough Concentration	
		Low	Adequate
Antidrug antibodies (ADA)	Undetectable Low titers	Dose optimize Switch within class or Consider dose optimization or Consider addition of immunomodulator (transient ADA)	Switch out of class
	High titers	Switch within class	

SUMMARY

This update has served to illustrate the significant progress made in the treatment of UC during the anti-TNF era. Considered together, this group of trials has demonstrated the value of an effective class of UC therapy. The results have brought about an increasingly widespread use of anti-TNF agents for UC and may yet see these agents being used earlier in the disease course.[9] The evidence gained from them, along with growing clinical experience, has opened up multiple new avenues of investigation. The predominant thrust of more recent research has concerned maximizing the benefit of these agents and has centered on treat-to-target strategies and the use of TDM. However, there is a lack of prospective trials comparing the efficacy of anti-TNF agents in clinical trials. Meta-analysis techniques may be attempted to compare therapies across trials; however, these are limited by not only the difference in inclusion criteria in the placebo arms but also the different pharmacokinetic properties of each anti-TNF agent, which may require unique dosing for their optimal efficacy in UC. Cluster randomization trials in UC will provide large-scale tests of the effectiveness of anti-TNF agent treatment strategies and their effect on outcomes such as costs, hospitalizations, and surgeries. Along with these well-established long-term outcomes, it may now be time also to consider additional outcomes, such as improvement in function or disability scores.[9,63]

The focus of anti-TNF research should now broaden to include comparative effectiveness trials.[64] The potential benefits of trials designed to compare these medications directly include the identification of optimal treatments, a better understanding of their relative economic impacts, and greater applicability to everyday practice.[65] The fact these issues remain unresolved demonstrates that, although anti-TNF agents have delivered on their early promise, there remains significant progress still to be made.

CONFLICTS OF INTEREST PAST 12 MONTHS

M.A. Samaan, P. Bagi: none.

N. Vande Casteele is a Postdoctoral Fellow of the Research Foundation-Flanders (FWO), Belgium. He has served as a consultant for MSD and Janssen Biologics. He has received payment for development of educational presentations, including service on speakers bureaus from AbbVie.

G. D'Haens has received consulting fees from Abbott/Abbvie, ActoGeniX NV, Amgen, AM-Pharma BV, Boehringer Ingelheim, ChemoCentryx, Centocor/Jansen Biologics, Cosmo Technologies, Elan/Biogen, EnGene Inc, Ferring Pharmaceuticals, Gilead Sciences, Given Imaging, GSK, Merck Research Laboratories, Merck Serono, Millenium Pharmaceuticals, Novo Nordisk, NPS Pharmaceuticals, PDL Biopharma, Pfizer, Receptos, Salix Pharmaceuticals, Schering Plough, Shire Pharmaceuticals, Sigmoid Pharma Ltd, Teva Pharmaceuticals, Tillotts Pharma AG, UCB Pharma; research grants from Abbvie, GSK, Falk, Janssen, Merck, Given Imaging; payments for lectures/speakers bureaus from Abbvie, Jansen, Merck, Takeda, UCB, Shire.

B.G. Levesque has received consulting fees from Prometheus Laboratories, Santarus Inc.

REFERENCES

1. Schroeder KW. Role of mesalazine in acute and long-term treatment of ulcerative colitis and its complications. Scand J Gastroenterol Suppl 2002;(236): 42–7.

2. Sninsky CA, Cort DH, Shanahan F, et al. Oral mesalamine (Asacol) for mildly to moderately active ulcerative colitis. A multicenter study. Ann Intern Med 1991; 115(5):350–5.
3. Rogler G. Medical management of ulcerative colitis. Dig Dis 2009;27(4):542–9.
4. Rutgeerts P, Sandborn WJ, Feagan BG, et al. Infliximab for induction and maintenance therapy for ulcerative colitis. N Engl J Med 2005;353(23):2462–76.
5. Reinisch W, Sandborn WJ, Hommes DW, et al. Adalimumab for induction of clinical remission in moderately to severely active ulcerative colitis: results of a randomised controlled trial. Gut 2011;60(6):780–7.
6. Sandborn WJ, Feagan BG, Marano C, et al. Subcutaneous golimumab induces clinical response and remission in patients with moderate-to-severe ulcerative colitis. Gastroenterology 2014;146(1):85–95.
7. Panaccione R, Rutgeerts P, Sandborn WJ, et al. Review article: treatment algorithms to maximize remission and minimize corticosteroid dependence in patients with inflammatory bowel disease. Aliment Pharmacol Ther 2008;28(6):674–88.
8. Bouguen G, Levesque BG, Pola S, et al. Feasibility of endoscopic assessment and treating to target to achieve mucosal healing in ulcerative colitis. Inflamm Bowel Dis 2014;20:231–9.
9. Danese S, Colombel JF, Peyrin-Biroulet L, et al. Review article: the role of anti-TNF in the management of ulcerative colitis – past, present and future. Aliment Pharmacol Ther 2013;37(9):855–66.
10. Rutgeerts P, Van Assche G, Vermeire S. Optimizing anti-TNF treatment in inflammatory bowel disease. Gastroenterology 2004;126(6):1593–610.
11. Wilhelm SM, McKenney KA, Rivait KN, et al. A review of infliximab use in ulcerative colitis. Clin Ther 2008;30(2):223–30.
12. Truelove SC, Witts LJ. Cortisone in ulcerative colitis; final report on a therapeutic trial. Br Med J 1955;2(4947):1041–8.
13. Blackstone MO. Endoscoppic interpretation. New York: Raven Press; 1984.
14. Sands BE, Tremaine WJ, Sandborn WJ, et al. Infliximab in the treatment of severe, steroid-refractory ulcerative colitis: a pilot study. Inflamm Bowel Dis 2001;7(2):83–8.
15. Chey WY, Hussain A, Ryan C, et al. Infliximab for refractory ulcerative colitis. Am J Gastroenterol 2001;96(8):2373–81.
16. Kohu A, Prantera C, Pera A, et al. Anti-tumor necrosis factor alpha (infliximab) in the treatment of severe ulcerative colitis: result of an open study on 13 patients. Dig Liver Dis 2002;34:626–30.
17. Jarnerot G, Hertervig E, Friis-Liby I, et al. Infliximab as rescue therapy in severe to moderately severe ulcerative colitis: a randomized, placebo-controlled study. Gastroenterology 2005;128(7):1805–11.
18. Seo M, Okada M, Yao T, et al. An index of disease activity in patients with ulcerative colitis. Am J Gastroenterol 1992;87(8):971–6.
19. Lindgren SC, Flood LM, Kilander AF, et al. Early predictors of glucocorticosteroid treatment failure in severe and moderately severe attacks of ulcerative colitis. Eur J Gastroenterol Hepatol 1998;10(10):831–5.
20. Armuzzi A, De Pascalis B, Lupascu A, et al. Infliximab in the treatment of steroid-dependent ulcerative colitis. Eur Rev Med Pharmacol Sci 2004;8(5):231–3.
21. Schroeder KW, Tremaine WJ, Ilstrup DM. Coated oral 5-aminosalicylic acid therapy for mildly to moderately active ulcerative colitis. A randomized study. N Engl J Med 1987;317(26):1625–9.
22. Pineton de Chambrun G, Peyrin-Biroulet L, Lemann M, et al. Clinical implications of mucosal healing for the management of IBD. Nat Rev Gastroenterol Hepatol 2010;7(1):15–29.

23. Neurath MF, Travis SP. Mucosal healing in inflammatory bowel diseases: a systematic review. Gut 2012;61(11):1619–35.
24. Rutgeerts P. Landmark data in early IBD patients: time to change your practice? BMJ Satellite Symposium. 2009:3–5.
25. Sandborn WJ, Rutgeerts P, Feagan BG, et al. Colectomy rate comparison after treatment of ulcerative colitis with placebo or infliximab. Gastroenterology 2009; 137(4):1250–60 [quiz: 1520].
26. Reinisch W, Sandborn WJ, Rutgeerts P, et al. Long-term infliximab maintenance therapy for ulcerative colitis: the ACT-1 and -2 extension studies. Inflamm Bowel Dis 2012;18(2):201–11.
27. Panaccione R, Ghosh S, Middleton S, et al. Combination therapy with infliximab and azathioprine is superior to monotherapy with either agent in ulcerative colitis. Gastroenterology 2014;146(2):392–400.e3.
28. Reich K, Wozel G, Zheng H, et al. Efficacy and safety of infliximab as continuous or intermittent therapy in patients with moderate-to-severe plaque psoriasis: results of a randomized, long-term extension trial (RESTORE2). Br J Dermatol 2013;168(6):1325–34.
29. Lichtenstein GR, Feagan BG, Cohen RD, et al. Serious infection and mortality in patients with Crohn's disease: more than 5 years of follow-up in the TREAT registry. Am J Gastroenterol 2012;107(9):1409–22.
30. Ali T, Yun L, Rubin DT. Risk of post-operative complications associated with anti-TNF therapy in inflammatory bowel disease. World J Gastroenterol 2012;18(3): 197–204.
31. Yang Z, Wu Q, Wu K, et al. Meta-analysis: pre-operative infliximab treatment and short-term post-operative complications in patients with ulcerative colitis. Aliment Pharmacol Ther 2010;31(4):486–92.
32. Selvasekar CR, Cima RR, Larson DW, et al. Effect of infliximab on short-term complications in patients undergoing operation for chronic ulcerative colitis. J Am Coll Surg 2007;204(5):956–62 [discussion: 962–3].
33. Schluender SJ, Ippoliti A, Dubinsky M, et al. Does infliximab influence surgical morbidity of ileal pouch-anal anastomosis in patients with ulcerative colitis? Dis Colon Rectum 2007;50(11):1747–53.
34. Mor IJ, Vogel JD, da Luz Moreira A, et al. Infliximab in ulcerative colitis is associated with an increased risk of postoperative complications after restorative proctocolectomy. Dis Colon Rectum 2008;51(8):1202–7 [discussion: 1207–10].
35. Kunitake H, Hodin R, Shellito PC, et al. Perioperative treatment with infliximab in patients with Crohn's disease and ulcerative colitis is not associated with an increased rate of postoperative complications. J Gastrointest Surg 2008; 12(10):1730–6 [discussion: 1736–7].
36. Ferrante M, Vermeire S, Fidder H, et al. Long-term outcome after infliximab for refractory ulcerative colitis. J Crohns Colitis 2008;2(3):219–25.
37. Arts J, D'Haens G, Zeegers M, et al. Long-term outcome of treatment with intravenous cyclosporin in patients with severe ulcerative colitis. Inflamm Bowel Dis 2004;10(2):73–8.
38. Laharie D, Bourreille A, Branche J, et al. Ciclosporin versus infliximab in patients with severe ulcerative colitis refractory to intravenous steroids: a parallel, open-label randomised controlled trial. Lancet 2012;380(9857):1909–15.
39. Lichtiger S. Cyclosporine therapy in inflammatory bowel disease: open-label experience. Mt Sinai J Med 1990;57(5):315–9.
40. Levesque BG, Sandborn WJ. Infliximab versus ciclosporin in severe ulcerative colitis. Lancet 2012;380(9857):1887–8.

41. Kevans D, Murthy S, Iacono A, et al. Accelerated clearance of infliximab during induction therapy for acute ulcerative colitis is associated with treatment failure. Gastroenterology 2012;142(5 Suppl 1):S384–5.
42. Reinisch W, Feagan BG, Rutgeerts PJ, et al. Infliximab concentration and clinical outcome in patients with ulcerative colitis. Gastroenterology 2012;142(5 Suppl 1): S114.
43. Afif W, Leighton JA, Hanauer SB, et al. Open-label study of adalimumab in patients with ulcerative colitis including those with prior loss of response or intolerance to infliximab. Inflamm Bowel Dis 2009;15(9):1302–7.
44. Barreiro-de Acosta M, Lorenzo A, Dominguez-Munoz JE. Adalimumab in ulcerative colitis: two cases of mucosal healing and clinical response at two years. World J Gastroenterol 2009;15(30):3814–6.
45. Peyrin-Biroulet L, Laclotte C, Roblin X, et al. Adalimumab induction therapy for ulcerative colitis with intolerance or lost response to infliximab: an open-label study. World J Gastroenterol 2007;13(16):2328–32.
46. Taxonera C, Estelles J, Fernandez-Blanco I, et al. Adalimumab induction and maintenance therapy for patients with ulcerative colitis previously treated with infliximab. Aliment Pharmacol Ther 2011;33(3):340–8.
47. Hanauer SB, Sandborn WJ, Rutgeerts P, et al. Human anti-tumor necrosis factor monoclonal antibody (adalimumab) in Crohn's disease: the CLASSIC-I trial. Gastroenterology 2006;130(2):323–33 [quiz: 591].
48. Colombel JF, Sandborn WJ, Rutgeerts P, et al. Adalimumab for maintenance of clinical response and remission in patients with Crohn's disease: the CHARM trial. Gastroenterology 2007;132(1):52–65.
49. Sandborn WJ, van Assche G, Reinisch W, et al. Adalimumab induces and maintains clinical remission in patients with moderate-to-severe ulcerative colitis. Gastroenterology 2012;142(2):257–65.e1–3.
50. Sandborn WJ, Colombel JF, D'Haens G, et al. One-year maintenance outcomes among patients with moderately-to-severely active ulcerative colitis who responded to induction therapy with adalimumab: subgroup analyses from ULTRA 2. Aliment Pharmacol Ther 2013;37(2):204–13.
51. D'Haens G, Reinisch W, Satsangi J, et al. PYRAMID registry: an observational study of adalimumab in Crohn's disease: results at year 3. Inflamm Bowel Dis 2011;17:S21.
52. Sandborn WJ, Feagan BG, Marano C, et al. Subcutaneous golimumab maintains clinical response in patients with moderate-to-severe ulcerative colitis. Gastroenterology 2014;146(1):96–109.e1.
53. Hanauer SB. Still in pursuit. Gastroenterology 2014;146(1):13–5.
54. Bitton A, Peppercorn MA, Antonioli DA, et al. Clinical, biological, and histologic parameters as predictors of relapse in ulcerative colitis. Gastroenterology 2001; 120(1):13–20.
55. Riley SA, Mani V, Goodman MJ, et al. Microscopic activity in ulcerative colitis: what does it mean? Gut 1991;32(2):174–8.
56. Peyrin-Biroulet L, Bressenot A, Kampman W. Histologic remission: the ultimate therapeutic goal in ulcerative colitis? Clin Gastroenterol Hepatol 2014;12:929–34.e2.
57. Bouguen G, Levesque BG, Feagan BG, et al. Treat to target: a proposed new paradigm for the management of crohn's disease. Clin Gastroenterol Hepatol 2013. [Epub ahead of print].
58. Seow CH, Newman A, Irwin SP, et al. Trough serum infliximab: a predictive factor of clinical outcome for infliximab treatment in acute ulcerative colitis. Gut 2010; 59(1):49–54.

59. Murthy S, Kevans D, Seow CH, et al. Association of serum infliximab and anti-bodies to infliximab to long-term clinical outcome in acute ulcerative colitis. Gastroenterology 2012;142(5 Suppl 1):S-388.

60. Roblin X, Marotte H, Rinaudo M, et al. Association between pharmacokinetics of adalimumab and mucosal healing in patients with inflammatory bowel diseases. Clin Gastroenterol Hepatol 2014;12(1):80–4.e2.

61. Velayos FS, Kahn JG, Sandborn WJ, et al. A test-based strategy is more cost effective than empiric dose escalation for patients with Crohn's disease who lose responsiveness to infliximab. Clin Gastroenterol Hepatol 2013;11(6): 654–66.

62. Steenholdt C, Brynskov J, Thomsen OO, et al. Individualised therapy is more cost-effective than dose intensification in patients with Crohn's disease who lose response to anti-TNF treatment: a randomised, controlled trial. Gut 2014; 63:919–27.

63. Peyrin-Biroulet L, Cieza A, Sandborn WJ, et al. Development of the first disability index for inflammatory bowel disease based on the international classification of functioning, disability and health. Gut 2012;61(2):241–7.

64. Cheifetz AS, Melmed GY, Spiegel B, et al. Setting priorities for comparative effectiveness research in inflammatory bowel disease: results of an international provider survey, expert RAND panel, and patient focus groups. Inflamm Bowel Dis 2012;18(12):2294–300.

65. Roland M, Torgerson DJ. What are pragmatic trials? BMJ 1998;316(7127):285.

The Use of Biologic Agents in Pregnancy and Breastfeeding

Sara Horst, MD[a], Sunanda Kane, MD, MSPH[b],*

KEYWORDS

- Inflammatory bowel disease • Crohn disease • Ulcerative colitis • Biologic
- Pregnancy • Breastfeeding

KEY POINTS

- Treatment of patients with inflammatory bowel disease in pregnancy is of utmost importance.
- The safety of biologic medications in pregnancy (anti-TNF medications and natalizumab) is a prominent issue.
- The safety of biology medications during breastfeeding is a key concern.

INTRODUCTION

Inflammatory bowel disease (IBD), including Crohn disease (CD) and ulcerative colitis (UC), often affects women during their peak reproductive years. Indeed, 50% of patients are younger than 35 years old at diagnosis.[1,2] Disease treatment and medication effects on the patient's health, current and future pregnancies, and the health of the child after pregnancy are very important issues for patients who are pregnant or considering pregnancy in the future. Determining the risks of medications during pregnancy versus the benefits of these medications to help with disease control is a complex equation. Therefore, it is imperative for a comprehensive review of the available data and literature to help physicians and patients who may require biologic therapy during and after pregnancy. No randomized studies exist for medications in patients with IBD who are pregnant, given the ethical considerations. This article focuses on the available data regarding anti–tumor necrosis factor (TNF)-α therapy, including infliximab, adalimumab, certolizumab pegol, and golimumab, and the anti-integrin antibody, natalizumab, because these medications have become a mainstay of therapy in patients with moderate to severe UC and CD.

[a] Vanderbilt University Medical Center, 1211 21st Avenue, South 220 Medical Arts Building, Nashville, TN 37232, USA; [b] Mayo Clinic, 200 First Street Southwest, Rochester, MN 55905, USA
* Corresponding author.
E-mail address: Kane.Sunanda@mayo.edu

Gastroenterol Clin N Am 43 (2014) 495–508
http://dx.doi.org/10.1016/j.gtc.2014.05.005
0889-8553/14/$ – see front matter © 2014 Elsevier Inc. All rights reserved.

IBD, DISEASE ACTIVITY, AND PREGNANCY

It is important to consider several issues when considering medication therapy in patients who have IBD.

Pregnancy Impact on IBD

Several studies, including large population-based studies, have shown that females with CD and UC may have greater risk for adverse pregnancy outcomes, including preterm birth and low birth weight.[3–10] Most of these data have been retrospective; however, a recent prospective 1:1 case control study evaluating 332 pregnant women with IBD found that women with IBD had similar pregnancy outcomes to women without IBD.[11]

Disease activity at conception is an important determinant of disease activity throughout pregnancy, because studies have found that only one-third of patients with quiescent IBD at conception have a flare, whereas most of those with active disease at conception continue to have active disease through pregnancy.[12–15] In a large population-based cohort study from Northern California, most patients with CD and UC had inactive or mild disease at conception, and had good outcomes throughout pregnancy.[10] However, more recent data suggest that patients with UC have an increased risk of disease flare during pregnancy as compared with nonpregnant patients with IBD. A prospective multicenter case-control study followed 209 pregnant patients with IBD and found that pregnant patients with UC were significantly more likely to have a disease flare than nonpregnant patients with UC.[16] Only 65% of patients with UC in remission at conception remained in remission.

Disease Activity Impact on Pregnancy

The effect of disease activity on pregnancy outcomes is a key issue to consider. Studies have suggested that increased disease activity can lead to worse pregnancy outcomes, including fetal loss, preterm birth, and low birth weight.[17–22] A more recent large cohort study of women with CD found that disease activity during pregnancy was associated with preterm birth.[23] Another population-based case-control study evaluating 1209 women with UC and 787 women with CD found that the risk of venous thromboembolism was increased in patients with UC, particularly in those with flaring disease. Furthermore, women with IBD had increased risk for an emergency cesarean section, and in patients with CD, the risk increased with disease activity.[24] In a prospective case-control study in pregnant women with and without IBD, patients with UC who required hospitalizations had a higher risk of preterm birth, small-for-gestational-age birth, and cesarean section compared with those who only required ambulatory care.[8]

In summary, significant evidence exists to suggest that the most important factor for an expectant mother with IBD and her unborn child is to have adequate disease control before conception. This may be especially important in patients with UC. With this in mind, physicians and patients should focus on disease response and remission, and in patients with moderate to severe IBD, biologic therapy may be required.

BIOLOGIC THERAPY DURING PREGNANCY
Anti-TNF Medications in Pregnancy

Anti–TNF-α medications are monoclonal antibodies or antibody fragments to TNF, an important cytokine in pathogenesis of inflammation in IBD. Infliximab is a chimeric mouse/human IgG1 monoclonal antibody against TNF, and in large clinical trials was found to be effective for induction and maintenance of remission in UC and

CD.[25] Adalimumab is a fully human IgG1 anti-TNF monoclonal antibody, and in large clinical trials was found to be effective for induction and maintenance of remission in UC and CD.[26,27] Certolizumab pegol is a polyethylene glycolylated Fab' fragment of humanized anti–TNF-α monoclonal antibody, and in large clinical trials has been shown to have clinical efficacy in CD.[28,29] Golimumab is a fully human monoclonal antibody to TNF, and in large clinical trials found to be effective for induction and maintenance of remission in UC.[30,31]

Anti–TNF-α Antibodies and Placental Transfer

An important consideration in the evaluation of the safety of anti-TNF antibodies administered during pregnancy is when the fetus will be exposed to the medication. IgG antibodies are the main subclass of antibodies that are transferred across the placenta, with selective binding of the Fc gamma portion of the IgG at the surface of the syncytiotrophioblast layer.[32] Additionally, an Fc receptor neonatal molecule is bound to the IgG and is responsible for the transfer of the IgG from mother and neonate.[33] Studies have shown that IgG1 subclass antibodies likely increase linearly through pregnancy, with fetal blood concentrations steadily increasing from second trimester until delivery, with most antibodies being transferred in the third trimester.[34–36]

Infliximab, adalimumab, and golimumab are complete anti-TNF antibodies with an intact Fc portion of IgG1 subclass, and should therefore cross the placenta through the previously described mechanisms. These anti-TNF medications have been shown to cross the placenta, because studies have shown detectable umbilical cord blood concentrations of anti-TNF medication at delivery.[37–40] A recent study evaluating the outcomes of pregnant patients with IBD on infliximab or adalimumab found detectable cord blood levels in most patients, even those who stopped anti-TNF medication greater than 10 weeks from delivery.[39] Recently, a prospective multicenter observational study evaluated pregnant patients with IBD treated with infliximab or adalimumab. Infliximab levels from mother at delivery and cord blood in 11 newborns and 8 mothers (last dose given at mean gestational week 28; range, 24–31 weeks) were higher in the cord blood than the mother, with a mean ratio of 3.8 (range, 0.9–10.7). Adalimumab levels were drawn in five mothers and newborn cord blood at delivery, and similar levels were found in the mothers and newborn. Mahadevan and colleagues[40] evaluated 31 pregnant women on infliximab, adalimumab, and certolizumab. The median level of infliximab in the cord blood was 160% that of the mother, and the adalimumab median drug level was 153% that of the mother. Drug levels could be detected up to 6 months after delivery in the infants. Because certolizumab is a polyethylene glycolylated Fab' fragment, it does not have an Fc portion, and therefore should not be transported actively across the placenta. The only transfer of the antibody fragment that occurs will likely be passive, and in a much smaller amount than actively transported antibodies.[40] In the previously mentioned study by Mahadevan and colleagues,[40] infants of 10 pregnant women on certolizumab were found to have very low drug levels, with a median level of 3.9% of the mother.

Anti–TNF-α Medications in Pregnancy

Although newborns will likely be exposed to certain anti-TNF medications in utero, all anti-TNF medications are Food and Drug Administration (FDA) pregnancy class B (**Table 1**). In evaluation of available animal data, toxicity studies using doses several hundred times higher than the recommended human dosing of infliximab and adalimumab showed no evidence of teratogenic effects.[41,42] Data available from each individual medication are presented next, and further studies combining data from all anti-TNF medication use in pregnancy are then summarized.

Infliximab

Although early case reports documented adverse outcomes in a patient with active IBD on infliximab, a growing body of evidence supports that infliximab use in patients with IBD who are pregnant is low risk.[43] The Crohn's Therapy, Resource, Evaluation, and Assessment Tool registry is a large prospective registry of more than 6000 patients with CD on differing medication regimens or no medications. Sixty-six pregnancies were reported, with 36 patients exposed to infliximab. Rates of spontaneous abortion (11% vs 7.1%) and neonatal complications (8.3% vs 7.1%) were not significantly different between cases who were exposed to infliximab and those not exposed to infliximab. No congenital anomalies were noted.[44] The Infliximab Safety Database is a retrospective data collection set up by the manufacturer of infliximab (Janssen Biotech, Horsham, PA) using voluntary reports of adverse events. The outcomes of women with CD or rheumatoid arthritis exposed to infliximab in pregnancy were no different from the general population. Two major fetal structural abnormalities were noted (tetralogy of Fallot and intestinal malrotation).[45] Mahadevan and colleagues[46] reported on a series of 10 women intentionally on maintenance infliximab throughout pregnancy. All infants were liveborn with no congenital abnormalities. Three infants were preterm and two had neonatal illnesses not thought to be related to infliximab use.

Adalimumab

A registry study from the Organization for Teratology Information Specialists reported on 38 women with autoimmune diseases (not exclusively IBDs) enrolled in a prospective study of adalimumab in pregnancy and 133 pregnant women exposed to adalimumab from case series. There were similar rates of spontaneous abortion (13%) compared with a control group and the general population, and no increased rates of congenital malformation (6.1%).[47] A recent review regarding adalimumab use during pregnancy for disease states not limited to IBD found 85 pregnancies reported from registry studies and case reports, with no increased risk of adalimumab use during pregnancy.[48]

Certolizumab pegol

There have been case reports in the literature regarding certolizumab use in pregnancy.[49] Recently, a certolizumab safety database was queried, and of 139 pregnant women exposed to certolizumab in pregnancy, no increased adverse outcomes compared with the US National Vital Statistics data were noted.[50]

Table 1	
Food and Drug Administration categories for use of medications in pregnancy	
FDA Pregnancy Category	**Interpretation**
A	Controlled studies in animals and women have shown no risk in the first trimester, and possible fetal harm is remote
B	Either animal studies have not demonstrated a fetal risk but no controlled studies in pregnant women exist, or animal studies have shown an adverse effect that was not confirmed in controlled studies in women in their first trimester
C	No controlled studies in humans have been performed, and animal studies have shown adverse events, or studies in humans and animals are not available; give if potential benefit outweighs the risk
D	Positive evidence of fetal risk is available, but the benefits may outweigh the risk if life-threatening or serious disease
X	Studies in animals or humans show fetal abnormalities; drug contraindicated

Summary of anti-TNF medication use in pregnancy

As experience continues to increase with use of anti-TNF medications in pregnancy, studies recently have coalesced all anti-TNF medications into a class and evaluated the effects of their use in pregnancy. A recent systematic review has synthesized much of the available data regarding anti-TNF therapy and use in pregnancy for autoimmune disease states including IBD.[51] A total number of 471 patients (infliximab = 195, adalimumab = 259, and certolizumab = 17) were evaluated. Approximately 6% of live births had reported congenital abnormalities, with no pattern of specific birth defects seen. Thirty-seven fetal deaths (35 spontaneous abortions and 2 stillbirths) were recorded, which per the review is similar to rates in the US general population. Thirty-nine preterm or premature births were recorded, which is higher than expected in the general population, but this has been previously documented for patients with IBD in general. Overall, the authors highlight the growing body of evidence of low risk of use of anti-TNF medications in pregnancy; however, data are still insufficient given the lack of controlled studies to prove absolute safety of anti-TNF medications during pregnancy with the review.

Gisbert and Chaparro[52] recently published a critical review of the literature regarding anti-TNF medication use in pregnancy. They summarized data from more than 462 women exposed to anti-TNF medications and all outcomes including such complications as spontaneous abortion, congenital anomalies, intrauterine growth retardation, and preterm birth did not seem to differ from other patients with IBD not on anti-TNF medication. They calculated the rate of spontaneous abortion to be 11%, a figure similar to that reported in the general population and in patients with IBD not exposed to anti-TNF medications. A 2013 systematic review of 58 reports on the safety of TNF-α inhibitors during pregnancy concluded that there was no association between administration of TNF inhibitors and adverse pregnancy outcomes or congenital abnormalities.[53]

Recently, several additional studies have added to the knowledge of safety of anti-TNF medications in pregnancy. An observational study by Schnitzler and colleagues[54] compared pregnant women with and without IBD in the following groups: 42 pregnancies with known anti-TNF exposure (35 infliximab, 7 adalimumab; all were stopped before third trimester), 23 pregnancies before diagnosis of IBD, 78 pregnancies before the start of anti-TNF, 53 pregnancies with indirect exposure to infliximab, and 56 matched healthy pregnant women. Pregnancy outcomes after known anti-TNF exposure were not different from the other groups. A retrospective multicenter study by Casanova and colleagues[55] evaluated pregnancies in patients with IBD exposed to thiopurines (N = 187) compared with those exposed to anti-TNF medications (N = 66) and those without exposure to these medications (N = 318). A global pregnancy outcome was evaluated, and neither anti-TNF medications nor thiopurine medications were associated with complications in pregnancy or newborn. Bortlik and colleagues[56] conducted a prospective three-center observational study in which consecutive patients with IBD on anti-TNF medications were followed. Forty-one pregnancies (27 CD, 14 UC) were followed and exposed to either infliximab (N = 32) or adalimumab (N = 9). Five pregnancies (12%) ended in spontaneous abortions, and two had elective abortions. No congenital abnormalities were noted except for one case of hip dysplasia. No serious perinatal complications were noted.

The Pregnancy IBD and Neonatal Outcomes (PIANO) study, currently in abstract form, is the largest study evaluating the safety of anti-TNF therapy during pregnancy.[57] This prospective study, performed in 30 IBD centers in the United States, follows patients through pregnancy and children to age 4 years. There are currently 1115 women being followed, with 366 with exposure to biologics and 279 with exposure to thiopurines. The use of thiopurines and anti-TNF agents has not been associated with increased rates of complications, including congenital abnormalities, preterm birth, or overall rates of infection, when controlling for preterm birth and developmental milestones at months 4, 9, and 12. When adjusting for disease activity, patients exposed to biologics had increased rates of spontaneous abortion (relative risk [RR], 2.56; 95% confidence interval [CI], 1.07–6.12). Patients on combination therapy had a slightly increased risk of preterm birth, and an increased rate of infection in infants at 9 to 12 months (RR, 1.35; 95% CI, 1.01–1.80) when certolizumab pegol was excluded from the analysis, because it does not likely cross the placenta.[57]

Several position statements have addressed this issue. The World Congress of Gastroenterology recommends that anti-TNF medications are low risk and compatible with use at least in the first two trimesters and certolizumab is compatible with use in pregnancy.[58] The American Gastroenterological Association also notes that anti-TNF medications infliximab and adalimumab are low risk in pregnancy and benefits likely outweigh known risks.[59] The European Crohn's and Colitis Organization noted limited data on the safety of anti-TNF medications in pregnancy, but suggest that they are low risk.[60]

Effect of Anti-TNF Medication on Newborns

As noted, anti-TNF levels have been detected in umbilical cord blood in multiple studies, often at levels higher than maternal anti-TNF levels. Although most data have not shown deleterious effects of this, immunosuppression of the mother can lead to adverse outcomes. A recent case report documented a fatal case of disseminated bacille Calmette-Guérin (BCG) infection after BCG vaccination in an infant born to a mother treated with infliximab throughout her pregnancy.[61] However, nonlive vaccines are likely safe, and it is currently recommended that infants exposed to anti-TNF therapy in utero can undergo vaccinations according to regular schedule, because no adverse effects have been noted and vaccination responses seem appropriate.[60] A few recent case reports have documented appropriate vaccine responses in infants exposed to anti-TNF medications in utero.[38,62]

Bortlik and colleagues[63] recently prospectively evaluated the long-term impact of maternal anti-TNF medication on 25 exposed children (infliximab = 22, adalimumab = 3) until median gestational age 26 weeks (range, 17–37 weeks). Twelve mothers (48%) were on concomitant thiopurines. All children had normal growth and all but one had normal psychomotor development. Twenty-three (92%) had normal vaccination according to protocol, and 15 children had tuberculosis vaccination (BCG vaccine within 1 week of birth) without serious complication. Immunologic evaluation was performed in 17 children, cellular immunity was normal in all infants, and all had detectable serologic response to vaccination. Additionally, the largest amount of data available, from the large prospective PIANO registry, shows no increased risk of infections from biologic therapy exposure in infants to 1 year. There was a small but significant increase in infections in children detected at 12 months in the combination therapy–treated group (excluding certolizumab pegol–treated patients given the minimal placental transfer; RR, 1.35; 95% CI, 1.01–1.80). These infants will be followed prospectively for 4 years, and further data are forthcoming.[57,64]

Therefore, with limited data that are available, children exposed to anti-TNF therapy likely will have normal development and minimally increased risk of immunodeficiency syndromes. Children exposed to combination therapy, however, may be at slight increased risk of infections in the first and second year of life, although documented infections were mild. Given the recent data regarding improved outcomes in patients on combination therapy (both an immunomodulator and anti-TNF medication) compared with either medication alone in patients with moderate to severe IBD,[65] more patients will likely become pregnant while on combination therapy with thiopurine and anti-TNF medications. More data regarding combination therapy throughout pregnancy are needed.

Based on available data, infants exposed to anti-TNF medications in utero will likely mount appropriate immune response to inactivated vaccinations and these can be given according to regular schedule. Live vaccines, however, should be avoided for at least the first 6 months in infants.[52]

How Long to Continue Anti-TNF Therapy During Pregnancy

Opinions in the literature regarding this question differ. Because most placental transfer of immunoglobulins, and thus anti-TNF medications, occurs in the third trimester, it had been suggested in the literature to stop anti-TNF medication before gestational week 30.[66,67] However, older studies have suggested cessation of therapy could worsen patient outcomes in pregnancy, but this was before the era of biologics.[17,18] Also, it has been well documented that stopping anti-TNF medications is associated with a high risk of recurrence of luminal and perianal disease.[52] To answer this question, a previously mentioned study was conducted to evaluate if patients with IBD in remission could safely stop their anti-TNF medication in the second trimester.[39] Five women had active disease in their second trimester and continued infliximab to weeks 30 to 34. Twelve women were in remission and stopped infliximab in the second trimester (between weeks 18 and 27; average, week 23), and 11 patients on adalimumab were in remission and stopped in their second trimester (stopped between weeks 21 and 27; average, week 22). Only two women, both in the adalimumab-treated group, had a flare in their third trimester (at weeks 30 and 36). Those who stopped the anti-TNF inhibitor greater than 10 weeks before delivery still had detectable cord blood levels. However, the cord blood levels were significantly lower in the patients who had their infliximab stopped greater than 10 weeks before delivery compared with those who continued through delivery.[39]

However, stopping anti-TNF medication in the second or third trimester leads to continued exposure of medication for the fetus, because the previously mentioned studies have shown cord blood levels persist if mothers last received the medication as early as gestational weeks 16 to 20.[56,68] Certainly, if a patient has active disease, she should continue her biologic therapy throughout pregnancy, because much of the available literature detailed now supports the medications' safety in pregnancy. Also, newer literature showing that patients with UC have an increased risk of flare, even if they are in remission at conception, compared with nonpregnant patients with UC, would cause more hesitation for medication cessation in this group. However, if a patient is in clinical remission, it may be reasonable to consider cessation of anti-TNF medications in the second trimester, and physicians and patients should consider options carefully.[69]

Anti-integrin Antibody Therapy in Pregnancy

Natalizumab is an IgG4 antibody that inhibits the α_4 integrin adhesion molecule. IgG4 antibodies cross the placenta in the second and third trimester, although not as preferentially as IgG1.[33] There is limited knowledge of the use of natalizumab during pregnancy and lactation. In a small study of pregnant guinea pigs given seven times the human dose based on body weight, there was a small reduction in pup survival.[70] A primate study showed hematologic effects on the fetus (mild anemia, decreased platelet count, reduced weight of the liver and thymus, and increased splenic weight) at a dose of natalizumab that was 2.3-fold higher than typical clinical dosing in humans. No teratogenic effects were noted in either animal study.[71]

In one study of 143 pregnancies reported in patients with CD or multiple sclerosis who received natalizumab in their first trimester, no increased numbers of birth defects were noted.[72] A preliminary data review of the prospective Tysabri (natalizumab) Pregnancy Exposure Registry in 2011 following patients on natalizumab showed 277 known pregnancy outcomes. The rate of spontaneous abortions (11%) was consistent with the expected rate in the US population. Malformations occurred in 23 pregnancies in 21 of the 277 women, but they were isolated, some were confounded by other risk factors, and they did not suggest a drug-related pattern.[73] The ongoing multi-center PIANO study includes a cohort of six women with natalizumab exposure in pregnancy with no increased rates of adverse events of congenital anomalies or abnormal infant growth or development.[57,74] Recently, a study evaluated two pregnant women with relapsing multiple sclerosis treated with natalizumab until pregnancy week 34. Both newborns had uneventful deliveries with normal birth weights and were followed to week 12 of age. One infant had no adverse events. One infant had a possible minor intracerebral hemorrhage detected on a screening ultrasound, which normalized by week 12. This infant also had mild anemia and thrombocytopenia, which normalized by week 12. Blood was evaluated in both infants at weeks 2 and 12 of age and found impaired in vitro CXCL-12–induced T-lymphocyte chemotaxis rate, which normalized by week 12.[75] The authors noted that similar effects on in vivo chemotaxis of T lymphocytes have been demonstrated in adults treated with natalizumab,[76] but the clinical significance of this is yet unclear.

Currently, natalizumab has an FDA pregnancy category class C. A recent World Congress of Gastroenterology position statement highlights that the safety of natalizumab in pregnancy is unknown, with available human data showing no increased risk of birth defects. The authors state that physicians and patients should judge the risk versus the individual patient needs with use of natalizumab during pregnancy.[58]

BREASTFEEDING WHILE ON BIOLOGIC THERAPY

Many patients on anti-TNF or other biologic medications who have a successful pregnancy will also be interested in breastfeeding. IgA is the predominant immunoglobulin in human milk. Anti-TNF medications are IgG subclass, so secretion is likely to be limited, and given that they are large protein molecules, are likely to be broken down by infant gastrointestinal tract digestive enzymes.[52] In a study evaluating IgG levels in breast milk, total IgG subclass levels were not detectable.[77] A few case reports evaluating infliximab levels in breast milk found them to be below detectable levels.[37,78] One small case series prospectively evaluated three pregnant patients with CD receiving infliximab (5 mg/kg) at regular dosing until approximately gestational week 30, and resumed after delivery. Maternal sera showed detectable infliximab levels, but no infliximab was detected in the maternal breast milk or infant sera.[79] However, a few other case reports evaluating infliximab levels in breast milk used a different technique to calibrate the standard curve, using control breast milk samples instead of blood levels. These case reports did show detectable levels of infliximab and adalimumab, although the amounts were very small (1/100 to 1/200th of the level in mother's sera).[80–82] One study evaluated certolizumab pegol levels in the breast milk of a patient with CD treated with certolizumab through pregnancy and after delivery. The five breastmilk samples evaluated had undetectable certolizumab levels.[40] Most recently, the previously mentioned large prospective PIANO registry study has captured information regarding mothers who were treated

Table 2
Biologic therapy in pregnant patients with inflammatory bowel disease

Medication	Structure	FDA Pregnancy Category	Placental Transfer	Recommendations for Pregnancy	Breast Milk Transfer
Infliximab	Chimeric mouse/human IgG1 monoclonal anti-TNF antibody	B	Active placental transfer; detectable in infant cord blood	Low risk: possible increased risk of newborn infection if given with azathioprine	Limited human data; probably compatible
Adalimumab	Fully human IgG1 monoclonal anti-TNF antibody	B	Active placental transfer; detectable in infant cord blood	Low risk: possible increased risk of newborn infection if given with azathioprine	Limited human data; probably compatible
Certolizumab	Polyethylene glycolylated Fab' fragment of a humanized IgG1 monoclonal anti-TNF antibody	B	Limited to no placental transfer	Low risk: possibly no increased risk of newborn infections	Limited human data; probably compatible
Natalizumab	Recombinant humanized IgG4 monoclonal antibody	C	Limited human data	Low risk: limited human data	Limited human data

with anti-TNF medication (N = 102) throughout pregnancy. Most of these newborns were breastfed (72%), but breastfeeding was not associated with an increased risk of infant infections.[57] So although very small amounts of the anti-TNF medications infliximab and adalimumab have been detected in some case reports in breast milk, these tiny amounts are very unlikely to result in immunosuppression, and the infant's gastrointestinal tract will likely breakdown these large protein molecules before they become systemically absorbed.[52] The World Congress of Gastroenterology recommends that infliximab and adalimumab are compatible with breastfeeding, and the American Gastroenterological Association noted that infliximab was likely compatible with breastfeeding.[58,59]

SUMMARY AND PATIENT COUNSELING

In summary, mounting evidence exists that anti-TNF medications are low risk in pregnancy and members of this drug class are currently FDA pregnancy category B (**Table 2**). Several issues, such as how long to continue the medication in pregnancy, and if other medications including thiopurines can be used concomitantly, are still in debate and remain decisions to be made on a case-by-case basis. Breastfeeding while patients are maintained on anti-TNF medications is likely safe given low amounts of antibody transfer to breast milk (see **Table 2**).

As physicians who care for patients with IBD are well aware, each patient is on a wide spectrum of disease severity, and treatment decisions are highly individualized. However, it is important to remember several factors when counseling patients when pregnancy is encountered or considered. First and foremost, it is important to have a discussion about medication safety before a patient is pregnant if possible to avoid unnecessary anxiety when a pregnancy occurs. It is imperative that patients understand that active disease overall may be the worst contributor to a possible adverse pregnancy outcome. If a patient with CD requires an anti-TNF medication and is of child-bearing age, physicians and patients may want to consider future pregnancy wishes when considering which anti-TNF medication to use. For example, certolizumab pegol is not likely to be transferred across the placenta in pregnancy, and therefore may be a reasonable option for some patients.[69] Breastfeeding while on anti-TNF medication is likely safe. The newborn exposed to anti-TNF medications in utero can safely take nonlive vaccines in the first year of life, but live vaccines should be avoided.

REFERENCES

1. Andres PG, Friedman LS. Epidemiology and the natural course of inflammatory bowel disease. Gastroenterol Clin North Am 1999;28:255–81, vii.
2. Munkholm P. Crohn's disease–occurrence, course and prognosis. An epidemiologic cohort-study. Dan Med Bull 1997;44:287–302.
3. Cornish J, Tan E, Teare J, et al. A meta-analysis on the influence of inflammatory bowel disease on pregnancy. Gut 2007;56:830–7.
4. Baird DD, Narendranathan M, Sandler RS. Increased risk of preterm birth for women with inflammatory bowel disease. Gastroenterology 1990;99:987–94.
5. Dominitz JA, Young JC, Boyko EJ. Outcomes of infants born to mothers with inflammatory bowel disease: a population-based cohort study. Am J Gastroenterol 2002;97:641–8.
6. Fonager K, Sorensen HT, Olsen J, et al. Pregnancy outcome for women with Crohn's disease: a follow-up study based on linkage between national registries. Am J Gastroenterol 1998;93:2426–30.

7. Kornfeld D, Cnattingius S, Ekbom A. Pregnancy outcomes in women with inflammatory bowel disease: a population-based cohort study. Am J Obstet Gynecol 1997;177:942–6.
8. Stephansson O, Larsson H, Pedersen L, et al. Congenital abnormalities and other birth outcomes in children born to women with ulcerative colitis in Denmark and Sweden. Inflamm Bowel Dis 2011;17:795–801.
9. Stephansson O, Larsson H, Pedersen L, et al. Crohn's disease is a risk factor for preterm birth. Clin Gastroenterol Hepatol 2010;8:509–15.
10. Mahadevan U, Sandborn WJ, Li DK, et al. Pregnancy outcomes in women with inflammatory bowel disease: a large community-based study from Northern California. Gastroenterology 2007;133:1106–12.
11. Bortoli A, Pedersen N, Duricova D, et al. Pregnancy outcome in inflammatory bowel disease: prospective European case-control ECCO-EpiCom study, 2003-2006. Aliment Pharmacol Ther 2011;34:724–34.
12. Khosla R, Willoughby CP, Jewell DP. Crohn's disease and pregnancy. Gut 1984;25:52–6.
13. Willoughby CP, Truelove SC. Ulcerative colitis and pregnancy. Gut 1980;21:469–74.
14. Mogadam M, Korelitz BI, Ahmed SW, et al. The course of inflammatory bowel disease during pregnancy and postpartum. Am J Gastroenterol 1981;75:265–9.
15. Agret F, Cosnes J, Hassani Z, et al. Impact of pregnancy on the clinical activity of Crohn's disease. Aliment Pharmacol Ther 2005;21:509–13.
16. Pedersen N, Bortoli A, Duricova D, et al. The course of inflammatory bowel disease during pregnancy and postpartum: a prospective European ECCO-EpiCom study of 209 pregnant women. Aliment Pharmacol Ther 2013;38:501–12.
17. Nielsen OH, Andreasson B, Bondesen S, et al. Pregnancy in Crohn's disease. Scand J Gastroenterol 1984;19:724–32.
18. Nielsen OH, Andreasson B, Bondesen S, et al. Pregnancy in ulcerative colitis. Scand J Gastroenterol 1983;18:735–42.
19. Morales M, Berney T, Jenny A, et al. Crohn's disease as a risk factor for the outcome of pregnancy. Hepatogastroenterology 2000;47:1595–8.
20. Reddy D, Murphy SJ, Kane SV, et al. Relapses of inflammatory bowel disease during pregnancy: in-hospital management and birth outcomes. Am J Gastroenterol 2008;103:1203–9.
21. Norgard B, Fonager K, Sorensen HT, et al. Birth outcomes of women with ulcerative colitis: a nationwide Danish cohort study. Am J Gastroenterol 2000;95:3165–70.
22. Bush MC, Patel S, Lapinski RH, et al. Perinatal outcomes in inflammatory bowel disease. J Matern Fetal Neonatal Med 2004;15:237–41.
23. Norgard B, Hundborg HH, Jacobsen BA, et al. Disease activity in pregnant women with Crohn's disease and birth outcomes: a regional Danish cohort study. Am J Gastroenterol 2007;102:1947–54.
24. Broms G, Granath F, Linder M, et al. Complications from inflammatory bowel disease during pregnancy and delivery. Clin Gastroenterol Hepatol 2012;10:1246–52.
25. Hanauer SB, Feagan BG, Lichtenstein GR, et al. Maintenance infliximab for Crohn's disease: the ACCENT I randomised trial. Lancet 2002;359:1541–9.
26. Colombel JF, Sandborn WJ, Rutgeerts P, et al. Adalimumab for maintenance of clinical response and remission in patients with Crohn's disease: the CHARM trial. Gastroenterology 2007;132:52–65.

27. Sandborn WJ, Hanauer SB, Rutgeerts P, et al. Adalimumab for maintenance treatment of Crohn's disease: results of the CLASSIC II trial. Gut 2007;56: 1232–9.
28. Sandborn WJ, Feagan BG, Stoinov S, et al. Certolizumab pegol for the treatment of Crohn's disease. N Engl J Med 2007;357:228–38.
29. Schreiber S, Khaliq-Kareemi M, Lawrance IC, et al. Maintenance therapy with certolizumab pegol for Crohn's disease. N Engl J Med 2007;357:239–50.
30. Sandborn WJ, Feagan BG, Marano C, et al. Subcutaneous golimumab maintains clinical response in patients with moderate-to-severe ulcerative colitis. Gastroenterology 2014;146:96–109.e1.
31. Sandborn WJ, Feagan BG, Marano C, et al. Subcutaneous golimumab induces clinical response and remission in patients with moderate-to-severe ulcerative colitis. Gastroenterology 2014;146:85–95.
32. Wood WG, Fricke H, von Klitzing L, et al. Solid phase antigen luminescent immunoassays (SPALT) for the determination of insulin, insulin antibodies and gentamicin levels in human serum. J Clin Chem Clin Biochem 1982;20: 825–31.
33. Kane SV, Acquah LA. Placental transport of immunoglobulins: a clinical review for gastroenterologists who prescribe therapeutic monoclonal antibodies to women during conception and pregnancy. Am J Gastroenterol 2009;104: 228–33.
34. Malek A, Sager R, Schneider H. Maternal-fetal transport of immunoglobulin G and its subclasses during the third trimester of human pregnancy. Am J Reprod Immunol 1994;32:8–14.
35. Palmeira P, Quinello C, Silveira-Lessa AL, et al. IgG placental transfer in healthy and pathological pregnancies. Clin Dev Immunol 2012;2012:985646.
36. Simister NE. Placental transport of immunoglobulin G. Vaccine 2003;21:3365–9.
37. Vasiliauskas EA, Church JA, Silverman N, et al. Case report: evidence for transplacental transfer of maternally administered infliximab to the newborn. Clin Gastroenterol Hepatol 2006;4:1255–8.
38. Zelinkova Z, de Haar C, de Ridder L, et al. High intra-uterine exposure to infliximab following maternal anti-TNF treatment during pregnancy. Aliment Pharmacol Ther 2011;33:1053–8.
39. Zelinkova Z, van der Ent C, Bruin KF, et al. Effects of discontinuing anti-tumor necrosis factor therapy during pregnancy on the course of inflammatory bowel disease and neonatal exposure. Clin Gastroenterol Hepatol 2013;11:318–21.
40. Mahadevan U, Wolf DC, Dubinsky M, et al. Placental transfer of anti-tumor necrosis factor agents in pregnant patients with inflammatory bowel disease. Clin Gastroenterol Hepatol 2013;11:286–92 [quiz: e24].
41. Rychly DJ, DiPiro JT. Infections associated with tumor necrosis factor-alpha antagonists. Pharmacotherapy 2005;25:1181–92.
42. Baker DE. Adalimumab: human recombinant immunoglobulin g1 anti-tumor necrosis factor monoclonal antibody. Rev Gastroenterol Disord 2004;4:196–210.
43. Mahadevan U. Fertility and pregnancy in the patient with inflammatory bowel disease. Gut 2006;55:1198–206.
44. Lichtenstein GR, Feagan BG, Cohen RD, et al. Serious infections and mortality in association with therapies for Crohn's disease: TREAT registry. Clin Gastroenterol Hepatol 2006;4:621–30.
45. Katz JA, Antoni C, Keenan GF, et al. Outcome of pregnancy in women receiving infliximab for the treatment of Crohn's disease and rheumatoid arthritis. Am J Gastroenterol 2004;99:2385–92.

46. Mahadevan U, Kane S, Sandborn WJ, et al. Intentional infliximab use during pregnancy for induction or maintenance of remission in Crohn's disease. Aliment Pharmacol Ther 2005;21:733–8.

47. Johnson DL, Jones KL, Chambers CD, et al. Pregnancy outcomes in women exposed to adalimumab: the OTIC autoimmune diseases in pregnancy project. Gastroenterology 2009;136:A27.

48. Jurgens M, Brand S, Filik L, et al. Safety of adalimumab in Crohn's disease during pregnancy: case report and review of the literature. Inflamm Bowel Dis 2010; 16:1634–6.

49. Oussalah A, Bigard MA, Peyrin-Biroulet L. Certolizumab use in pregnancy. Gut 2009;58:608.

50. Mahadevan U, Wolf D, Stach C, et al. Outcomes of pregnancy in subjects exposed to certolizumab pegol. Am J Gastroenterol 2012;107:S621.

51. Marchioni RM, Lichtenstein GR. Tumor necrosis factor-alpha inhibitor therapy and fetal risk: a systematic literature review. World J Gastroenterol 2013;19: 2591–602.

52. Gisbert JP, Chaparro M. Safety of anti-TNF agents during pregnancy and breastfeeding in women with inflammatory bowel disease. Am J Gastroenterol 2013;108:1426–38.

53. Nielson OH, Loftus EV Jr, Jess T. Safety of TNF-α inhibitors during IBD pregnancy: a systematic review. BMC Med 2013;11:174.

54. Schnitzler F, Fidder H, Ferrante M, et al. Outcome of pregnancy in women with inflammatory bowel disease treated with antitumor necrosis factor therapy. Inflamm Bowel Dis 2011;17:1846–54.

55. Casanova MJ, Chaparro M, Domenech E, et al. Safety of thiopurines and anti-TNF-alpha drugs during pregnancy in patients with inflammatory bowel disease. Am J Gastroenterol 2013;108:433–40.

56. Bortlik M, Machkova N, Duricova D, et al. Pregnancy and newborn outcome of mothers with inflammatory bowel diseases exposed to anti-TNF-alpha therapy during pregnancy: three-center study. Scand J Gastroenterol 2013;48:951–8.

57. Mahadevan U, Martin C, Sandler R, et al. PIANO: a 1000 patient prospective registry of pregnancy outcomes in women with IBD exposed to immunomodulators and biologic therapy. Gastroenterology 2012;142:S149.

58. Mahadevan U, Cucchiara S, Hyams JS, et al. The London Position Statement of the World Congress of Gastroenterology on Biological Therapy for IBD with the European Crohn's and Colitis Organisation: pregnancy and pediatrics. Am J Gastroenterol 2011;106:214–23 [quiz: 224].

59. Mahadevan U, Kane S. American gastroenterological association institute technical review on the use of gastrointestinal medications in pregnancy. Gastroenterology 2006;131:283–311.

60. van der Woude CJ, Kolacek S, Dotan I, et al. European evidenced-based consensus on reproduction in inflammatory bowel disease. J Crohns Colitis 2010;4:493–510.

61. Cheent K, Nolan J, Shariq S, et al. Case report: fatal case of disseminated BCG infection in an infant born to a mother taking infliximab for Crohn's disease. J Crohns Colitis 2010;4:603–5.

62. Vasiliauskas E, Barry M, Dubinsky M. High serum levels of infliximab detected in the newborn of a mother receiving during pregnancy. Gastroenterology 2005; 128:P33.

63. Bortlik M, Duricova D, Machkova N, et al. Impact of anti-tumor necrosis factor alpha antibodies administered to pregnant women with inflammatory bowel

disease on long-term outcome of exposed children. Inflamm Bowel Dis 2014; 20(3):495–501.

64. Friedman S, McElrath TF, Wolf JL. Management of fertility and pregnancy in women with inflammatory bowel disease: a practical guide. Inflamm Bowel Dis 2013;19:2937–48.

65. Colombel JF, Sandborn WJ, Reinisch W, et al. Infliximab, azathioprine, or combination therapy for Crohn's disease. N Engl J Med 2010;362:1383–95.

66. Gisbert JP. Safety of immunomodulators and biologics for the treatment of inflammatory bowel disease during pregnancy and breast-feeding. Inflamm Bowel Dis 2010;16:881–95.

67. Van Assche G, Dignass A, Reinisch W, et al. The second European evidence-based consensus on the diagnosis and management of Crohn's disease: special situations. J Crohns Colitis 2010;4:63–101.

68. Julsgaard M, Brown S, Gibson P, et al. Adalimumab levels in an infant. J Crohns Colitis 2013;7:597–8.

69. Kane S. Anti-tumor necrosis factor agents and placental transfer: relevant clinical data for rational decision-making. Clin Gastroenterol Hepatol 2013;11: 293–4.

70. Wehner NG, Shopp G, Rocca MS, et al. Effects of natalizumab, an alpha4 integrin inhibitor, on the development of Hartley guinea pigs. Birth Defects Res B Dev Reprod Toxicol 2009;86:98–107.

71. Tysabri; (natalizumab) prescribing information. Available at: http://www.tysabri.com/pdfs/l61061-13_PI.pdf. Accessed March 2014.

72. Nazareth M, Christiano L, Kooijmans M, et al. Natalizumab use during pregnancy. Am J Gastroenterol 2008;103:S449.

73. Cristiano L, Bozic C, Bloomgren G. Preliminary evaluation of pregnancy outcomes from the Tysabri (natalizumab) pregnancy exposure registry. Mult Scler 2011;17:S457.

74. Ng SW, Mahadevan U. Management of inflammatory bowel disease in pregnancy. Expert Rev Clin Immunol 2013;9:161–73 [quiz: 174].

75. Schneider H, Weber CE, Hellwig K, et al. Natalizumab treatment during pregnancy: effects on the neonatal immune system. Acta Neurol Scand 2013;127: e1–4.

76. Niino M, Bodner C, Simard ML, et al. Natalizumab effects on immune cell responses in multiple sclerosis. Ann Neurol 2006;59:748–54.

77. Gasparoni A, Avanzini A, Ravagni Probizer F, et al. IgG subclasses compared in maternal and cord serum and breast milk. Arch Dis Child 1992;67:41–3.

78. Stengel JZ, Arnold HL. Is infliximab safe to use while breastfeeding? World J Gastroenterol 2008;14:3085–7.

79. Kane S, Ford J, Cohen R, et al. Absence of infliximab in infants and breast milk from nursing mothers receiving therapy for Crohn's disease before and after delivery. J Clin Gastroenterol 2009;43:613–6.

80. Ben-Horin S, Yavzori M, Katz L, et al. Adalimumab level in breast milk of a nursing mother. Clin Gastroenterol Hepatol 2010;8:475–6.

81. Ben-Horin S, Yavzori M, Kopylov U, et al. Detection of infliximab in breast milk of nursing mothers with inflammatory bowel disease. J Crohns Colitis 2011;5: 555–8.

82. Fritzsche J, Pilch A, Mury D, et al. Infliximab and adalimumab use during breast-feeding. J Clin Gastroenterol 2012;46:718–9.

Risk of Infections with Biological Agents

Uri Kopylov, MD, Waqqas Afif, MD*

KEYWORDS

- Inflammatory bowel disease • Biologics • Anti–tumor necrosis factor α • Infection
- Opportunistic infections • Vaccinations

KEY POINTS

- Biological medications are generally safe in patients with inflammatory bowel disease.
- Biological medications may increase the risk of certain opportunistic infections.
- The increased risk of opportunistic infections can be minimized with screening, close surveillance, and adherence to immunization guidelines.

INTRODUCTION

The treatment of inflammatory bowel disease (IBD) has rapidly evolved over the last 15 years since the introduction of the first biological medication, a monoclonal anti–tumor necrosis factor α (anti-TNF-α) agent. Since then, several other anti-TNF-α agents and other monoclonal antibodies targeting interleukin 12 (IL-12), IL-23, and cellular adhesion molecule ligands α_4 integrin and $\alpha_4\beta_7$ integrin have been approved, or are near approval, for the treatment of IBD. Biological medications have shown improved clinical efficacy over older therapies and are being used earlier in the disease course, in an attempt to alter the natural history of IBD. Given the increasing use of these biological medications, it is important to review the safety profile of these agents. One of the main safety issues with biological agents is the risk of infectious complications, particularly the risk of opportunistic infections.

This article contains an overview of the infectious complications of biological medications in the treatment of IBD. The first section of this article assesses the risk of serious infections with individual biological agents, and the second section focuses on specific infectious diseases. The final section deals with screening and immunization for vaccine-preventable diseases. Throughout this article, serious infections are defined as those that lead to prolonged hospitalizations, result in significant disability, are opportunistic in nature, or are life threatening or fatal.[1] Opportunistic infections

Division of Gastroenterology, McGill University Health Center, 687 Pine Avenue West, Ross 2.28, Montreal, Quebec H3A 1A1, Canada
* Corresponding author.
E-mail address: waqqas.afif@mcgill.ca

Gastroenterol Clin N Am 43 (2014) 509–524
http://dx.doi.org/10.1016/j.gtc.2014.05.001
0889-8553/14/$ – see front matter © 2014 Elsevier Inc. All rights reserved.

gastro.theclinics.com

include viral infections (eg, cytomegalovirus [CMV], Epstein-Barr virus, herpes simplex virus, and varicella zoster); bacterial infections (tuberculosis [TB] and streptococcal); and fungal infections (histoplasmosis, aspergillosis, candidiasis, and blastomycosis).[2]

RISK OF INFECTIONS IN PATIENTS WITH IBD

Several factors may predispose patients with IBD to infections. Although the most important predisposing factor is immunosuppressive therapy, additional factors include ongoing inflammatory disease, increasing age, malnutrition, increased exposure to nosocomial pathogens, and abdominal surgery.[3]

Several classes of medications have been associated with systemic immunosuppression and possible increased infectious risk (**Table 1**). A large case-control study showed that treatment with corticosteroids, azathioprine, or infliximab was associated with an odds ratio (OR) for infectious complications of 3.4, 3.1, and 4.4, respectively, and the combination of 2 or more of these agents increased the risk up to 14.5-fold.[2] However, the increased risk of infectious complications with the combination of agents was driven mainly by the use of corticosteroids. A recent Cochrane review, with a meta-analysis of randomized controlled trials, controlled clinical trials, and open-label extension studies of biologics for several indications, reported an OR of 1.28 (95% confidence interval [CI], 1.09–1.50) for serious infections for patients on any biologic.[4] However, a subgroup analysis of IBD trials only did not show a significantly increased risk of infection (OR, 1.28; 95% CI, 0.67–2.44).[2] Biological medications are a heterogeneous group of agents, targeting different areas of the inflammatory cascade; the risk of opportunistic infections may be increased and seems to be biologic-class specific.

BIOLOGICAL MEDICATIONS
Anti-TNF-α Monoclonal Antibodies

Several anti-TNF-α agents have been approved by the US Food and Drug Administration (FDA) for treatment of IBD. Infliximab (Janssen Biotech, Malvern, PA) and adalimumab (Humira, Abbvie, North Chicago, IL) have been approved for both Crohn disease (CD) and ulcerative colitis (UC). Certolizumab pegol (Cimzia, UCB, Smyrna, GA) is approved for use in only CD, and golimumab (Simponi, Janssen Biotech, Malvern, PA) was recently approved for patients with UC.

In addition to IBD, anti-TNF-α medications are approved for use in other inflammatory conditions, including rheumatoid arthritis (RA), psoriatic arthritis, ankylosing spondylitis, and psoriasis, and, therefore, abundant safety data are available. In RA, the association of anti-TNF-α medications with increased risk of infections has been clearly shown. A meta-analysis of 9 placebo-controlled trials of infliximab and adalimumab in RA[5] yielded a pooled OR for serious infection of 2.01 (95% CI, 1.31–3.09). In a Cochrane review,[4] a subgroup analysis stratified by type of medication

Table 1 Medications associated with systemic immunosuppression in patients with IBD	
Corticosteroids	≥20 mg of prednisone for ≥2 wk
Immunomodulators	Thiopurines (azathioprine, 6-mercaptopurine) Methotrexate
Biologics	Anti-TNF-α (infliximab, adalimumab, certolizumab pegol, golimumab) Leukocyte adhesion inhibitors (natalizumab, vedolizumab) IL-12/23 receptor antagonist (ustekinumab)

reported an increased risk of serious infections with certolizumab (OR, 2.82; 95% CI, 1.27–6.29) and infliximab (OR, 1.97; 95% CI, 1.41–2.75), but not with other biologics. No increased risk was identified in patients with IBD, indicating that the risk may be specifically related to patients with RA, who are usually older and have more comorbid disease. Older patients with IBD (>65 years of age) on anti-TNF-α medications may have an increased risk of serious infections, compared with younger patients (11% vs 2.6%), further supporting the implication that increasing age is an independent risk factor.[6] In a US-based large cohort study,[7] initiation of an anti-TNF-α treatment was not associated with an increased risk of serious infection hospitalization rates in the first year for any indication, including in IBD (2323 patients, adjusted hazard ratio [HR], 1.10; 95% CI, 0.83–1.46). Highlighting the importance of glucocorticoid use, baseline use was associated with a dose-dependent increase in infection rate, and there was a trend toward an increased risk of infections in those patients who received concomitant anti-TNF-α with greater than 10 mg/d of glucocorticoids (adjusted HR, 1.38; 95% CI, 0.98–1.95).

More specific to IBD, a recent update to the Crohn's TREAT (Therapy, Resource, Evaluation, and Assessment Tool) registry assessed 6723 patients with CD (3420 treated with infliximab) treated for a mean duration of 5.2 years. An increased risk of serious infections with corticosteroid therapy was again reported (HR, 1.57; 95% CI, 1.17–2.10). Infliximab was associated with an increased risk of serious infection (HR, 1.43; 95%, CI, 1.11–1.84), but the study did not evaluate whether this risk was modified by other risk factors, including disease severity and concomitant immunomodulator or corticosteroid therapy.[8] Without this assessment, it is difficult to attribute the increased risk to anti-TNF-α therapy alone. In this cohort of patients, 4 cases of mycobacteria and 5 cases of systemic fungal infections were reported in patients treated with anti-TNF. No cases of mycobacteria and only 1 single fungal infection were reported in the patients not treated with anti-TNF-α medications.[9]

In the largest single-center experience (Leuven, Belgium) to date, the long-term safety of anti-TNF-α agents was assessed in 1400 patients with CD.[10] Half of the patients received infliximab, and they were followed for a median of approximately 5 years. The incidence rate of serious infections in the 2 groups was not significantly different (1.6 per 100 patient-years in the infliximab group versus 1.1 per 100 patient-years in the control group). In the largest population-based cohort study (British Columbia, Canada), the association between serious bacterial infections and infliximab and other immunosuppressive agents was assessed in 10,662 patients with IBD.[11] The event rate of serious bacterial infection was 4.28 per 1000 patient-years (95% CI, 0.11–23.8), but this was not significantly increased compared with patients receiving corticosteroids or immunomodulators.

The risk of infectious complications with anti-TNF-α monotherapy in patients with IBD does not seem to be increased in terms of overall infections. However, these studies may not be large enough to detect rare opportunistic infections (see specific infection section).

IL-12/23 Monoclonal Antibody (Ustekinumab)

Ustekinumab (Stelara, Janssen Biotech, Malvern, PA) is a fully human IgG1κ monoclonal antibody that blocks the biological activity of IL-12 and IL-23 through their common p40 subunit.[12] Ustekinumab is approved for the treatment of plaque psoriasis and has been extensively evaluated for this indication, with long-term (≤5 years) follow-up safety data available. The most common infectious complications reported include respiratory tract infections, mainly nasopharyngitis, but the rate was not different from the placebo group.[13] There has been no reported increased risk of serious infections, including TB, compared with placebo.[13]

Ustekinumab is being studied for the treatment of CD and is not yet approved, but it has been used off-label in patients in anti-TNF-refractory patients. In a randomized controlled trial of ustekinumab, in patients with anti-TNF-resistant CD,[12] serious infections were reported in 5 patients receiving 6 mg of ustekinumab per kg body weight (*Clostridium difficile* infection, viral gastroenteritis, urinary tract infection, anal abscess, and vaginal abscess), in 1 patient receiving 1 mg/kg (staphylococcal infection in a central catheter), and in 1 patient receiving placebo (anal abscess) during the induction phase. During the maintenance phase, there were no major adverse infectious events, including TB or other serious opportunistic infections.

Overall, there does not seem to be an increased risk of serious infections or TB reactivation with ustekinumab. However, the IL-12/23 pathways are important for host protection against mycobacterial infection and reactivation. Therefore, the decreased risk of TB reactivation with ustekinumab may be secondary to better screening for latent TB.[14]

Cellular Adhesion Molecule α_4 Integrin Monoclonal Antibody (Natalizumab)

Natalizumab (Tysabri, Biogen Idec, Cambridge, MA and Elan Pharmaceuticals, South San Francisco, CA) is a humanized IgG4 monoclonal antibody against α_4-integrin–mediated leukocyte migration. It was first approved by the FDA for use in multiple sclerosis (MS) but was withdrawn from the market in 2005 because of several reports of progressive multifocal leukoencephalopathy (PML) caused by John Cunningham (JC) virus reactivation. It was reapproved in 2008 under a specialized surveillance program (TOUCH [Tysabri Outreach: Unified Commitment to Health]). In 2008, natalizumab was also approved for CD, in patients with evidence of active inflammation who did not respond or could not tolerate anti-TNF-α therapy.[15]

The largest available data on the risk of PML, in patients on natalizumab, comes from studies in MS. Among 99,571 patients with MS treated with natalizumab, 212 cases of PML were recorded (2.1 cases per 1000 patients).[16] Patients who were positive for anti-JC virus antibodies, had taken immunosuppressive medications before the initiation of natalizumab therapy, and had received 25 to 48 months of natalizumab treatment had the highest estimated risk (incidence, 11.1 cases per 1000 patients; 95% CI, 8.3–14.5), whereas patients lacking antibodies to JC virus had a significantly lower risk of PML (0.09 cases or less per 1000 patients; 95% CI, 0–0.48).[16]

Natalizumab is less frequently used in CD compared with MS. Reports of PML in patients with CD treated with natalizumab have been rare since its reintroduction in 2008. As of October 2011, 1 case had been reported in CD.[17] In 2 recently published series,[17,18] including a total of 113 patients with CD treated with natalizumab, no cases of PML occurred. The results of JC serology were not reported in these series. It is unclear whether the risk factors for PML reported for MS can be extrapolated to CD, but JC serology should be completed, and treatment should be reserved for seronegative patients. In addition, immunosuppressive medications should be discontinued, and the treatment duration should be limited, because almost all the cases of PML have occurred after longer durations of treatment. The value of monitoring anti-JC virus antibody titers in patients already on the treatment is unclear.

Natalizumab is not associated with a significant risk of other serious infections (excluding JC virus reactivation). In the induction and maintenance trial of natalizumab for CD,[19] which included 905 patients in the induction phase and 339 in a 1-year maintenance phase, serious infections were rare. Influenza and influenzalike illness were significantly more frequent in the actively treated patients (12% vs 5%, $P<.05$). In addition, 1 case each of varicella pneumonia and CMV hepatitis were reported in the natalizumab group. In a recently published case series,[17,18] 24% (13/54) to 37% (13/30) had experienced at least 1 serious infectious adverse event, including bacteremia, catheter-related infections, pneumonia, *Clostridium difficile* infection, fungal infection, or herpes zoster. It seems unlikely that natalizumab poses a specific risk of reactivation of latent TB; however, at least 2 cases of TB in patients with MS treated with natalizumab have been published.[20,21]

Overall, the use of natalizumab in CD is limited by the risk of PML, and newer agents that are gut specific are likely favored (see later discussion).

Cellular Adhesion Molecule $\alpha_4\beta_7$ Integrin Monoclonal Antibody (Vedolizumab)

Vedolizumab (Entyvio, Takeda Pharmaceuticals, Cambridge, MA) is a humanized monoclonal antibody that exclusively targets the $\alpha_4\beta_7$ integrin, blocking the migration of the lymphocytes to the bowel. The mode of action of this agent is similar to that of natalizumab, but the lymphocyte trafficking inhibition of vedolizumab is gut specific. Vedolizumab has proved to be effective for induction and maintenance of remission in UC and, to a lesser extent, in CD.[22,23] In the CD trial,[23] the prevalence of serious infectious adverse effects between the treatment and placebo arms was not significantly different (5.5% and 3%, respectively). The most commonly reported infectious adverse effect was nasopharyngitis in both the treatment and placebo groups (12.3% and 8%). Single cases of sepsis, septic shock, and latent TB were reported among the 814 patients who received at least 1 dose of vedolizumab. In the UC trial,[22] the incidence of serious infections in the active treatment arm and the placebo arm was similar (1.9% and 2.9%, respectively), and the most commonly reported adverse effect was again nasopharyngitis (12.9% vs 9.5%). In these trials, with 1186 patients exposed to vedolizumab, no cases of PML were reported. Given the gut-specific mechanism of action of vedolizumab, it is important to note that an increased risk of enteric infections was not reported. In an open-label extension study including 72 patients with CD and UC treated for 549 ($\pm$ 191) days, serious infections were rare, with the most serious being 1 case of *Salmonella enterica* sepsis. The risk of serious infections does not seem to be increased with vedolizumab, and, given its gut selectivity, the risk of PML seems negligible.

SPECIFIC INFECTIONS
Bacterial Infections

TB

There is an increased risk of reactivating TB with all currently used anti-TNF-α medications (**Table 2**). Mycobacteria (and other granulomatous infections) are sequestered within granulomas, and because TNF-α is required for the continued maintenance of granuloma structure, there is an increased risk of reactivation with this class of medications.[24] This risk is now incorporated as a black-box warning for all medications in this class.[15] A Swedish study[25] that included patients with RA reported that anti-TNF-α agents were associated with a 4-fold increase in the risk of TB, whereas in a US study[26] including more than 10,000 patients with RA, the incidence of TB was 8-fold to 10-fold higher in patients treated with infliximab. In 70 cases of TB (patients with IBD and RA) reported under the MedWatch FDA program,[27] TB was diagnosed shortly after the start of treatment (a median of 12 weeks or 3 infusions) and in areas of low prevalence, suggesting reactivation of a latent disease rather than a new onset. TB presented mainly as extrapulmonary disease (57%) and was reported to be associated with a mortality risk of up to 13%. For biologics other than TNF-α inhibitors, data on the risk of TB are limited.

Table 2 Frequent infections in patients with IBD	
Bacterial	*Clostridium difficile* *Legionella pneumophila* *Nocardia* species *Salmonella* species *Streptococcus pneumoniae* TB
Viral	CMV Epstein-Barr virus Hepatitis B (reactivation) Herpes simplex virus Human papillomavirus Influenza JC virus reactivation with natalizumab
Fungal and parasitic infections	Aspergillosis *Candida* species Coccidiomycosis Cryptococcosis Cryptosporidiosis Histoplasmosis

Screening for latent TB There is a consensus concerning the need for screening for latent TB infection (LTBI), albeit the optimal screening strategy still needs to be clarified. In all patients, the risk of LTBI should be assessed by medical history, physical examination, and tuberculin skin test (TST).[3] A TST is considered to be positive when the induration is at least 5 mm in diameter. In addition, suspicious radiologic findings, such as calcifications, linear opacities, and pleural thickening, should also be considered suggestive of TB.[3] In patients considered to have latent TB, chemoprophylaxis should be administered. The therapeutic guidelines may vary between geographic regions as a result of variations in drug susceptibility and prevalence of multidrug-resistant strains.[28]

The common prophylactic regimen consists of oral isoniazid (INH) for 6 to 9 months. If there is a need for a prompt initiation of a biological treatment, INH should precede the biological treatment of at least 3 weeks, unless there is a truly urgent clinical need for biological therapy.[3]

Even although pretreatment screening and prophylactic treatment reduce the risk of active TB significantly, patients treated with anti-TNF-α medications are still susceptible to TB. Patients with an initial negative LTBI screening may develop active TB, as well as patients who have been treated with a prophylactic treatment.[29,30]

Screening for LTBI with TST has multiple limitations, such as a high rate of interobserver variability, false positivity secondary to BCG vaccination, and repeated TST testing. Moreover, the sensitivity of TST is low in immune-compromised patients or patients receiving immunosuppressive therapy, especially systemic corticosteroids.[30]

In 2008, an additional screening modality was introduced into clinical practice. Interferon γ release assays (IGRA) (QuantiFERON Gold In-Tube, QFT-GIT, Cellestis, Carnegie, VIC, Australia and T-SPOT.TB, Oxford Immunotec, Abingdon, UK) measure interferon γ response to *Mycobacterium tuberculosis* proteins. This assay does not require recurrent visits and provides a quantitative readout not susceptible to operator influence. The specificity is significantly better compared with TST, and the sensitivity may be improved in immunosuppressed patients.[30] The concordance between the TST and QFT-GIT was found to be only moderate (K = 0.4152, P = .0041) in a large

American cohort with IBD.[31] Immunomodulator or anti-TNF-α treatments do not seem to significantly interfere with the IGRA results; however, systemic corticosteroid treatment, with doses of prednisone of 10 mg/d or greater, severely depress the accuracy of both IGRA and TST.[31] Because IGRA testing is associated with higher costs, it is unclear whether it should be routinely incorporated into the screening strategy or whether it should be offered as an alternative or a complementary test for TST. Given the increased risk of false-negative results with both tests, in the context of immunosuppression, it is recommended to test for latent TB early in the course of disease, before the need for systemic immunosuppressive therapy arises.

Other granulomatous infections

Listeria monocytogenes *Listeria monocytogenes* is a gram-positive food-borne pathogen that is resistant to most cooking techniques. In immune-competent individuals, it frequently leads to mild gastroenteritis, but in immunosuppressed individuals, the infection may result in sepsis, as well as meningoencephalitis, arthritis, and cholecystitis. *L monocytogenes* infection is associated with a 30% risk of spontaneous abortion in pregnant patients.[32] More than 40 cases of listeriosis (15 with IBD) associated with anti-TNF-α therapy have been published. Most patients were older than 50 years and were treated with at least 2 immunosuppressive medications.[32] Prevention measures include avoidance of unpasteurized milk or cheese, uncooked meat, and raw vegetables, especially during pregnancy. Anti-TNF-α treatment should be discontinued as soon as suspicion of infection arises.[3]

Nocardiosis *Nocardia* species may lead to severe systemic infection, associated with significant mortality and morbidity, usually from central nervous system involvement. At least 7 cases of nocardiosis (4 with IBD) in anti-TNF-treated patients have been described in the literature,[33] with most receiving concomitant immunosuppressive therapy at the time of diagnosis.

Clostridium difficile

IBD is an independent risk factor for development of *Clostridium difficile*–associated diarrhea (CDAD), with a risk ratio of 2.9 compared with control individuals without IBD.[34] The incidence of CDAD is steadily increasing in patients with IBD.[35] Immunosuppressive therapy is an established risk factor for development of CDAD; however, it is not clear whether biologics pose any specific risk.[34] In a large cohort of more than 10,000 patients with IBD, infliximab was not associated with a risk of CDAD, whereas corticosteroid-treated patients had at least a 3-fold increase in the incidence of CDAD.[11] Continued immunosuppressive treatment in patients with IBD with CDAD seems to be associated with an increased risk of colectomy.[36]

Additional bacterial infections

Several bacterial infections, such as *Streptococcus pneumoniae*, *Legionella pneumophila*, and *Salmonella* species, pose an increased risk to patients with IBD on immunosuppressive therapy, but there are no specific data in patients on biological agents.[3,37–42]

Fungal Infections

Pneumocystis carinii

Immunosuppression is the main risk factor associated with *Pneumocystis carinii* pneumonia (PCP) infection. As of 2009, at least 119 cases of PCP in patients on biologics had been published.[3,43,44] PCP prophylaxis should be considered in all patients receiving triple immunosuppression (corticosteroids, immunomodulators, and biological therapy).

Granulomatous fungal infections

Anti-TNF-α therapy is associated with an increased risk of granulomatous fungal infections, such as histoplasmosis and coccidioidomycosis. In 2008, a black-box FDA warning was issued on the TNF-α blockers regarding this risk. Up to 2008, more than 240 cases of histoplasmosis in patients on anti-TNFs were published.[15,45,46] Most of the afflicted patients were living in the endemic areas and were receiving concomitant immunosuppression.[46,47]

Other fungal infections

More than 20 cases of *Cryptococcus neoformans* infection in patients treated with anti-TNF-α medications for various indications have been published, mostly in patients on concomitant immunosuppression.[48] Several cases of aspergillosis, systemic candidiasis, and cryptococcal and cryptosporidial infections have been reported in anti-TNF-treated patients as well.[48–54]

Viral Infections

Hepatitis B

The prevalence of hepatitis B virus (HBV) in patients with IBD is similar to that of the general population.[55] Chronic immunosuppressive therapy may lead to reactivation of latent hepatitis B infection, potentially resulting in fulminant hepatitis.[56] Although more common in patients receiving systemic chemotherapy, cases of reactivation of the virus under TNF-α inhibitors have been published.[3,56] Screening for HBV should be undertaken on diagnosis, preferably before the need for immunosuppressive therapy arises. Cases of reactivation have been described not only in hepatitis B surface antigen (HBsAg)-positive patients but also in HBsAg-negative/anti-HBC (hepatitis B core antigen)-positive patients.[57] In anti-TNF-α patients, reactivation has been described as early as after the second infusion and as late as 2 years from the start of therapy.[56] Patients receiving concomitant immunosuppressives or corticosteroids have the highest risk of reactivation. Hepatitis B reactivation is associated with significant morbidity and mortality. In the largest case series to date, two-thirds of the patients with HBV reactivation (HBsAg-positive patients) developed hepatic failure.[58] HBV chemoprophylaxis is recommended in HBsAg-positive patients receiving immunomodulatory therapy; however, no clear recommendation exists in regards to anti-HBC-positive patients. In chronic HBsAg-positive carriers, antiviral prophylaxis with nucleotide/nucleoside analogues is recommended before administering immunosuppressive agents. Patients with high baseline HBV DNA levels (>2000 IU/mL) should continue antiviral treatment until end points applicable to nonimmunosuppressed patients are reached. If immunosuppressive therapy is expected to last more than 1 year, nucleotide/nucleoside analogues with a lower propensity than lamivudine for generating drug-resistant mutations may be preferred.[3] Preferably, a hepatologist should be involved in the initiation and monitoring of antiviral therapy in these patients. All seronegative (negative or low-titer HBsAb) patients should be vaccinated at diagnosis; however, this occurs in less than half of the patients.[59] It is safe to administer the standard vaccination protocol to patients with IBD on immunosuppressive medications, but the response may be significantly reduced, and an intensified vaccination protocol may be required. Postvaccination HBsAb titers should be monitored, and, if nonprotective (<10 mIU/mL), a booster dose or revaccination should be administered.[56]

Hepatitis C

The prevalence of hepatitis C virus (HCV) in patients with IBD is similar to that of the general population.[55] There are no data to suggest that biologics are associated with reactivation or exacerbation of the course of HCV.[60,61] Anti-TNF-α medications are generally considered safe in patients with HCV.[62,63]

CMV

CMV infection is common in the healthy adult population. Reported seropositivity rates for CMV-IgG range within 87% to 100%, depending on the age and geographic location.[64] In immunocompromised patients, CMV infection or reactivation may lead to a systemic disease or end-organ involvement, manifesting as severe pneumonitis, hepatitis, or colitis.[65,66] In patients with acute severe UC, CMV has been reported to be present in the colonic tissue of 21% to 34% of patients, and it is present in 33% to 36% of steroid-refractory cases.[67] The clinical significance of detecting CMV in patients with UC remains debatable.[68,69] Many of these CMV biopsy-positive patients have been treated with anti-TNF-α medications without obvious complication, but it is still unclear whether these agents pose any specific risk in the context of an active CMV infection.

Varicella zoster virus

Varicella zoster virus (VZV) can be associated with a significant morbidity and mortality in immunocompromised patients. Severe multidermatomal shingles and disseminated varicella infection with end-organ involvement (meningoencephalitis, pneumonitis, hepatitis, colitis) have been reported.[70–72] However, the increased risk of VZV reactivation is not specific only to biologics. In a recent large cohort study,[73] including more than 33,000 patients treated with anti-TNF-α medications and 27,000 control individuals treated with nonbiological anti-inflammatory medications for various indications (3850 patients with IBD), the risk of herpes zoster was similar in patients with IBD treated with anti-TNF-α agents and with thiopurines. VZV-related complications can be easily prevented by vaccination. A live attenuated VZV vaccine has been

Table 3
Infectious screening in newly diagnosed patients with IBD (before immunosuppression)

	History	Diagnostic Tests
TB	History of exposure Travel/habitation in endemic areas	Chest radiography (in all patients prebiologic) TST or IGRA (in all patients prebiologic)
Varicella	History of illness or vaccination	Serology (if no clear history of illness/vaccination)
MMR	History of vaccination/illness	Serology (if no clear history of illness/vaccination)
HPV	History of vaccination	None
Hepatitis B	History of vaccination/illness	Anti-HBs, HBsAg, Anti-HBc (in all patients prebiologic) Liver enzymes HBV DNA if there is a history of chronic disease or carrier state
Hepatitis A	History of vaccination	Serology
Diphtheria and pertussis	History of vaccination	None
Meningococcal meningitis	History of vaccination	None
Pneumococcal pneumonia	History of vaccination	None

Abbreviation: MMR, measles, mumps, and rubella.

Table 4
Recommended routine vaccinations for patients with IBD

Vaccine	Live/ Inactive	Serology Before Vaccination?	Timing	Need for Revaccination	Strategy During Active Immunosuppressive Treatment
MMR	Live	Yes	Once, if never vaccinated	No	Avoid
Varicella	Live	Yes	If no clear history of disease/ vaccination, negative VZV IgG	No	Avoid
Zoster	Live	—	>60 y	No	Avoid
Td/Tdap	Inactive	No	Administer vaccine if not given over the past 10 y or give Tdap if Td ≥2 y	See timing	Allowed
HPV	Inactive	No	Females 9–26 y old	3 Doses (0, 2, 6 mo)	Allowed
Influenza	Inactive	No	Annual	Annual	Allowed Live vaccine (Flumist) should be avoided (including household)
Pneumococcal	Inactive	No	Every 5 y	Every 5 y	Allowed
Hepatitis A	Inactive	Yes	2 doses at 0, 6–12 mo; or 0, 6–18 mo	Booster >10 y	Allowed
Hepatitis B	Inactive	Yes	3 doses at 1, 1–2, 4–6 mo	Check postvaccine titers 1 mo after finishing last dose. If no response, then revaccinate with double dose. If low-titer anti-HBs, administer booster	Allowed
Meningococcal vaccine	Inactive	No	Persons at risk,[a] if not previously vaccinated	Every 5 y	Allowed

Abbreviations: MMR, measles, mumps, and rubella vaccine; Td/Tdap, tetanus-diphtheria or tetanus-diphtheria-pertussis vaccine.

[a] Asplenic, terminal complement deficiencies, college students living in dormitories before first year at school, military recruits, and persons who travel to areas endemic for meningococcal disease.

Adapted from Wasan SK, Baker SE, Skolnik PR, et al. A practical guide to vaccinating the inflammatory bowel disease patient. Am J Gastroenterol 2010;105:1231–8.

associated with a 61% reduction in the burden of VZV-related illness in children, and a 51% reduction in the risk of shingles.[74] Because this vaccine should not be administered after onset of systemic immunosuppression, VZV-IgG status should be checked as early as possible in the course of the disease, with prompt vaccination of the seronegative patients.[75]

Human immunodeficiency virus

Several case series and case reports describing patients who are infected with human immunodeficiency virus (HIV) and were treated with anti-TNF-α medications for various indications have been published.[76–78] There is no evidence of an adverse impact with these agents on the course of HIV.

Human papillomavirus

There is an increased incidence of human papillomavirus (HPV)-associated warts or condylomata in patients taking immunosuppressants; however, no data suggesting a specific association with biologics are available.[79] Routine prophylactic immunization starting at 9 to 11 years of age is now recommended routinely.[80] Because this is not a live vaccine, immunomodulator or anti-TNF-α therapy is not a contraindication for vaccination. Current or previous infection with HPV is not a contraindication for initiation of immunomodulator or biological therapy.[3]

SCREENING AND PROPHYLAXIS OF PREVENTABLE INFECTIONS

Screening for potentially preventable infections should be a routine part of the evaluation of every patient with IBD. Ideally, such evaluation should be undertaken as early as possible in the course of disease, preceding the need for systemic immunosuppression (**Table 3**). In general, live vaccines are contraindicated for patients on immunosuppressive therapy and should be administered either before the onset of treatment or after discontinuation (≥3 months for immunomodulators and biologics and 1 month for corticosteroids). For influenza and pneumococcal infections, periodic vaccination is required. The suggested vaccination schedule for patients on biological medications is described in **Table 4**.

SUMMARY

Biological medications are generally safe but may be associated with an increased risk of opportunistic infectious complications. A careful screening, surveillance, and immunization strategy, in accordance with the available guidelines, is important to minimize the potential morbidity and mortality from infectious complications. Data are limited in regards to the newer biological agents, but until further information is available, the same guidelines should apply.

REFERENCES

1. Colombel JF, Loftus EV, Tremaine WJ, et al. The safety profile of infliximab in patients with Crohn's disease: the Mayo Clinic experience in 500 patients. Gastroenterology 2004;126:19–31.
2. Toruner M, Loftus EV Jr, Harmsen WS, et al. Risk factors for opportunistic infections in patients with inflammatory bowel disease. Gastroenterology 2008;134: 929–36.
3. Rahier JF, Ben-Horin S, Chowers Y, et al. European evidence-based consensus on the prevention, diagnosis and management of opportunistic infections in inflammatory bowel disease. J Crohns Colitis 2009;3:47–91.

4. Singh JA, Wells GA, Christensen R. Adverse effects of biologics: a network meta-analysis and Cochrane overview. Cochrane Database Syst Rev 2011;(2):CD008794.

5. Bongartz T, Sutton AJ, Sweeting MJ, et al. Anti-TNF antibody therapy in rheumatoid arthritis and the risk of serious infections and malignancies–systematic review and meta-analysis of rare harmful effects in randomized controlled trials. JAMA 2006;295:2275–85.

6. Cottone M, Kohn A, Daperno M, et al. Advanced age is an independent risk factor for severe infections and mortality in patients given anti-tumor necrosis factor therapy for inflammatory bowel disease. Clin Gastroenterol Hepatol 2011;9: 30–5.

7. Grijalva CG, Chen L, Delzell E, et al. Initiation of tumor necrosis factor-alpha antagonists and the risk of hospitalization for infection in patients with autoimmune diseases. JAMA 2011;306:2331–9.

8. Lichtenstein GR, Feagan BG, Cohen RD, et al. Serious infection and mortality in patients with Crohn's disease: more than 5 years of follow-up in the TREAT registry. Am J Gastroenterol 2012;107:1409–22.

9. Reddy JG, Loftus EV Jr. Safety of infliximab and other biologic agents in the inflammatory bowel diseases. Gastroenterol Clin North Am 2006;35:837–55.

10. Fidder H, Schnitzler F, Ferrante M, et al. Long-term safety of infliximab for the treatment of inflammatory bowel disease: a single-centre cohort study. Gut 2009;58:501–8.

11. Schneeweiss S, Korzenik J, Solomon DH, et al. Infliximab and other immunomodulating drugs in patients with inflammatory bowel disease and the risk of serious bacterial infections. Aliment Pharmacol Ther 2009;30:253–64.

12. Sandborn WJ, Gasink C, Gao LL, et al. Ustekinumab induction and maintenance therapy in refractory Crohn's disease. N Engl J Med 2012;367:1519–28.

13. Toussirot E, Michel F, Bereau M, et al. Ustekinumab in chronic immune-mediated diseases: a review of long term safety and patient improvement. Patient Prefer Adherence 2013;7:369–77.

14. Flynn JL, Chan J. Immunology of tuberculosis. Annu Rev Immunol 2001;19: 93–129.

15. Afif W, Loftus EV. Safety profile of IBD therapeutics: infectious risks. Med Clin North Am 2010;94:115–33.

16. Bloomgren G, Richman S, Hotermans C, et al. Risk of natalizumab-associated progressive multifocal leukoencephalopathy. N Engl J Med 2012;366:1870–80.

17. Kane SV, Horst S, Sandborn WJ, et al. Natalizumab for moderate to severe Crohn's disease in clinical practice: the Mayo Clinic Rochester experience. Inflamm Bowel Dis 2012;18:2203–8.

18. Juillerat P, Wasan SK, Fowler SA, et al. Efficacy and safety of natalizumab in Crohn's disease patients treated at 6 Boston academic hospitals. Inflamm Bowel Dis 2013;19:2457–63.

19. Sandborn WJ, Colombel JF, Enns R, et al. Natalizumab induction and maintenance therapy for Crohn's disease. N Engl J Med 2005;353:1912–25.

20. Mulero P, Caminero AB, Neri Crespo MJ, et al. Latent tuberculosis seems not to reactivate in multiple sclerosis patients on natalizumab. J Neuroimmunol 2012; 243:103–5.

21. Dahdaleh D, Altmann DM, Malik O, et al. Breathlessness, night sweats, and weight loss on natalizumab. Lancet 2012;380:726–7.

22. Feagan BG, Rutgeerts P, Sands BE, et al. Vedolizumab as induction and maintenance therapy for ulcerative colitis. N Engl J Med 2013;369:699–710.

23. Sandborn WJ, Feagan BG, Rutgeerts P, et al. Vedolizumab as induction and maintenance therapy for Crohn's disease. N Engl J Med 2013;369:711–21.
24. Gardam MA, Keystone EC, Menzies R, et al. Anti-tumour necrosis factor agents and tuberculosis risk: mechanisms of action and clinical management. Lancet Infect Dis 2003;3:148–55.
25. Askling J, Fored CM, Brandt L, et al. Risk and case characteristics of tuberculosis in rheumatoid arthritis associated with tumor necrosis factor antagonists in Sweden. Arthritis Rheum 2005;52:1986–92.
26. Wolfe F, Michaud K, Anderson J, et al. Tuberculosis infection in patients with rheumatoid arthritis and the effect of infliximab therapy. Arthritis Rheum 2004; 50:372–9.
27. Sichletidis L, Settas L, Spyratos D, et al. Tuberculosis in patients receiving anti-TNF agents despite chemoprophylaxis. Int J Tuberc Lung Dis 2006;10: 1127–32.
28. Broekmans JF, Migliori GB, Rieder HL, et al. European framework for tuberculosis control and elimination in countries with a low incidence. Recommendations of the World Health Organization (WHO), International Union Against Tuberculosis and Lung Disease (IUATLD) and Royal Netherlands Tuberculosis Association (KNCV) working group. Eur Respir J 2002;19:765–75.
29. Jauregui-Amezaga A, Turon F, Ordas I. Risk of developing tuberculosis under anti-TNF treatment despite latent infection screening. J Crohns Colitis 2013;7: 208–12.
30. Theis VS, Rhodes JM. Review article: minimizing tuberculosis during anti-tumour necrosis factor-alpha treatment of inflammatory bowel disease. Aliment Pharmacol Ther 2008;27:19–30.
31. Qumseya BJ, Ananthakrishnan AN, Skaros S, et al. QuantiFERON TB gold testing for tuberculosis screening in an inflammatory bowel disease cohort in the United States. Inflamm Bowel Dis 2011;17:77–83.
32. Abreu C, Magro F, Vilas-Boas F, et al. Listeria infection in patients on anti-TNF treatment: report of two cases and review of the literature. J Crohns Colitis 2013;7:175–82.
33. Ali T, Chakraburtty A, Mahmood S, et al. Risk of nocardial infections with anti-tumor necrosis factor therapy. Am J Med Sci 2013;346:166–8.
34. Issa M, Vijayapal A, Graham MB, et al. Impact of *Clostridium difficile* on inflammatory bowel disease. Clin Gastroenterol Hepatol 2007;5:345–51.
35. Rodemann JF, Dubberke ER, Reske KA, et al. Incidence of *Clostridium difficile* infection in inflammatory bowel disease. Clin Gastroenterol Hepatol 2007;5: 339–44.
36. Ben-Horin S, Margalit M, Bossuyt P, et al. Combination immunomodulator and antibiotic treatment in patients with inflammatory bowel disease and *Clostridium difficile* infection. Clin Gastroenterol Hepatol 2009;7:981–7.
37. Beigel F, Jurgens M, Filik L, et al. Severe *Legionella pneumophila* pneumonia following infliximab therapy in a patient with Crohn's disease. Inflamm Bowel Dis 2009;15:1240–4.
38. Epping G, van der Valk PD, Hendrix R. *Legionella pneumophila* pneumonia in a pregnant woman treated with anti-TNF-alpha antibodies for Crohn's disease: a case report. J Crohns Colitis 2010;4:687–9.
39. Vinter H, Nielsen HI. *Legionella pneumonia* in patients treated with infliximab. Ugeskr Laeger 2009;171:247 [in Danish].
40. Katsarolis I, Tsiodras S, Panagopoulos P, et al. Septic arthritis due to *Salmonella enteritidis* associated with infliximab use. Scand J Infect Dis 2005;37:304–5.

41. Rijkeboer A, Voskuyl A, Van Agtmael M. Fatal *Salmonella enteritidis* septicaemia in a rheumatoid arthritis patient treated with a TNF-alpha antagonist. Scand J Infect Dis 2007;39:80–3.

42. Rim JY, Tenorio AR. *Salmonella* septic arthritis in a patient with Crohn's disease on infliximab. Inflamm Bowel Dis 2010;16:545–7.

43. Kaur N, Mahl TC. *Pneumocystis carinii* pneumonia with oral candidiasis after infliximab therapy for Crohn's disease. Dig Dis Sci 2004;49:1458–60.

44. Kaur N, Mahl TC. *Pneumocystis jiroveci (carinii)* pneumonia after infliximab therapy: a review of 84 cases. Dig Dis Sci 2007;52:1481–4.

45. Wood KL, Hage CA, Knox KS, et al. Histoplasmosis after treatment with anti-tumor necrosis factor-alpha therapy. Am J Respir Crit Care Med 2003;167:1279–82.

46. Lee JH, Slifman NR, Gershon SK, et al. Life-threatening histoplasmosis complicating immunotherapy with tumor necrosis factor alpha antagonists infliximab and etanercept. Arthritis Rheum 2002;46:2565–70.

47. Bergstrom L, Yocum DE, Ampel NM, et al. Increased risk of coccidioidomycosis in patients treated with tumor necrosis factor alpha antagonists. Arthritis Rheum 2004;50:1959–66.

48. Fraison JB, Guilpain P, Schiffmann A, et al. Pulmonary cryptococcosis in a patient with Crohn's disease treated with prednisone, azathioprine and adalimumab: exposure to chicken manure as a source of contamination. J Crohns Colitis 2013;7:e11–4.

49. De Rosa FG, Shaz D, Campagna AC, et al. Invasive pulmonary aspergillosis soon after therapy with infliximab, a tumor necrosis factor-alpha-neutralizing antibody: a possible healthcare-associated case? Infect Control Hosp Epidemiol 2003;24:477–82.

50. Alderson JW, Van Dinter TG Jr, Opatowsky MJ, et al. Disseminated aspergillosis following infliximab therapy in an immunosuppressed patient with Crohn's disease and chronic hepatitis C: a case study and review of the literature. MedGenMed 2005;7:7.

51. Belda A, Hinojosa J, Serra B, et al. Systemic candidiasis and infliximab therapy. Gastroenterol Hepatol 2004;27:365–7 [in Spanish].

52. Hage CA, Wood KL, Winer-Muram TH, et al. Pulmonary cryptococcosis after initiation of anti-tumor necrosis factor-alpha therapy. Chest 2003;124:2395–7.

53. Osawa R, Singh N. Colitis as a manifestation of infliximab-associated disseminated cryptococcosis. Int J Infect Dis 2010;14:e436–40.

54. True DG, Penmetcha M, Peckham SJ. Disseminated cryptococcal infection in rheumatoid arthritis treated with methotrexate and infliximab. J Rheumatol 2002;29:1561–3.

55. Loras C, Saro C, Gonzalez-Huix F, et al. Prevalence and factors related to hepatitis B and C in inflammatory bowel disease patients in Spain: a nationwide, multicenter study. Am J Gastroenterol 2009;104:57–63.

56. Gisbert JP, Chaparro M, Esteve M. Review article: prevention and management of hepatitis B and C infection in patients with inflammatory bowel disease. Aliment Pharmacol Ther 2011;33:619–33.

57. Madonia S, Orlando A, Scimeca D, et al. Occult hepatitis B and infliximab-induced HBV reactivation. Inflamm Bowel Dis 2007;13:508–9.

58. Loras C, Gisbert JP, Minguez M, et al. Liver dysfunction related to hepatitis B and C in patients with inflammatory bowel disease treated with immunosuppressive therapy. Gut 2010;59:1340–6.

59. Melmed GY, Ippoliti AF, Papadakis KA, et al. Patients with inflammatory bowel disease are at risk for vaccine-preventable illnesses. Am J Gastroenterol 2006;101:1834–40.
60. Brunasso AM, Puntoni M, Gulia A, et al. Safety of anti-tumour necrosis factor agents in patients with chronic hepatitis C infection: a systematic review. Rheumatology (Oxford) 2011;50:1700–11.
61. Vauloup C, Krzysiek R, Greangeot-Keros L, et al. Effects of tumor necrosis factor antagonist treatment on hepatitis C-related immunological abnormalities. Eur Cytokine Netw 2006;17:290–3.
62. Vigano M, Degasperi E, Aghemo A, et al. Anti-TNF drugs in patients with hepatitis B or C virus infection: safety and clinical management. Expert Opin Biol Ther 2012;12:193–207.
63. Papa A, Felice C, Marzo M, et al. Prevalence and natural history of hepatitis B and C infections in a large population of IBD patients treated with anti-tumor necrosis factor-alpha agents. J Crohns Colitis 2013;7:113–9.
64. Lawlor G, Moss AC. Cytomegalovirus in inflammatory bowel disease: pathogen or innocent bystander? Inflamm Bowel Dis 2010;16:1620–7.
65. Kopylov U, Eliakim-Raz N, Szilagy A, et al. The impact of antiviral therapy in patients with ulcerative colitis complicated by cytomegalovirus: a systematic review and meta-analysis. World J Gastroenterol 2014;20:2695–703.
66. Manuel O, Perrottet N, Pascual M. Valganciclovir to prevent or treat cytomegalovirus disease in organ transplantation. Expert Rev Anti Infect Ther 2011;9: 955–65.
67. Kandiel A, Lashner B. Cytomegalovirus colitis complicating inflammatory bowel disease. Am J Gastroenterol 2006;101:2857–65.
68. Hommes DW, Sterringa G, van Deventer SJ, et al. The pathogenicity of cytomegalovirus in inflammatory bowel disease: a systematic review and evidence-based recommendations for future research. Inflamm Bowel Dis 2004;10:245–50.
69. Domenech E, Vega R, Ojanguren I, et al. Cytomegalovirus infection in ulcerative colitis: a prospective, comparative study on prevalence and diagnostic strategy. Inflamm Bowel Dis 2008;14:1373–9.
70. Shale MJ. The implications of anti-tumour necrosis factor therapy for viral infection in patients with inflammatory bowel disease. Br Med Bull 2009;92:61–77.
71. Ricart E, Panaccione R, Loftus EV, et al. Infliximab for Crohn's disease in clinical practice at the Mayo Clinic: the first 100 patients. Am J Gastroenterol 2001;96: 722–9.
72. Vergara M, Brullet E, Campo R, et al. Fulminant infection caused by varicella herpes zoster in patient with Crohn disease undergoing treatment with azathioprine. Gastroenterol Hepatol 2001;24:47 [in Spanish].
73. Winthrop KL, Baddley JW, Chen L, et al. Association between the initiation of anti-tumor necrosis factor therapy and the risk of herpes zoster. JAMA 2013; 309:887–95.
74. Oxman MN. Zoster vaccine: current status and future prospects. Clin Infect Dis 2010;51:197–213.
75. Kopylov U, Levin A, Mendelson E, et al. Prior varicella zoster virus exposure in IBD patients treated by anti-TNFs and other immunomodulators: implications for serological testing and vaccination guidelines. Aliment Pharmacol Ther 2012; 36:145–50.
76. Beltran B, Nos P, Bastida G, et al. Safe and effective application of anti-TNF-alpha in a patient infected with HIV and concomitant Crohn's disease. Gut 2006;55:1670–1.

77. Calabrese LH, Zein N, Vassilopoulos D. Safety of antitumour necrosis factor (anti-TNF) therapy in patients with chronic viral infections: hepatitis C, hepatitis B, and HIV infection. Ann Rheum Dis 2004;63:18–24.

78. Cepeda EJ, Williams FM, Ishimori ML, et al. The use of anti-tumour necrosis factor therapy in HIV-positive individuals with rheumatic disease. Ann Rheum Dis 2008;67:710–2.

79. Seksik P, Cosnes J, Sokol H, et al. Incidence of benign upper respiratory tract infections, HSV and HPV cutaneous infections in inflammatory bowel disease patients treated with azathioprine. Aliment Pharmacol Ther 2009;29:1106–13.

80. Saslow D, Castle PE, Cox JT, et al. American Cancer Society guideline for human papillomavirus (HPV) vaccine use to prevent cervical cancer and its precursors. CA Cancer J Clin 2007;57:7–28.

The Risk of Malignancy Associated with the Use of Biological Agents in Patients with Inflammatory Bowel Disease

Parambir S. Dulai, MBBS, Corey A. Siegel, MD, MS*

KEYWORDS

- Malignancy • Lymphoma • Skin cancer • Biologics • Inflammatory bowel disease

KEY POINTS

- The risk of lymphoma and skin cancer with anti–tumor necrosis factor (anti-TNF) therapy is largely driven by the use of concomitant immunomodulator therapy, particularly thiopurines.
- The risk of lymphoma and skin cancer with newer biologics seems to be similar to that seen with anti-TNF therapy, but this is largely based on either non–inflammatory bowel disease (IBD) data or IBD data with short follow-up.
- Tofacitinib has a measurable risk of malignancy when used in patients with rheumatoid arthritis, and further long-term data are needed in patients with IBD.
- In patients at particular risk for developing a malignancy while on therapy, there should be an effort to focus on modifiable risk factors.
- The optimal approach to the use of biologics in patients with IBD with a previous history of malignancy remains unclear.

INTRODUCTION

The pathogenesis of inflammatory bowel disease (IBD) is multifactorial and involves a complex interaction between genetic, environmental, microbial, and immune factors.[1] The ensuing pathologic response affects both the innate and adaptive immune systems, with the net result of these cellular mechanisms being granulocyte

Disclosures: C.A. Siegel serves on the advisory board and as a consultant for AbbVie, Janssen, Takeda, and UCB, and has received grant support from AbbVie, Janssen, and UCB. He has delivered continuing medical education lectures for AbbVie, Janssen, and Merck. Dr C.A. Siegel is supported by grant number 1R01HS021747-01 from the Agency for Healthcare Research and Quality.
Inflammatory Bowel Disease Center, Dartmouth-Hitchcock Medical Center, One Medical Center Drive, Lebanon, NH 03756, USA
* Corresponding author.
E-mail address: corey.a.siegel@hitchcock.org

accumulation, cytokine production, and intestinal inflammation.[2,3] This complex immune response has provided the opportunity for the development of biological agents that target specific components of the immune cascade.[4] These biological drugs have dramatically changed the manner in which the treatment of IBD is approached and the outcomes that may be expected. Despite the proven efficacy of these agents and the shifting of treatment goals toward early aggressive use of these drugs,[5–7] concerns surrounding toxicity have posed a significant emotional barrier to their use. Infectious complications remain the most common side effect, but the fear of developing cancer poses the greatest obstacle for patients and providers to overcome.[8–10]

Patients with IBD are at an increased baseline risk for intestinal and extra-intestinal malignancies,[11–13] but the 2 cancers that have gained the most attention are lymphoma and skin cancer. Although there are some conflicting data,[12,14] several studies suggest that IBD alone is not associated with an increased risk for lymphoma.[11,15,16] In contrast, there seems to be a clear association between IBD and the development of melanoma and nonmelanoma skin cancers (NMSC).[13,17,18] There is also much evidence implicating IBD-related medications, particularly thiopurines, in the development of these malignancies.[18–21] It is difficult to determine the risk of malignancy with biologics on their own, because most patients with IBD treated with biologics have also previously been exposed to thiopurines.

In this review, the available evidence regarding the risk of malignancy when using biological agents for the treatment of IBD are highlighted, with a particular focus on lymphoma and skin cancer. This risk is compared with that seen with other treatment options in IBD and with the general population. The approach to managing these medications in patients who have a history of malignancy is further highlighted. We anticipate that this review will help providers better understand how best to broadly approach the difficult conversation of biological therapy and cancer with their patients.

ANTI–TUMOR NECROSIS FACTOR THERAPY
Risk of Lymphoma

The hallmark of active IBD is infiltration of the lamina propria by innate (neutrophils, macrophages, dendritic, and natural killer T cells) and adaptive immune cells (B and T cells). The increased number of these activated cells in the intestinal mucosa leads to enhanced local levels of proinflammatory cytokines, which play important roles in the interaction between immune and nonimmune cells.[22] One of these cytokines, tumor necrosis factor α (TNF-α), has been shown to play a key role in the pathogenesis of IBD, and has therefore served as the prototypical target for biologics in both Crohn disease (CD) and ulcerative colitis (UC). Around the time that infliximab was approved from use in CD, there was already increasing concern over a potential increase in risk of lymphoma with these agents.[23] Since then, the evidence surrounding the potential association between anti-TNF therapy and lymphoma occurrence has increased significantly.

Initial attempts at understanding the risk of lymphoma with anti-TNF therapy used pooled analyses of randomized controlled trials (RCTs). The first meta-analysis to look at this subject[24] pooled data from 21 RCTs and assessed the efficacy and safety of anti-TNF agents for the treatment of CD. This study examined 3341 patients exposed to anti-TNF with a median follow-up period of 24 weeks per patient and did not find an increased risk for lymphoma occurrence with anti-TNF use. In most of these RCTs, many of the controls also had some exposure to anti-TNF therapy. The investigators performed a sensitivity analysis of studies with unexposed controls, but this was an exploratory subanalysis and was likely underpowered to address this outcome. A more recent meta-analysis looking specifically at the risk of lymphoma with adalimumab therapy[25] included 6 RCTs with 1594 patients with CD and 3050 patient-years (PY) of exposure (PYE) to adalimumab. These investigators reported that patients treated with anti-TNF therapy in combination with an immunomodulator had a significantly higher risk of lymphoma occurrence when compared with the general population (**Table 1**). This increase in lymphoma risk with anti-TNF combination therapy had previously been reported in a meta-analysis by Siegel and colleagues.[26] This group pooled data from 26 studies, including 8905 patients with 21,178 patient years of follow-up (PYF), and reported that the risk of lymphoma with anti-TNF combination therapy was increased when compared with the general population (standardized incidence ratio [SIR], 3.23; 95% confidence interval [CI], 1.5–6.9), but when compared with immunomodulator monotherapy in CD, the use of anti-TNF combination therapy seemed to have no incremental increase in risk of lymphoma occurrence (SIR, 1.7; 95% CI, 0.5–7.1). When examining the pediatric gastroenterology literature, a recent systematic review by our group[10] studied 5528 patients with 9516 PYF and reported that the risk of lymphoma with anti-TNF therapy in pediatric IBD was similar to that seen in the general pediatric population (SIR, 3.5; 95% CI, 0.35–19.6), a population of pediatric patients receiving thiopurine monotherapy (SIR, 0.47; 95% CI, 0.03–6.44), and among adult patients with IBD treated with anti-TNF agents (SIR, 0.34; 95% CI, 0.04–1.51).

Although these RCT data seem reassuring, data from observational studies are conflicting. The claims-based population study by Marehbian and colleagues[27] reported

Table 1 Risk of lymphoma with anti-TNF therapy			
	Incidence Rate (per 10,000 PYF)	SIR	95% CI
Current Thiopurine Without Anti-TNF Exposure			
Herrinton et al,[16] 2011	4.1	1.4	1.2–1.7
CESAME[20,a]	8.8	6.5	3.5–11.2
Khan et al,[77] 2013	14.6	7.5	4.7–12.0
Current Thiopurine with Previous Anti-TNF Exposure			
CESAME[20,a]	8.8	6.5	3.5–11.2
Herrinton et al,[16] 2011	15.1	5.3	3.5–7.0
Current Anti-TNF Therapy with Current Thiopurine Therapy			
Dulai et al,[10] 2014	2.1	3.5	0.35–19.6
TREAT[29]	4.5	2.0	0.87–3.95
Siegel et al,[26] 2009	6.1	3.2	1.5–6.9
CESAME[20]	10.4	10.2	1.2–36.9
Osterman et al,[25] 2014	14.3	8.0	0.97–29.0
Herrinton et al,[16] 2011	19.1	6.6	4.4–8.8
Current Anti-TNF Therapy with Previous Thiopurine Exposure			
Herrinton et al,[16] 2011	14.9	5.2	3.5–6.8
Current Anti-TNF Therapy Without Thiopurine Exposure			
n/a	—	—	—

Abbreviations: CI, confidence interval; n/a, data not available to calculate rate; PYF, patient-years of follow-up; SIR, standardized incidence ratio.
  [a] Analysis included patients who had who had never received anti-TNF therapy and those who had discontinued anti-TNF therapy.
Data from Refs.[10,16,20,25,26,29,77]

that the odds of developing a lymphoma was numerically, but not statistically, higher with anti-TNF monotherapy (odds ratio [OR], 2.1; 95% CI, 0.82–5.40) than with immunomodulator monotherapy (OR, 1.66; 95% CI, 0.95–2.88). A later population-based study using the Kaiser Permanente IBD Registry[16] evaluated lymphoma risk among 16,023 patients with IBD followed for an average of 5.8 years. This study similarly found that when compared with the general non-IBD Kaiser population, the risk of lymphoma with anti-TNF therapy (SIR, 4.4; 95% CI, 3.4–5.4) was higher than the risk of lymphoma with thiopurine monotherapy (SIR, 1.4; 95% CI, 1.2–1.7). These studies therefore suggest that in contrast to RCT, the use of anti-TNF therapy outside clinical trials increases the risk of lymphoma above that seen with immunomodulators. This theory may be explained by the strict selection of patients and exclusion of high-risk populations (elderly) in clinical trials,[28] but there are several key points to consider when interpreting these data. The study by Marehbian and colleagues used a claims-based method for data collection, and therefore is at risk for underreporting or over-reporting certain outcomes based on claims submissions and follow-up. Furthermore, the use of pharmacy-based claims is limited by the lack of confirmation regarding medication usage and inability to accurately quantify the residual effects of treatments after discontinuation. These factors may help account for the fact that this study is the only one to have ever reported a lower odds of lymphoma with anti-TNF and immuno-modulator combination therapy when compared with monotherapy for either agent (OR, 0.63; 95% CI, 0.08–4.64). Although the Kaiser study by Herrinton and colleagues also noted that anti-TNF therapy was associated with an increased risk of lymphoma, the comparison with control individuals who did not have IBD and use of pharmacy-based confirmation for medication usage similarly limits the conclusions that can be drawn from these data. Given the inherit limitations within RCT and claims-based population studies, perhaps the most compelling evidence comes from prospective observational cohort studies specifically aimed at addressing the question of malignancy risk with IBD treatments.

We have 2 such studies to consider: the Cancers Et Surrisque Associé aux Maladies inflammatoires intestinales En France (CESAME) trial and the Crohn's Therapy, Resource, Evaluation, and Assessment Tool (TREAT) registry.[20,29] The TREAT registry enrolled 6273 patients with an average follow-up of 5.2 years/patient and found that neither immunomodulator monotherapy (hazard ratio [HR], 1.43; 95% CI, 0.92–2.21), nor infliximab monotherapy (HR, 0.59; 95% CI, 0.28–1.22), nor their combination (HR, 1.22; 95% CI, 0.81–1.86) was independently associated with an increased risk of malignancy. When looking specifically at the risk of lymphoma, there appeared to be no statistical difference in incidence between patients treated with infliximab (SIR, 2.01; 95% CI, 0.87–3.95) or immunosuppressants (SIR, 2.06; 95% CI, 0.99–3.80), when compared with the general population. In contrast, the CESAME trial reported that patients continuing thiopurine therapy in combination with anti-TNF therapy (SIR, 10.2; 95% CI, 1.24–36.9) were at a higher risk for lymphoma when compared with patients continuing thiopurine therapy without anti-TNF therapy (SIR, 6.5; 95% CI, 3.48–11.2).

Hepatosplenic T-Cell Lymphoma

A subtype of lymphoma, hepatosplenic T-cell lymphoma (HSTCL), has raised the greatest amount of concern when using biologics, given the aggressiveness and fatality rate of this malignancy. A study to address this concern pooled data from published literature and the US Food and Drug Administration (FDA) Adverse Event Registry System (AERS).[30] At the time of their publication in 2011, there had been 36 cases reported, with all but 2 occurring in male patients (12–58 years of age). All 36 patients had received thiopurine therapy alone (n = 16) or in combination with an anti-TNF agent (n = 20). A subsequent review of the FDA AERS 2 years later[31] identified only 1 additional case in a patient with CD. This study used 3 causality assessment tools and noted that establishing a causative effect between anti-TNF therapy and HSTCL beyond possible was not feasible. A more recent study using AERS and a literature search[32] examined the risk of subtypes of all T-cell lymphomas across different disease entities (IBD n = 45, rheumatoid arthritis [RA] n = 38, psoriasis n = 11, ankylosing spondylitis n = 6). These investigators found that the risk of T-cell lymphoma was highest in patients receiving thiopurine monotherapy and combination therapy with an anti-TNF agent and thiopurines. A single case of HSTCL was reported with anti-TNF monotherapy, which was not statistically significantly increased when compared with a control population. Although these studies give us the best information currently available for HSTCL, they all use the AERS system, which has inherent biases, which are difficult to overcome. More information is still needed to better understand the absolute incidence of these nearly universally fatal malignancies and how much of an influence anti-TNFs play (or do not play) in their genesis. Similar to the standard lymphomas reported earlier, it is likely that most, if not all, of the risk is associated with thiopurine therapy.

Risk of Skin Cancer

NMSC

NMSC includes both basal cell carcinoma (BCC) and squamous cell carcinoma (SCC), and this cancer ranks among the most common malignancies reported in the United States, with an annual incidence of more than 3 million cases.[33] Although most NMSC have a low metastatic potential and can be easily treated with topical and surgical therapies, those occurring in high-risk areas may have up to a 30% risk of metastasis, and the treatment of these lesions may be costly and lead to permanent disfiguration.[34] Given the increased baseline risk of NMSC in patients with IBD,[13,18] and the impact that this malignancy has on patient outcomes, it is important to understand how IBD therapy may affect this risk.

The first study to directly address this question was a nested case-control retrospective cohort analysis in which 742 patients with IBD with NMSC were matched to 4 patients with IBD without NMSC to understand the impact of immunomodulators and biologics on malignancy risk.[35] This group reported that the recent (<90 days) and persistent (>365 days) use of biological monotherapy increased the risk of NMSC 2-fold to 3-fold, but this risk was still lower than the 3-fold to 4-fold increase in risk seen with thiopurine monotherapy and the 5-fold to 6-fold increase in risk seen with combination therapy (**Table 2**). However, a later study by the same group using similar methodology[18] found the risk of NMSC with biologics to be limited to only those patients with persistent (>365 days) use of biologics. These investigators again reported that the use of an immunomodulator, alone or in combination with a biologic, carried a higher risk for NMSC than biological therapy alone. When comparing this risk with the general population, a recent meta-analysis[25] pooled data across all adalimumab RCTs and found that the use of adalimumab monotherapy was not associated with an increased risk of NMSC (SIR, 1.20; 95% CI, 0.39–2.80), whereas the use of adalimumab combination therapy with an immunomodulator was associated with an increased risk of NMSC when compared with the general population (SIR, 4.59; 95% CI, 2.51–7.70).

Melanoma

In contrast to NMSC, melanomas are not so easily cured, and the mortality secondary to these cancers has been largely unchanged in the United States despite efforts to

Table 2			
Risk of NMSC with anti-TNF therapy			
	Treatment	OR	95% CI
Long et al,[35] 2010	Recent use (<90 d)		
	Biologics	2.47	1.29–4.73
	Immunomodulators	3.71	2.74–5.02
	Combination therapy	5.85	3.2–10.8
	Persistent use (>365 d)		
	Biologics	3.23	1.24–8.45
	Immunomodulators	4.45	2.94–6.75
	Combination therapy	6.75	2.74–16.65
Long et al,[18] 2012	Overall risk		
	Biologics	1.14	0.95–1.36
	Immunomodulators	1.85	1.66–2.05
	Persistent use (>365 d)		
	Biologics	1.63	1.12–2.36
	Immunomodulators	2.72	2.27–3.26
	Combination therapy	3.89	2.33–6.46
Osterman et al,[25] 2014	Combination therapy	3.46	1.08–11.06

Data from Refs.[18,25,35]

enhance early detection of these lesions.[17] Patients with IBD are at a higher baseline risk for the development of melanoma skin cancer,[17] but when attempting to understand the added risk of melanoma with anti-TNF therapy, there are few data on which to base decisions. The nested case-control study by Long and colleagues[18] reported that, unlike NMSC, the risk of melanoma was increased with biologics (OR, 1.88; 95% CI, 1.08–3.29) but not immunomodulators (OR 1.10; 95% CI, 0.72–1.67). In an effort to understand this association, the investigators performed an exploratory subgroup analysis and identified that patients undergoing long-term therapy with anti-TNF agents were at higher risk than those not exposed to long-term therapy (OR, 3.93; 95% CI, 1.82–8.50). In contrast to this study, the CESAME group reported that the risk of melanoma was not increased in patients with IBD who were receiving thiopurines (SIR, 1.09; 95% CI, 0.13–3.94) or anti-TNF treatment (SIR, 2.57; 95% CI, 0.06–14.33).[36] Less than 10% of patients in the CESAME trial were prescribed nonthiopurine medications, and the investigators therefore commented that a reliable risk of melanoma with anti-TNF therapy could not be determined.

OTHER BIOLOGICS

Although anti-TNF agents now represent an integral component of the treatment algorithm for IBD, less than a third of patients initially responding to these medications maintain remission beyond 1 year of therapy.[22,37,38] Researchers have therefore also turned their attention toward several other therapeutic targets, including proinflammatory cytokines (interleukin 12 [IL-12]/IL-23), the downstream effects of cytokine stimulation (leukocyte trafficking), and the cytokine signaling pathways (Janus kinase [JAK]) responsible for the altered immune response and inflammation seen in IBD. These newer biologics represent a new article in the treatment paradigm of IBD, and it is therefore imperative to understand any associated risk of malignancy with these agents to better optimize the long-term management of patients, particularly given the role that these drug targets have in immune function and neoplastic transformation.[39] Data regarding the risk of malignancy with these agents are largely limited to non-IBD populations or early phase RCTs used for drug approval in patients with IBD.

Anti-Integrins (Natalizumab and Vedolizumab)

Natalizumab is a recombinant humanized monoclonal IgG4 antibody directed against the integrin subunit α_4, which blocks both $\alpha_4\beta_7$ receptors in the gut and $\alpha_4\beta_1$ receptors in the central nervous system (CNS). Natalizumab was the first antiadhesion treatment developed and approved for use in IBD, but, despite its proven efficacy, its use has now largely been limited by the risk of developing progressive multifocal leukoencephalopathy, an opportunistic and usually fatal brain infection caused by reactivation of latent John Cunningham polyomavirus.[40] Long-term follow-up data are largely lacking in the population with IBD, but reports from patients who do not have IBD have raised concern that therapies targeting cell adhesion molecules may be associated with an increased risk of cancer progression.[41] Initial reports noted a possible association between natalizumab therapy and the development of primary CNS lymphoma in patients with multiple sclerosis,[42] but when looking at pooled cumulative clinical trial experience,[43] there appeared to be no clear association, and the rate of lymphoma with this therapy was quantified to be lower than that seen with other biologics (1.3/10,000 PYF). Similarly, case reports suggested that natalizumab may be associated with an increased risk for melanoma, but this was not supported by a later meta-analysis of clinical trials,[44] which reported that the rate of melanoma with natalizumab (4.2/10,000 PYF) was similar to that seen with placebo (8.2/10,000 PYF).

Vedolizumab is a humanized IgG1 monoclonal antibody that binds exclusively to the gut-specific $\alpha_4\beta_7$-integrin and inhibits leukocyte trafficking into the gastrointestinal mucosa. This selective blockade of gut-homing T lymphocytes allows it to avoid the CNS side effects noted with previous anti-integrins (ie, natalizumab). Two recent phase 3 RCTs have reported that vedolizumab was more effective than placebo in inducing and maintaining remission in both CD and UC.[45,46] An interesting observation within these studies was the differential effect of vedolizumab for inducing a clinical response in CD and UC, with patients with CD requiring a longer duration of therapy to show a significant benefit, which was postulated to be secondary to a time-dependent inhibition of leukocyte trafficking in CD or the more systemic nature of the disease.[47] These data support the use of vedolizumab in both CD and UC and support the long-term use of this agent in IBD, making an assessment of cancer risk important. Given that vedolizumab is not approved for any other indication, these phase 3 RCTs are the only data that determine the risk of malignancy with this agent. These RCTs in combination with ongoing long-term safety studies include a total of 3129 patients with 3096 PYF.[48] Within this cohort, 1 lymphoma (B-cell lymphoma), 3 NMSC (2 SCC, 1 BCC), and 2 melanomas have been reported (**Table 3**). This single lymphoma occurred in a 42-year-old man with CD who had received previous immunosuppressive therapy, including infliximab and azathioprine, and continued on azathioprine and corticosteroids while enrolled in the study. The patient had worsening CD despite therapy (21 doses of vedolizumab) and underwent colorectal surgery. Approximately 6 weeks later, the patient was found to have a solid mass in the lesser pelvis in the vicinity of the rectal stump, for which he was discontinued from the study, and received treatment with rituximab. Of the 5 skin cancers, only 2 were believed to be possibly related to vedolizumab when reviewed by independent study investigators or an FDA reviewer.

Anti-IL-12/23 (Ustekinumab)

Anti-TNF agents are generally regarded as safe agents, but these biologics are often associated with dermatologic adverse events, including the occurrence of psoriasiform skin lesions in up to 5% of patients with IBD treated with anti-TNF.[49] Intuitively,

Table 3
Overall rate of lymphoma and skin cancer with biologics

	Lymphoma	NMSC	Melanoma
Expected rate (general population)[a]	20/100,000 PYF	NR	21/100,000 PYF
Anti-TNF therapy (infliximab, adalimumab, certolizumab, golimumab)	6.1/10,000 PYF	5/10,000 PYF[b]	n/a
Anti-integrins (vedolizumab, natalizumab)	3.2/10,000 PYF	9.7/10,000 PYF[c]	6.5/10,000 PYF
Anti-IL-12/23 (ustekinumab)[d]	2.2/10,000 PYF	52/10,000 PYF[e]	6.7/10,000 PYF
Janus kinase inhibitors (tofacitinib)[d]	6.6/10,000 PYE	45/10,000 PYE	2.9/10,000 PYE

Abbreviations: PYE, patient years of exposure; PYF, patient years of follow-up; n/a, data not available to calculate rate; NR, not reported in SEER database.
[a] Based on Surveillance, Epidemiology, and End Results (SEER) Program.
[b] The rate of NMSC when looking specifically at adalimumab is 66/10,000 PYE,[25] with adalimumab monotherapy (20/10,000 PYE) carrying a lower risk than adalimumab combination therapy (80/10,000 PYE).
[c] Data presented for vedolizumab only.
[d] Non-IBD data.
[e] The use of PUVA (psoralen and ultraviolet A) therapy for psoriasis significantly affected the risk of NMSC in this cohort.
Adapted from Refs.[26,48,52,55,58]

this finding seems to be a paradoxic response, given that TNF-α plays a key role in the pathogenesis of psoriasis, and anti-TNF agents are used for the management of severe psoriatic lesions. Recently, it was noted[49] that these psoriasiform lesions in patients with IBD treated anti-TNF were characterized by Th17 and Th1 cellular infiltrates, and the use of anti-IL-12/23 agents directed against Th17 and Th1 cells is highly effective in treating these lesions. Furthermore, the use of these anti-IL-12/23 agents seems to have a significant impact on disease activity in patients suffering from CD.[50,51] Although these initial early phase clinical trials reported no serious adverse events, longer-term follow-up data are required to understand the risk of malignancy with these biologics.

Ustekinumab is approved for use in psoriasis, and long-term management with this agent is typical for patients suffering from moderate to severe psoriasis. Therefore, to better understand the potential malignancy risk with this agent when being used for IBD, the available safety data in psoriasis must be relied on. A recent systematic review and meta-analysis[52] evaluated the safety data of ustekinumab in patients with psoriasis treated for up to 5 years. This analysis included 3117 patients with 8998 PYF, approximately 48% (1482 patients) of whom had greater than 4 years of treatment exposure and 27% (838 patients) had greater than 5 years of treatment exposure. The observed rate of malignancies in patients treated with ustekinumab was comparable with that expected in the general US population (SIR, 0.98; 95% CI, 0.74–1.29). Within this cohort, 2 patients developed lymphomas, one with Hodgkin lymphoma and one with a cutaneous T-cell lymphoma, which had been misdiagnosed as psoriasis on study entry (see **Table 3**). The rate of skin cancer occurrence was significantly higher in this cohort when compared with other agents, with a total of 47 patients developing NMSC lesions (BCC, n = 40; SCC, n = 10) and 6 patients developing a melanoma (in situ, n = 5; invasive, n = 1) while on therapy. When compared with the general population, the rate of melanoma occurrence in this cohort was not significantly higher (SIR, 1.42; 95% CI, 0.52–3.09). Although the rate of NMSC with ustekinumab seems to be higher than that seen with other biologics (see **Table 3**), patients treated with ustekinumab and PUVA therapy (psoralen + ultraviolet A), a treatment used for psoriasis, were at a significantly higher risk for NMSC occurrence compared with patients treated with ustekinumab therapy alone (P<.001).

Janus Kinase Inhibitor (Tofacitinib)

In addition to inhibiting cytokine production and cytokine receptors, an alternative means of blunting inflammation under investigation is the blocking of downstream signaling pathways mediated by these cytokines. The Janus kinases (JAK) play a crucial role in cell growth, survival, development, and differentiation of immune cells. JAK 1 and JAK 2 are ubiquitously expressed, but JAK 3 is found only in hematopoietic cells and is part of the signaling pathway activated by several key cytokines.[4] Tofacitinib, a small molecule inhibitor of JAK3, is approved for use in RA and is undergoing phase 2 and 3 clinical trials for use in CD and UC. Its efficacy in CD clinical trials has been less substantial,[53] but this agent seems to be well tolerated and effective in patients suffering from moderate to severe UC.[54] These early phase clinical trials in IBD did not collect data beyond 12 weeks for adverse events, and therefore, a meaningful analysis of malignancy risk in IBD cannot be obtained. However, the data from RA have raised some possible concerns regarding the malignancy risk with this biologic.

A recent Advisory Committee Meeting study by Pfizer[55] pooled data from phase 2 and 3 clinical trials and pooled data from 2 ongoing long-term extension studies in RA. This study included a total of 4923 patients, 3515 of whom were entered into the long-term extension studies, with a total of 6921 PYE. The incidence rate for all malignancies (excluding NMSC) was 94/10,000 PYE, and the rate of malignancy occurrence appeared to be higher with higher doses and longer durations of exposure. For lymphoma specifically, a total of 6 cases were reported for patients RA treated with tofacitinib with 9071 PYE (see **Table 3**). These lymphomas included: primary CNS lymphoma (n = 1), Epstein-Barr virus + lymphoma or lymphoproliferative disorder (n = 2), diffuse large B-cell lymphoma (n = 1), high grade B-cell Burkitt-like lymphoma (n = 1), and T-cell chronic lymphocytic leukemia (n = 1). This rate seemed to be similar to that seen in the general population (SIR, 2.2; 95% CI, 0.81–4.79), and, unlike the overall risk of malignancy with tofacitinib, the risk of lymphoma appeared to be unaffected by dose or duration of therapy. However, compared with TNF inhibitors and other biological disease-modifying antirheumatic drugs (DMARDs), this rate is significantly higher (95% CI 1.1–9.7). When skin cancers were investigated, 2 patients developed malignant melanomas (5 mg, n = 1; 10 mg, n = 1) and 31 patients developed NMSC, with more patients developing NMSC in the 10-mg group (89/10,000 PYE) than the 5-mg group (37/10,000 PYE).

OTHER MALIGNANCIES

Although lymphoma and skin cancer are the most closely examined malignancies and represent the 2 cancers most well known to patients, there are several other notable extraintestinal malignancies that warrant further discussion. Patients with UC and CD both seem to be at an increased risk for hematologic malignancies, with leukemia accounting for most of this risk.[11,13,56] There also seems to be an association between IBD and the development of smoking-related cancers, predominately lung and bladder malignancy.[11–13] Because patients with IBD carry a significantly higher risk for several of these malignancies within the first year of diagnosis,[13] and given the changing of treatment strategies toward use of biologics early in the disease course, it is important to understand and discuss the risk of extraintestinal malignancies associated with these agents early in the disease course.

Anti-TNF Therapy

Initial data surrounding the use of anti-TNF therapy in RA suggested that these agents may increase the overall risk of malignancy, but later data did not support these findings.[57] When patients with IBD were specifically investigated, early pooled RCT data found no increase in malignancy risk, which was later supported by a large observational cohort study (TREAT).[24,29] A more recent meta-analysis investigating adalimumab therapy reported that although the use of anti-TNF therapy in combination with an immunomodulator carried an increased risk for malignancies (other than NMSC), the use of anti-TNF monotherapy did not have a greater than expected incidence of cancer.[25] This finding is further supported by another meta-analysis of RCT for all anti-TNF agents in IBD,[58] which yielded a relative risk of 0.77 (95% CI, 0.37–1.59) for malignancy with anti-TNF therapy in IBD when compared with within study placebo controls.

Other Biologics

The overall rate of malignancy and rates for notable extraintestinal malignancies with vedolizumab and ustekinumab seems to be similar to that seen with anti-TNF therapy and the general population (**Table 4**). When considering tofacitinib, there seems to be a slightly higher overall rate of malignancy, and specifically, a higher rate of lung cancer when compared with the general population (SIR, 2.35; 95% CI, 1.34–3.82) and when compared with other biological DMARDs used for RA (95% CI, 1.08–3.5).[55] Within the FDA report, a total of 16 patients developed lung cancer during therapy with tofacitinib (13 non–small cell lung cancers and 3 small–cell lung cancers), and, as expected, many of these patients were current (n = 9) or previous smokers

Table 4
Rate of notable extraintestinal malignancies with biologics

	Overall Rate	Lung	Bladder	Breast	Prostate	Leukemia
Expected rate (general population)[a]	463/100,000 PYF	61/100,000 PYF	21/100,000 PYF	124/100,000 PYF	152/100,000 PYF	13/100,000 PYF
Anti-TNF therapy (infliximab, adalimumab, certolizumab, golimumab)	69/10,000 PYF	8.6/10,000 PYF	4.3/10,000 PYF	4.3/10,000 PYF	4.3/10,000 PYF	3.3/10,000 PYE[b]
Anti-integrins (vedolizumab)	58/10,000 PYF	6.5/10,000 PYF	3.3/10,000 PYF	6.5/10,000 PYF	n/a	n/a
Anti-IL-12/23 (ustekinumab)[c]	67/10,000 PYF	1.1/10,000 PYF	2.2/10,000 PYF	4.5/10,000 PYF	15/10,000 PYF	2.2/10,000 PYF
JAK inhibitors (tofacitinib)[c]	94/10,000 PYE	23/10,000 PYE	2.2/10,000 PYE	19/10,000 PYE	2.2/10,000 PYE	n/a

Abbreviations: PYE, patient years of exposure; PYF, patient years of follow-up; n/a, data not available to calculate rate.
[a] Based on Surveillance, Epidemiology, and End Results (SEER) Program.
[b] Data presented for pooled analysis of adalimumab studies.
[c] Non-IBD data.
Adapted from Refs.[25,48,52,55,58]

(n = 4). Although breast cancer was among the most common malignancies in the FDA report, the rate of breast cancer with tofacitinib was comparable with that seen in the general population (SIR, 0.82; 95% CI, 0.41–1.46).

MANAGING RISK FACTORS
Combination Therapy with an Immunomodulator

There seems to be an increased risk of malignancy when adding an immunomodulator to an anti-TNF agent, but the debate surrounding the use of combination therapy still remains, given the clear impact that these medications have on disease outcomes.[59] Although most data are largely in support of the overall use of combination therapy, providers should take into consideration which patients are most likely to benefit from this strategy. A recent study[60] addressed this question across 134 clinical scenarios and determined that combination therapy was preferred in most patients. However, in young males with limited disease (short segment bowel involvement and no perianal disease), combination therapy was believed to be less appropriate because of the risk of HSTCL with thiopurines. In all patients, special consideration should be given to the duration of combination therapy necessary and the ideal immunomodulator for use. In patients achieving clinical remission with combination therapy, providers may consider stopping the immunomodulator and continuing biological monotherapy in patients at low risk for relapse.[61] These patients should be monitored carefully for decreasing trough levels, antibody development, and disease relapse, because this strategy has been shown to be associated with decreasing anti-TNF trough concentrations.[62] If continued immunomodulator use is believed to be most appropriate, consideration can be given to switching to methotrexate in higher-risk patients. This is becoming a popular strategy for mitigating the increased risk of malignancy seen with thiopurines, but a lack of data in IBD does not imply safety, and methotrexate has been associated with malignancy in patients with RA.[63,64] Furthermore, there are no supportive data to confirm that biological therapy in combination with methotrexate is clinically beneficial.[65]

Disease and Patient Characteristics

Several studies have identified specific patient and disease characteristics associated with an increased risk for the development of cancer in IBD (**Box 1**).[11–14]

Box 1
Risk factors for malignancy with biologics

Nonmodifiable risk factors

- Young males
- Older age
- Disease duration and subtype
- Extraintestinal manifestations

Modifiable risk factors

- Smoking
- Photoprotection
- Vitamin D deficiency
- Immunomodulators

Smoking and gender have been shown to correlate with an increased risk of malignancy, with male patients being at a higher overall risk.[11–14] Increasing age is also a predictor of malignancy risk independent of immunosuppressive use, with the greatest risk being in patients older than 65 years.[19,20,29] The CESAME trial quantified this risk at an HR of 1.06 per 1-year increase in age, and the TREAT registry quantified it at an HR of 1.59 per 10-year increase in age. A specific patient characteristic is the association between HSTCL and young males. This risk seems to be largely driven by thiopurine use, with duration of therapy being a strong predictor of risk.[30] The correlation between disease activity and malignancy risk has been well established, and patients at the greatest risk of malignancy are those with more extensive involvement, higher inflammatory markers, and extraintestinal manifestations of their disease.[11–14,66,67] Although clear supportive evidence is lacking, it seems intuitive to aggressively control disease activity early in the disease course to help reduce this increased risk.

Vitamin D Deficiency

Patients with IBD are commonly deficient in vitamin D, and this deficiency may even precede the diagnosis.[68] Several studies have also reported an association between vitamin D status and disease activity, risk of hospitalization, and surgery.[69] Recently, it was shown that patients with IBD with vitamin D deficiency had an increased risk of cancer (OR, 1.82; 95% CI, 1.25–2.65) when compared with those patients with normal vitamin D levels.[70] Within this study, each 1-ng/mL increase in plasma 25-hydroxy vitamin D was associated with a reduction in the risk of colorectal cancer by 6% (OR, 0.94; 95% CI, 0.88–0.96) and lung cancer by 5% (OR, 0.95; 95% CI, 0.90–0.99). Although this study has several limitations, and there is no clear association with a reduced risk when supplementing vitamin D in deficient patients, it seems prudent to ensure that patients are optimized in regards to vitamin D status.[71]

Previous History of Malignancy

An important scenario to consider is how best to manage these immunosuppressive medications in patients with a previous history of cancer or those developing a cancer while on therapy. The CESAME study group[72] recently evaluated the risk of new or recurrent cancer among patients with IBD with previous cancer. The rate of incidence cancer was 21.1/1000 PY and 6.1/1000 PY in patients with and without a previous cancer, respectively. On multivariate analysis, the adjusted HR for incident cancer between patients with and without previous cancer was 1.9 (95% CI, 1.2–3.0). When patients stratified according to immunosuppressant use were specifically studied, the risk of new different cancers was numerically, but not statistically, higher in patients taking immunosuppressants compared with those not taking immunosuppressants (23.1/1000 PY vs 13.2/1000 PY), but the risk of recurrent cancer was similar (3.9/1000 PY vs 6.0/1000 PY). This study largely assessed the risks with immunomodulator (thiopurine) therapy, because less than 10% were exposed to nonthiopurine immunosuppressants. Data regarding the risk of malignancy with biologics in patients with a previous history of cancer are largely lacking in the IBD population. Within the RA literature, studies have suggested that the use of anti-TNF therapy in patients with a history of cancer had no impact on the risk of a recurrent or new malignancy.[73,74] Given the lack of data and certainty regarding risk, current IBD guidelines indicate that anti-TNF therapy is contraindicated in patients with a history of lymphoma, and careful consideration should be given to initiating anti-TNF therapy in those with a history of nonhematopoietic cancer.[75,76]

SUMMARY

Taken together, these data show that the overall risk of malignancy with biologics is similar to that seen in the general population, and the specific risk of NMSC and lymphoma is largely driven by the use of thiopurines. When considering HSTCL, this risk seems to be exposure and patient (age and gender) dependent, with men younger than 35 years exposed to long-term (>2 years) thiopurine therapy being at the highest risk. The measurable cancer risk with tofacitinib in the RA literature is worth noting and needs to be monitored closely when using these agents for patients with IBD, particularly when considering the risk of lung cancer. When possible, providers should attempt to minimize the risk of malignancy through age-appropriate screening and modification of risk factors. The optimal approach to using biologics in patients with a previous history of cancer remains unclear.

REFERENCES

1. Baumgart DC, Carding SR. Inflammatory bowel disease: cause and immunobi-ology. Lancet 2007;369:1627–40.
2. Danese S, Fiocchi C. Ulcerative colitis. N Engl J Med 2011;365:1713–25.
3. Abraham C, Cho JH. Inflammatory bowel disease. N Engl J Med 2009;361:2066–78.
4. Danese S. New therapies for inflammatory bowel disease: from the bench to the bedside. Gut 2012;61:918–32.
5. Bouguen G, Levesque BG, Pola S, et al. Endoscopic assessment and treating to target increase the likelihood of mucosal healing in patients with Crohn's disease. Clin Gastroenterol Hepatol 2014;12(6):978–85.
6. Bouguen G, Levesque BG, Pola S, et al. Feasibility of endoscopic assessment and treating to target to achieve mucosal healing in ulcerative colitis. Inflamm Bowel Dis 2014;20(2):231–9.
7. Neurath MF, Travis SP. Mucosal healing in inflammatory bowel diseases: a systematic review. Gut 2012;61:1619–35.
8. Dulai PS, Siegel CA, Dubinsky MC. Balancing and communicating the risks and benefits of biologics in pediatric inflammatory bowel disease. Inflamm Bowel Dis 2013;19:2927–36.
9. Siegel CA. Shared decision making in inflammatory bowel disease: helping patients understand the tradeoffs between treatment options. Gut 2012;61:459–65.
10. Dulai PS, Thompson KD, Blunt HB, et al. Risks of serious infection or lymphoma with anti-tumor necrosis factor therapy for pediatric inflammatory bowel disease: a systematic review. Clin Gastroenterol Hepatol 2014. [Epub ahead of print].
11. Pedersen N, Duricova D, Elkjaer M, et al. Risk of extra-intestinal cancer in inflammatory bowel disease: meta-analysis of population-based cohort studies. Am J Gastroenterol 2010;105:1480–7.
12. Jess T, Horvath-Puho E, Fallingborg J, et al. Cancer risk in inflammatory bowel disease according to patient phenotype and treatment: a Danish population-based cohort study. Am J Gastroenterol 2013;108:1869–76.
13. Kappelman MD, Farkas DK, Long MD, et al. Risk of cancer in patients with inflammatory bowel diseases: a nationwide population-based cohort study with 30 years of follow-up evaluation. Clin Gastroenterol Hepatol 2014;12(2):265–73.e1.
14. Bernstein CN, Blanchard JF, Kliewer E, et al. Cancer risk in patients with inflammatory bowel disease: a population-based study. Cancer 2001;91:854–62.

15. Lewis JD, Bilker WB, Brensinger C, et al. Inflammatory bowel disease is not associated with an increased risk of lymphoma. Gastroenterology 2001;121:1080–7.

16. Herrinton LJ, Liu L, Weng X, et al. Role of thiopurine and anti-TNF therapy in lymphoma in inflammatory bowel disease. Am J Gastroenterol 2011;106:2146–53.

17. Singh S, Nagpal SJ, Murad MH, et al. Inflammatory bowel disease is associated with an increased risk of melanoma: a systematic review and meta-analysis. Clin Gastroenterol Hepatol 2014;12(2):210–8.

18. Long MD, Martin CF, Pipkin CA, et al. Risk of melanoma and nonmelanoma skin cancer among patients with inflammatory bowel disease. Gastroenterology 2012;143:390–9.e1.

19. Kandiel A, Fraser AG, Korelitz BI, et al. Increased risk of lymphoma among inflammatory bowel disease patients treated with azathioprine and 6-mercaptopurine. Gut 2005;54:1121–5.

20. Beaugerie L, Brousse N, Bouvier AM, et al. Lymphoproliferative disorders in patients receiving thiopurines for inflammatory bowel disease: a prospective observational cohort study. Lancet 2009;374:1617–25.

21. Peyrin-Biroulet L, Khosrotehrani K, Carrat F, et al. Increased risk for nonmelanoma skin cancers in patients who receive thiopurines for inflammatory bowel disease. Gastroenterology 2011;141:1621–8.e1–5.

22. Bouguen G, Chevaux JB, Peyrin-Biroulet L. Recent advances in cytokines: therapeutic implications for inflammatory bowel diseases. World J Gastroenterol 2011;17:547–56.

23. Sandborn WJ, Hanauer SB. Antitumor necrosis factor therapy for inflammatory bowel disease: a review of agents, pharmacology, clinical results, and safety. Inflamm Bowel Dis 1999;5:119–33.

24. Peyrin-Biroulet L, Deltenre P, de Suray N, et al. Efficacy and safety of tumor necrosis factor antagonists in Crohn's disease: meta-analysis of placebo-controlled trials. Clin Gastroenterol Hepatol 2008;6:644–53.

25. Osterman MT, Sandborn WJ, Colombel JF, et al. Increased risk of malignancy with adalimumab combination therapy, compared with monotherapy, for Crohn's disease. Gastroenterology 2014;146(4):941–9.

26. Siegel CA, Marden SM, Persing SM, et al. Risk of lymphoma associated with combination anti-tumor necrosis factor and immunomodulator therapy for the treatment of Crohn's disease: a meta-analysis. Clin Gastroenterol Hepatol 2009;7:874–81.

27. Marehbian J, Arrighi HM, Hass S, et al. Adverse events associated with common therapy regimens for moderate-to-severe Crohn's disease. Am J Gastroenterol 2009;104:2524–33.

28. Stallmach A, Hagel S, Gharbi A, et al. Medical and surgical therapy for inflammatory bowel disease in the elderly–prospects and complications. J Crohns Colitis 2011;5:177–88.

29. Lichtenstein GR, Feagan BG, Cohen RD, et al. Drug therapies and the risk of malignancy in Crohn's disease: results from the TREAT registry. Am J Gastroenterol 2014;109(2):212–23.

30. Kotlyar DS, Osterman MT, Diamond RH, et al. A systematic review of factors that contribute to hepatosplenic T-cell lymphoma in patients with inflammatory bowel disease. Clin Gastroenterol Hepatol 2011;9:36–41.e1.

31. Selvaraj SA, Chairez E, Wilson LM, et al. Use of case reports and the Adverse Event Reporting System in systematic reviews: overcoming barriers to assess the link between Crohn's disease medications and hepatosplenic T-cell lymphoma. Syst Rev 2013;2:53.

32. Deepak P, Sifuentes H, Sherid M, et al. T-cell non-Hodgkin's lymphomas reported to the FDA AERS with tumor necrosis factor-alpha (TNF-alpha) inhibitors: results of the REFURBISH study. Am J Gastroenterol 2013;108:99–105.
33. Rogers HW, Weinstock MA, Harris AR, et al. Incidence estimate of nonmelanoma skin cancer in the United States, 2006. Arch Dermatol 2010;146:283–7.
34. Long MD, Kappelman MD, Pipkin CA. Nonmelanoma skin cancer in inflammatory bowel disease: a review. Inflamm Bowel Dis 2011;17:1423–7.
35. Long MD, Herfarth HH, Pipkin CA, et al. Increased risk for non-melanoma skin cancer in patients with inflammatory bowel disease. Clin Gastroenterol Hepatol 2010;8:268–74.
36. Peyrin-Biroulet L, Chevaux JB, Bouvier AM, et al. Risk of melanoma in patients who receive thiopurines for inflammatory bowel disease is not increased. Am J Gastroenterol 2012;107:1443–4.
37. Gisbert JP, Panes J. Loss of response and requirement of infliximab dose intensification in Crohn's disease: a review. Am J Gastroenterol 2009;104:760–7.
38. Billioud V, Sandborn WJ, Peyrin-Biroulet L. Loss of response and need for adalimumab dose intensification in Crohn's disease: a systematic review. Am J Gastroenterol 2011;106:674–84.
39. Hynes RO. Integrins: bidirectional, allosteric signaling machines. Cell 2002;110:673–87.
40. Lobaton T, Vermeire S, Van Assche G, et al. Review article: anti-adhesion therapies for inflammatory bowel disease. Aliment Pharmacol Ther 2014;39(6):579–94.
41. Johnson JP. Cell adhesion molecules in the development and progression of malignant melanoma. Cancer Metastasis Rev 1999;18:345–57.
42. Schweikert A, Kremer M, Ringel F, et al. Primary central nervous system lymphoma in a patient treated with natalizumab. Ann Neurol 2009;66:403–6.
43. Bozic C, LaGuette J, Panzara MA, et al. Natalizumab and central nervous system lymphoma: no clear association. Ann Neurol 2009;66:261–2.
44. Panzara MA, Bozic C, Sandrock AW. More on melanoma with transdifferentiation. N Engl J Med 2008;359:99 [author reply: 99–100].
45. Sandborn WJ, Feagan BG, Rutgeerts P, et al. Vedolizumab as induction and maintenance therapy for Crohn's disease. N Engl J Med 2013;369:711–21.
46. Feagan BG, Rutgeerts P, Sands BE, et al. Vedolizumab as induction and maintenance therapy for ulcerative colitis. N Engl J Med 2013;369:699–710.
47. Cominelli F. Inhibition of leukocyte trafficking in inflammatory bowel disease. N Engl J Med 2013;369:775–6.
48. Takeda. FDA Briefing Document: Joint Meeting of the Gastrointestinal Drugs Advisory Committee and the Drug Safety and Risk Management Advisory Committee. Deerfield, September 9, 2013.
49. Tillack C, Ehmann LM, Friedrich M, et al. Anti-TNF antibody-induced psoriasiform skin lesions in patients with inflammatory bowel disease are characterised by interferon-gamma-expressing Th1 cells and IL-17A/IL-22-expressing Th17 cells and respond to anti-IL-12/IL-23 antibody treatment. Gut 2014;63(4):567–77.
50. Sandborn WJ, Feagan BG, Fedorak RN, et al. A randomized trial of ustekinumab, a human interleukin-12/23 monoclonal antibody, in patients with moderate-to-severe Crohn's disease. Gastroenterology 2008;135:1130–41.
51. Toedter GP, Blank M, Lang Y, et al. Relationship of C-reactive protein with clinical response after therapy with ustekinumab in Crohn's disease. Am J Gastroenterol 2009;104:2768–73.

52. Papp KA, Griffiths CE, Gordon K, et al. Long-term safety of ustekinumab in patients with moderate-to-severe psoriasis: final results from 5 years of follow-up. Br J Dermatol 2013;168:844–54.

53. Sandborn WJ, Ghosh S, Panes J, et al. A phase 2 study of tofacitinib, an oral Janus kinase inhibitor, in patients with Crohn's disease. Clin Gastroenterol Hepatol 2014. [Epub ahead of print].

54. Sandborn WJ, Ghosh S, Panes J, et al. Tofacitinib, an oral Janus kinase inhibitor, in active ulcerative colitis. N Engl J Med 2012;367:616–24.

55. Pfizer. FDA Report: Advisory Committee Meeting Briefing Document–Tofacitinib for the Treatment of Rheumatoid Arthritis NDA 203214. May 9, 2012.

56. Askling J, Brandt L, Lapidus A, et al. Risk of haematopoietic cancer in patients with inflammatory bowel disease. Gut 2005;54:617–22.

57. Targownik LE, Bernstein CN. Infectious and malignant complications of TNF inhibitor therapy in IBD. Am J Gastroenterol 2013;108:1835–42 [quiz: 1843].

58. Williams CJ, Peyrin-Biroulet L, Ford AC. Systematic review with meta-analysis: malignancies with anti-tumour necrosis factor-alpha therapy in inflammatory bowel disease. Aliment Pharmacol Ther 2014;39:447–58.

59. Colombel JF, Sandborn WJ, Reinisch W, et al. Infliximab, azathioprine, or combination therapy for Crohn's disease. N Engl J Med 2010;362:1383–95.

60. Melmed GY, Spiegel BM, Bressler B, et al. The appropriateness of concomitant immunomodulators with anti-tumor necrosis factor agents for Crohn's disease: 1 size does not fit all. Clin Gastroenterol Hepatol 2010;8:655–9.

61. Clarke K, Regueiro M. Stopping immunomodulators and biologics in inflammatory bowel disease patients in remission. Inflamm Bowel Dis 2012;18:174–9.

62. Van Assche G, Magdelaine-Beuzelin C, D'Haens G, et al. Withdrawal of immunosuppression in Crohn's disease treated with scheduled infliximab maintenance: a randomized trial. Gastroenterology 2008;134:1861–8.

63. Buchbinder R, Barber M, Heuzenroeder L, et al. Incidence of melanoma and other malignancies among rheumatoid arthritis patients treated with methotrexate. Arthritis Rheum 2008;59:794–9.

64. Solomon DH, Kremer JM, Fisher M, et al. Comparative cancer risk associated with methotrexate, other non-biologic and biologic disease-modifying anti-rheumatic drugs. Semin Arthritis Rheum 2014;43:489–97.

65. Feagan BG, McDonald JW, Panaccione R, et al. Methotrexate in combination with infliximab is no more effective than infliximab alone in patients with Crohn's disease. Gastroenterology 2014;146:681–8.e1.

66. Ananthakrishnan AN, Cagan A, Gainer VS, et al. Mortality and extraintestinal cancers in patients with primary sclerosing cholangitis and inflammatory bowel disease. J Crohns Colitis 2014. [Epub ahead of print].

67. Ananthakrishnan AN, Cheng SC, Cai T, et al. Serum inflammatory markers and risk of colorectal cancer in patients with inflammatory bowel diseases. Clin Gastroenterol Hepatol 2014. [Epub ahead of print].

68. Mouli VP, Ananthakrishnan AN. Review article: vitamin D and inflammatory bowel diseases. Aliment Pharmacol Ther 2014;39:125–36.

69. Ananthakrishnan AN, Cagan A, Gainer VS, et al. Normalization of plasma 25-hydroxy vitamin D is associated with reduced risk of surgery in Crohn's disease. Inflamm Bowel Dis 2013;19:1921–7.

70. Ananthakrishnan AN, Cheng SC, Cai T, et al. Association between reduced plasma 25-hydroxy vitamin D and increased risk of cancer in patients with inflammatory bowel diseases. Clin Gastroenterol Hepatol 2014;12(5):821–7.

71. Bernstein CN. Should patients with inflammatory bowel disease take vitamin D to prevent cancer? Clin Gastroenterol Hepatol 2014;12(5):828–30.
72. Beaugerie L, Carrat F, Colombel JF, et al. Risk of new or recurrent cancer less than immunosuppressive therapy in patients with IBD and previous cancer. Gut 2013. [Epub ahead of print].
73. Dixon WG, Watson KD, Lunt M, et al. Influence of anti-tumor necrosis factor therapy on cancer incidence in patients with rheumatoid arthritis who have had a prior malignancy: results from the British Society for Rheumatology Biologics Register. Arthritis Care Res (Hoboken) 2010;62:755–63.
74. Strangfeld A, Hierse F, Rau R, et al. Risk of incident or recurrent malignancies among patients with rheumatoid arthritis exposed to biologic therapy in the German biologics register RABBIT. Arthritis Res Ther 2010;12:R5.
75. Dignass A, Van Assche G, Lindsay JO, et al. The second European evidence-based consensus on the diagnosis and management of Crohn's disease: current management. J Crohns Colitis 2010;4:28–62.
76. Lichtenstein GR, Hanauer SB, Sandborn WJ. Management of Crohn's disease in adults. Am J Gastroenterol 2009;104:465–83 [quiz: 464, 484].
77. Khan N, Abbas AM, Lichtenstein GR, et al. Risk of lymphoma in patients with ulcerative colitis treated with thiopurines–a nationwide retrospective cohort study. Gastroenterology 2013;145:1007–15.e3.

Miscellaneous Adverse Events with Biologic Agents (Excludes Infection and Malignancy)

Joseph D. Feuerstein, MD, Adam S. Cheifetz, MD*

KEYWORDS

- Anti-tumor necrosis factor • Infliximab • Adalimumab • Golimumab
- Certolizumab pegol • Complications • Infusion reactions • Autoimmune disease

KEY POINTS

- The risks of nonmalignant, noninfectious complications secondary to anti-tumor necrosis factor (TNF) therapy are low.
- The most frequent complications are infusion reactions and injection site reactions.
- Autoantibodies are frequently found, but true drug-induced lupus erythematosus is rare.
- Paradoxic psoriasiform reactions to anti-TNF are being described more frequently and appear to be a class effect.
- Most complications do not require cessation of anti-TNF therapy.

INTRODUCTION

Anti-tumor necrosis factor-α (anti-TNF) agents are frequently used in the treatment of inflammatory bowel disease (IBD). Currently, there are 4 anti-TNF therapies that are Food and Drug Administration (FDA)-approved for moderate to severe IBD: infliximab and adalimumab for both Crohn disease and ulcerative colitis, golimumab for ulcerative colitis, and certolizumab pegol for Crohn disease. Although these agents are efficacious, they are associated with a low risk for adverse events, the most common of which are injection-site and infusion reactions. In most situations, the benefit of anti-TNF agents outweighs the rare risk of complications. For most noninfectious, nonmalignant adverse events, cessation of anti-TNF therapy typically leads to improvement or resolution of drug-induced complications.[1,2] In this article, the current knowledge

Division of Gastroenterology, Department of Medicine, Center for Inflammatory Bowel Diseases, Beth Israel Deaconess Medical Center, Harvard Medical School, 330 Brookline Avenue, Rabb 425, Boston, MA 02215, USA
* Corresponding author.
E-mail address: acheifet@bidmc.harvard.edu

Gastroenterol Clin N Am 43 (2014) 543–563
http://dx.doi.org/10.1016/j.gtc.2014.05.002
0889-8553/14/$ – see front matter © 2014 Elsevier Inc. All rights reserved.

regarding the noninfectious and nonmalignant toxicities associated with anti-TNF agents is summarized.

BODY

Infusion Reactions

Infusion reactions to infliximab can be categorized based on their timing, pathogenesis, and severity. Most reactions are acute, nonimmune, and mild-to-moderate. Infusion reactions are classified as acute or delayed based on the timing of onset in relation to the infusion. Acute infusion reactions develop within 24 hours of the infusion with most occurring during the infusion. Delayed infusion reactions develop more than 24 hours following the infusion, with most occurring 5 to 10 days after an infusion.[3] Several infusion reactions are likely related to the presence of antibodies against the anti-TNF compound. The main risk factor for the development of antibodies to infliximab (ATI) formation is the episodic dosing of infliximab. In contrast, concomitant therapy with immunosuppressive agents (eg, azathioprine, mercaptopurine, or methotrexate) decreases the risk of ATI formation, and similarly, lowers the risk of infusion reactions.[4,5]

Acute Infusion Reactions

Acute infusion reactions can be classified as allergic reactions, immunoglobulin E (IgE)-mediated type 1 anaphylactic reactions, or nonimmune, rate-related reactions. True anaphylactic reactions are very rare.[3] To determine the pathophysiology of infusion reactions to infliximab, Cheifetz and colleagues[3] studied a cohort of 11 patients who had a total of 14 acute infusion reactions. All patients had normal serum tryptase levels, and serum IgE levels were normal in the 7 cases in which they were measured, suggesting that these infusion reactions were not due to classical allergic type 1 IgE-mediated hypersensitivity.[6] Similarly, a Danish group found no anti-infliximab IgE in 20 cases following severe infusion reactions.[6]

Epidemiology

The prevalence of acute infusion reactions to infliximab varies widely in the literature, ranging from 3% to 20%.[3,7–11] In the Crohn's Therapy, Resource, Evaluation, and Assessment Tool (TREAT) registry, 3% of infliximab infusions resulted in an acute infusion reaction, most of which were mild.[11] Similarly, Cheifetz and colleagues[3] and Colombel and colleagues[8] reported acute infusion reactions in 5% of patients at Mt Sinai Medical Center and 3.8% of patients treated at Mayo Clinic, respectively.

Classification and symptoms

Infusion reactions can also be classified based on their severity. Cheifetz and colleagues[3] developed a classification scheme based on symptoms (**Table 1**). In their cohort, most infusion reactions were classified as mild (51%), with 21% considered

Table 1 Classification of acute infusion reactions	
Mild	Flushing, dizziness, diaphoresis, nausea, palpitations, hyperemia
Moderate	Chest pain, hypertension (>20 mm Hg increase in systolic blood pressure), hypotension, fever, urticaria, dyspnea, chills, rash
Severe	Hypertension (>40 mm Hg increase in systolic blood pressure), hypotension, significant dyspnea, bronchospasm, stridor, wheezing, rigors

moderate, and 17% considered severe.[3] However, in the TREAT study, serious infusion reactions were seen infrequently.[11]

Prevention
Multiple factors have been shown to influence the development of infusion reactions. Utilization of an induction regimen (0, 2, 6 weeks), use of regular-scheduled maintenance dosing (nonepisodic), and concomitant immunomodulator administration all have been shown to decrease the risk of infusion reactions to infliximab by reducing the incidence of antibody formation.[4–6,12,13] Some experts advocate the use of combination therapy for at least 6 months to help mitigate the immune response and prevent antibody formation. When possible, episodic therapy should be avoided, because it appears to increase the risk of antibody formation. Routine premedication with corticosteroids and antihistamines has not been shown to decrease the risk of infusion reactions.[14,15]

Treatment
Although infusion reactions can be severe and life-threatening, the need to discontinue anti-TNF therapy is rare. In the ACCENT 1 trial, less than 3% of patients with infusion reactions stopped infliximab.[16] Similarly, Schaible and others[7,16,17] reported cessation of infliximab in less than 2% of patients.

The treatment of acute infusion reactions depends on the cause and severity of the reaction. **Fig. 1** details an algorithm for managing acute infusion reactions. As most reactions are nonimmune and rate-related, the infusions typically can be successfully completed. Any patients experiencing an infusion reaction should be administered intravenous fluids (normal saline) and have frequent monitoring of vital signs. Mild reactions can be managed by temporarily reducing the infusion rate. Once the symptoms resolve, the infusion rate can be increased slowly back to baseline. However, some physicians prefer to temporarily discontinue the infusion until all symptoms have abated. If necessary, acetaminophen or antihistamine can also be used. In more moderate reactions, the infusion should be discontinued, and acetaminophen, an antihistamine, and a systemic steroid should be administered. The infusion can then be restarted at a lower rate and increased slowly as long as symptoms do not recur. When severe reactions develop, the infusion should be discontinued. Immediate treatment with acetaminophen, a histamine blocker, and systemic steroids are warranted. If there is no evidence of anaphylaxis (wheezing, angioedema), then the infusion can be restarted if necessary. If anaphylaxis is present, epinephrine is necessary and should be given before corticosteroids. Advanced life support measures may be needed.[3] No attempt should be made to restart the infusion in the case of a true type I hypersensitivity reaction (anaphylaxis).

Re-treatment
Once an infusion reaction to infliximab has occurred, premedication protocols can be used that allow for continued use of the medication.[3] **Fig. 2** provides an algorithm for pretreatment prophylaxis of patients following an infusion reaction. In the study by Cheifetz and colleauges,[3] all patients with mild to moderate reactions who received prophylactic medication before subsequent infusions were successfully reinfused. Following a severe infusion reaction, 3 patients were re-treated, one of whom developed a recurrent severe reaction despite prophylaxis.[3] Other groups have confirmed the efficacy of re-treatment protocols, with less than 3% of patients requiring discontinuation of infliximab because of infusion reactions.[10,15,18,19] Given that recurrent infusion reactions may occur despite prophylaxis, in severe infusion reactions, a very

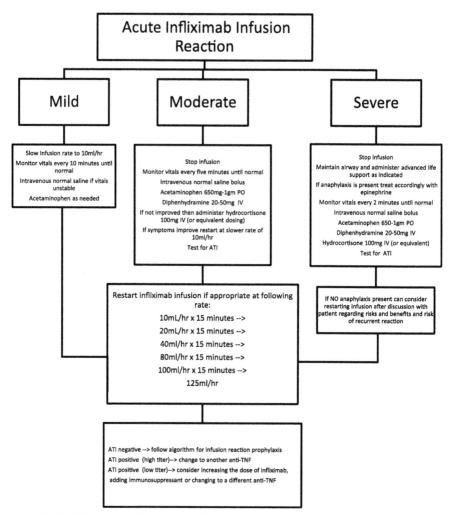

Fig. 1. Acute infusion reaction treatment protocol.

careful risk-benefit assessment must be made before considering continuation of infliximab.

Currently, if a patient has an acute infusion reaction, it is assessed if ATI are present. If ATI are present in significant concentration, the patient is switched to another anti-TNF. If ATIs are not present, then the infliximab infusions using the prophylaxis protocols are often continued.

Delayed Infusion Reactions

Epidemiology

Delayed infusion reactions typically occur 5 to 7 days (range, 1–14) after an infusion. They likely represent a mild type III immune complex reaction and have also been referred to as serum sickness-like reactions.[3,12] Delayed infusion reactions have been reported in 1% to 3% of patients treated with infliximab.[3,8,9,16] Although some older studies reported rates as high as 27%, this was likely attributable to use of a

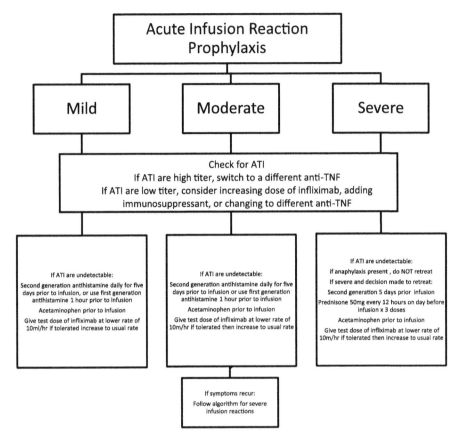

Fig. 2. Acute infusion reaction prophylaxis protocol.

liquid formulation of infliximab that is no longer available and to the use of episodic dosing protocols.[3,12,13] Similar to acute infusion reactions, delayed infusion reactions likely result from ATI formation. Risk factors include the episodic dosing of infliximab, delays in the routine infusion schedule of infliximab, and lack of a concomitant immunomodulator.[3,12,13,20]

Symptoms and treatment

Symptoms of delayed infusion reactions can be quite variable. The most common complaints include joint pains, rash, arthritis, myalgias, jaw pain, fatigue, headaches, edema, sore throat, and fever.[3,8] Delayed infusion reactions must be differentiated from viral syndromes, drug-induced lupus, and extra-intestinal manifestations of IBD.

Most delayed infusion reactions do not require specific treatment. For mild symptoms, acetaminophen can be administered. Patients with persistent, severe joint pains or arthritis may require a short course of corticosteroids. There are very little data regarding re-treatment of patients following a delayed infusion reaction, but some studies have shown that a delayed infusion reaction often leads to complete cessation of infliximab treatment. In one study, nearly 50% of patients who stopped infliximab did so because of a delayed infusion reaction.[21] In a separate study, the same group showed a discontinuation rate of 92% following a delayed infusion reaction.[10] As with acute infusion reactions, the authors' practice is to assess for ATI in this setting. There are very few data regarding re-treatment of patients following a delayed infusion reaction. In the authors' practice, they proceed with reinfusion so long as ATI are minimal or absent.

Prevention
Prevention of delayed infusion reactions is predicated on avoiding antibody development to infliximab (induction and maintenance infusions and use of concomitant immunomodulator) as described above.

Injection Site Reactions

Epidemiology
Injection site reactions are a frequent side effect of the self-injectable anti-TNF agents (adalimumab, golimumab, certolizumab pegol), with studies showing an incidence ranging from 1% to nearly 40%,[22–26] and most occur during the induction phase.[27] Higher rates of injection site reactions may be seen with adalimumab versus certolizumab pegol (2%–3%) or golimumab (3%–6%).[26,28–30] The pathophysiology of these reactions is usually traumatic but may also be related to a mild delayed hypersensitivity reaction.[31] Most of the injection site reactions are mild and do not lead to drug discontinuation.

Symptoms and treatment
Symptoms of injection site reactions include burning, pain, pruritus, erythema, swelling, bruising, irritation, and nonspecific complaints. Rarely, a hematoma may develop. Typically, the reactions last for 3 to 5 days and result in minor discomfort.[28] Symptomatic reactions can be treated with topical lidocaine and ice. In persistent cases, topical corticosteroids may be effective. If injection site reactions recur, pretreatment with ice and/or topical lidocaine can be prescribed, and the injection site location should be varied. Even in recurrent cases, injection site reactions rarely require cessation of anti-TNF.[28,32]

AUTOIMMUNE COMPLICATIONS

Anti-TNF agents have been associated with the development of autoantibodies and autoimmune conditions, which is discussed below.[33] Although autoantibodies alone do not cause alarm, in rare cases, autoimmune diseases may occur. However, given the rarity of these conditions and unclear significance of asymptomatic autoantibodies, routine testing for autoantibodies is not recommended.

Autoantibodies

Antinuclear antibody
Antinuclear antibody (ANA) is elevated at baseline in many of the conditions for which anti-TNF therapy is indicated. However, the prevalence of ANA positivity increases with the use of an anti-TNF. In patients with rheumatoid arthritis (RA), ANA-positive tests increased from 40% before infliximab therapy to 80% after therapy.[34,35] In seronegative spondyloarthropathies, the prevalence of ANA is only 8%, but treatment with infliximab has been shown to increase this prevalence to 46%.[34,35] Similarly, Vermeire and colleagues[33] reported a baseline prevalence of ANA in 7.2% of their 125 patients with IBD treated with infliximab. By 24 months of treatment with infliximab, 56.8% of patients had developed a positive ANA. In these cases, nearly 50% of the new ANA developed following the first infusion, and approximately 80% became ANA-positive within 3 infusions.[33] Beigel and colleagues[36] reported a prevalence of ANA positivity in 44% of patients with IBD treated with either infliximab or adalimumab. In contrast,

the CLASSIC II study reported new ANA in 19% after 56 weeks of therapy with adalimumab.[23] Schreiber and colleagues[30] noted 8% of patients developed new ANA at 26 weeks on certolizumab pegol compared with 1% in the placebo arm. Golimumab may have a lower rate of ANA development of only 3.5%.[29]

Anti-double-stranded DNA antibody

Anti-TNF therapy also appears to increase the rate of anti-double-stranded DNA antibody (anti-dsDNA) formation. Infliximab-associated anti-dsDNA ranges from 3% to more than 30%.[33,36–38] Although the rates for adalimumab-induced anti-dsDNA was 19%, both certizolizumab pegol and golimumab reported rates of 0.5% to 1%.[23,29,30]

Anti-cardiolipin and antihistone antibodies

Anticardiolipin antibodies (ACL) and antihistone antibodies may also be elevated because of anti-TNF therapy. In patients with RA treated with infliximab or etanercept, Jonsdottir and colleagues[39] reported an increase in ACL from 16% to 26%.

In refractory spondyloarthropathies treated with infliximab, Sellam and colleagues[40] found an increase in antihistone antibodies from 29% to 57%. In patients with IBD treated with either infliximab or adalimumab, 20.9% developed new-onset antihistone antibodies.[33]

Drug-induced Lupus Erythematosus

Despite how common autoantibody formation is, the development of drug-induced lupus erythematosus (DILE) is rare.

Epidemiology

DILE has been reported in patients treated with infliximab, etanercept, adalimumab, and golimumab.[41,42] In the BIOGEAS Spanish registry of biologics used to treat rheumatologic conditions, DILE was reported in 105 patients, of whom 43% were on infliximab, 35% on etanercept, and 21% on adalimumab.[41]

The incidence of DILE associated with anti-TNF is rare, ranging from 0.19% to 1.6%.[8,33,43,44] In Vermeire's cohort of 125 patients with IBD and a positive ANA, only 1.6% (n = 2) of patients on infliximab developed DILE.[33] In Colombel's series of 500 patients with Crohn disease on infliximab, DILE was reported in 0.6% (n = 3) of patients.[8] Recently, Yanai and colleagues[45] reported a higher rate of new-onset DILE (6.9%) in a cohort of 289 patients with IBD treated with infliximab or adalimumab. It is unclear if the higher rate is due to better reporting of DILE or to a referral bias.[45]

The mean time of onset of DILE is 14 to 16 months (range, 1–52 months).[46,47] DILE appears to be more prevalent in women.[45,46] Subramanian and coworkers[46] reported on 13 patients with IBD and DILE, of whom most were women with high titers of ANA and anti-dsDNA.

Symptoms

Symptoms of DILE include polyarthralgias, myalgias, serositis, fever, fatigue, or nonspecific rashes.[2,33,45,48] The most common presenting symptoms are symmetric polyarthralgias.[46,47] In contrast, typical lupus most commonly presents with a classic malar rash, discoid rash, alopecia, photosensitivity, and oral ulcers and may have systemic involvement of the kidneys and/or central nervous system (CNS).[45]

Diagnosis

Most patients with DILE do not fulfill the American College of Rheumatology diagnostic criteria for systemic lupus erythematosus, and there are no official diagnostic criteria for anti-TNF-induced lupus. However, De Bandt and colleagues[43] proposed a set of diagnostic criteria for DILE secondary to anti-TNF therapy (**Table 2**).[47] In

Table 2	
Proposed criteria for drug induced-lupus	
Patient currently being treated with anti-TNF	
Temporal relationship between clinical manifestations and anti-TNF therapy	
Presence of at least 1 serologic criteria for SLE per the American College of Rheumatology	ANA or anti-dsDNA
Presence of at least 1 nonserologic criteria for SLE per the American College of Rheumatology	Arthritis, serositis, hematologic disorder, malar rash

Data from De Bandt M, Sibilia J, Le Loët X, et al. Systemic lupus erythematosus induced by anti-tumour necrosis factor alpha therapy: a French national survey. Arthritis Res Ther 2005;7:R545; and Wetter DA, Davis MD. Lupus-Like Syndrome Attributable to Anti-Tumor Necrosis Factor α Therapy in 14 Patients During an 8-Year Period at Mayo Clinic. Mayo Clin Proc 2009;84(11):979–84.

Subramanian's cohort of patients on anti-TNF with DILE, positive autoantibodies and polyarthralgias followed by serositis were the most frequently present criteria.[46] The most commonly detected autoantibodies were ANA and anti-dsDNA; less frequently, anti-histone Ab titers are elevated, a finding typically associated with classic DILE.[43,45,46]

Treatment

The mainstay of therapy for DILE is cessation of the anti-TNF agent.[33,45–47] If symptoms persist, use of steroids or immunosuppressive therapy is effective.[43,45–47] Once symptoms resolve, re-treatment with another anti-TNF seems reasonable, although this recommendation is based on a small number of cases. In the Mayo Clinic series, 5 patients were rechallenged with an anti-TNF (adalimumab or etanercept) and 80% did well. The one patient who developed recurrent DILE was rechallenged with infliximab rather than with a different anti-TNF agent.[47] In Subramanian's cohort of patients, 8 were rechallenged with a second anti-TNF, 6 with certolizumab pegol, and 2 with adalimumab. Of the 6 patients on certolizumab pegol, only one developed a recurrence of DILE, whereas 1 of the 2 patients treated with adalimumab developed a recurrence.[46] Similarly, Yanai's study reported rechallenging 14 patients with a different anti-TNF, of whom only one patient developed recurrent DILE.[45] Nevertheless, the follow-up in these studies was short. Thus, it remains unclear if DILE is a true class effect or a reaction to a specific anti-TNF agent. If, after discussion with the patient regarding the risks and benefits, a decision is made to restart an anti-TNF, then a second anti-TNF agent should be tried. However, the agent that led to the initial DILE should be avoided. Based on Subramanian's findings, certolizumab pegol may be the anti-TNF agent of choice for rechallenge following a DILE.

Vasculitis

Over 200 cases of vasculitis attributed to anti-TNF therapy have been reported in the literature or to the FDA Adverse Events Reporting System.[27,48–51] The largest cohort of anti-TNF-related vasculitis consists of 113 cases published by Ramos-Casals and colleagues[48]: 59 patients received etanercept, 47 received infliximab, 5 received adalimumab, and 2 received other agents. Other series have indicted multiple anti-TNF agents and, thus, vasculitis is presumed to be a class effect.[50,51]

The exact pathophysiology is unknown, but the leading theory is that anti-TNF and circulating TNF form immune complexes that deposit in smaller capillaries and lead to a type III hypersensitivity reaction and resulting vasculitis.[27,51]

Cutaneous Vasculitis

Epidemiology
Cutaneous vasculitis is the most frequent form of anti-TNF-associated vasculitis, but is extremely rare.[41,48,50] Approximately 90% of the vasculitis associated with anti-TNF is a cutaneous leukocytoclastic vasculitis.[41,48] The mean duration of anti-TNF therapy before developing vasculitis ranges from 9 to 38 weeks.[2,48,50,51]

Symptoms
Palpable purpura is the most common symptom and occurs in 80% of cases.[50,51] Other symptoms include ulcerated skin lesions, nodules, and a maculopapular rash.[48]

Treatment
Cessation of anti-TNF leads to resolution of the vasculitis in more than 60% to 70% of cases.[2,41,48–51] If symptoms persist, most cases appear to be responsive to systemic steroids with or without immunosuppressive therapy.[2,41,48]

It is unclear if anti-TNF therapy can be reinstituted after an anti-TNF-associated vasculitis. In one study, 67% (n = 6/9) of patients rechallenged with the same anti-TNF developed a recurrent vasculitis.[49] In contrast, in the cohort of Saint Marcoux and De Bandt of 9 patients who were rechallenged with a different anti-TNF, 67% tolerated the second agent without difficulty.[51] As with DILE, any attempt at retreatment should be done with a different anti-TNF agent.

Other Vasculitis

Although uncommon, other forms of vasculitis associated with anti-TNF therapy have been described in the literature. Rarely, glomerulonephritis has been reported after starting anti-TNF therapy. Stopping the anti-TNF and treating with combined steroids and immunosuppressive agents has resulted in improved kidney function.[51,52] If vasculitis is suspected, renal function and a urinalysis should be checked to rule out renal involvement. There have also been case reports of anti-TNF-induced Henoch-Schönlein purpura, discoid systemic lupus erythematosus, necrotizing cutaneous vasculitis, granulomatosis with polyangiitis, and cerebral thrombophlebitis.[1,34,50]

Joint Inflammation

Epidemiology
De novo joint pains without any other criteria for DILE have been reported in patients receiving anti-TNF therapy without an obvious flare of the underlying IBD. In a series of 1300 patients who received anti-TNF, 21 developed new disabling polyarthralgias.[37] The mean onset of arthralgias was 12 months from onset of therapy. However, it remains unclear if these represent unique symptoms or if they are related to extraintestinal manifestations of IBD, delayed infusion reactions, or DILE.

Symptoms
Symptoms include morning stiffness of the hands and wrists, but no synovitis. In 11 of the patients, ANA titer was greater than 1:280, but other criteria for DILE were lacking.

Treatment
Treatment involves changing to a different anti-TNF, corticosteroids, or immunomodulator therapy.[37]

DERMATOLOGIC COMPLICATIONS

Multiple dermatologic conditions have been associated with anti-TNF therapy. The most frequent complications are a paradoxic psoriasiform reaction and eczema. It is unclear how many dermatologic conditions are truly anti-TNF-induced or incidentally noted. Fortunately, most conditions respond to topical agents and do not require discontinuation of anti-TNF therapy. Only when symptoms are persistent and severe is cessation of anti-TNF warranted.

Psoriasis

Epidemiology

There are numerous reports of psoriasis developing during anti-TNF therapy. Because patients with IBD are at an increased risk of psoriasis, it may be difficult to ascertain how many cases of psoriasis are truly secondary to the anti-TNF therapy versus the underlying disease.[53] The reported prevalence of psoriasis on anti-TNF ranges from 0.6% to 5.3%.[10,54,55] In one study from France, 2% of patients with IBD on anti-TNF developed new-onset psoriasis over a period of 4 years.[56]

Psoriasis can occur at any time during anti-TNF therapy. The onset of psoriasis ranges from several days to up to 4 years after starting therapy.[37,54,57–59] In the study of patients with IBD by Rahier and colleagues,[56] the median time to onset of psoriasis was 17 months for infliximab, 12 months for adalimumab, and 4.5 months for certolizumab pegol. In contrast, in Cullen's review of the literature of anti-TNF-induced psoriasis in patients with IBD, the median time to onset of rash was 5 months for infliximab, 2.5 months for adalimumab, and 5 months for certolizumab pegol.[60] Patients who developed anti-TNF-related psoriasis were more likely to have a personal history of psoriasis, family history of psoriasis, or family/personal history of atopy, and Crohn disease and be female.[56,58–61]

Pathophysiology

The exact pathogenesis of anti-TNF-induced psoriasis is unknown. Given that changing to a different anti-TNF does not improve the psoriasis in most cases, it is likely a class effect.[32] One hypothesis is that in genetically predisposed individuals, anti-TNF therapy may act as the "second hit" phenomenon.[32] Studies have shown that TNF inhibition causes an increase in the production of interferon-α by dendritic cells, ultimately resulting in the development of psoriatic lesions.[56,60]

Symptoms

Although the appearance of idiopathic psoriasis is typically characterized by plaques symmetrically involving the scalp and extensor surfaces, anti-TNF-induced psoriasis has been described as pustular and localized to the palms and soles of the feet in more than 40% of cases.[28,32,59,60] Rahier and colleagues[56] and Cullen and colleagues[60] report other areas of involvement, including the scalp and the flexures. The psoriatic lesions can be painful and pruritic.[27] They can appear as scaly erythematous plaques or pustules on examination. Multiple other forms of psoriasis have also been reported, including plaque-type, guttate, and forms with nail involvement.[27,59,61]

Treatment

We recommend dermatologic consultation for cases of anti-TNF-induced psoriasis. Initial therapy involves the use of topical therapies: steroids, keratolytics, emollients, or ultraviolet lights.[27,56,62] However, topical therapies only are effective in 25% to 50% of cases.[56,58–60] If these therapies fail and the psoriasis is severe, cessation of anti-TNF is warranted.[27,37,57,59,60,62] Following anti-TNF withdrawal, the median time to complete resolution of psoriasis is 3 months.[56] Although changing to a different anti-TNF can be attempted, this often leads to recurrence of the psoriasis and is only successful in 15% of cases.[32,57,61,62]

Eczema

Epidemiology

In a review of patients with RA on anti-TNF therapy, 7% of patients developed new-onset eczema.[63] In patients with IBD, the incidence of anti-TNF-induced eczema was 3%.[56] Eczema occurred a median 12 months after initiation of infliximab and 6 months after adalimumab. It appeared to be more common in men, active smokers, and patients with a history of atopy.[56] The most common types of eczema included dyshidrotic eczema, contact dermatitis, nummular eczema, atopic dermatitis, or nonspecific.[63]

Pathophysiology

The exact pathogenesis of anti-TNF-induced eczema is unknown but presumed to be the same as that described for psoriasis.

Symptoms

The lesions are typically red, scaly, and crusted and involve the scalp, trunk, genitals, face, and flexures.[10,56] Symptoms are usually pruritus and pain as classically seen with eczema.[10]

Treatment

Most cases of eczema appear to respond to topical therapy.[56] If this fails, then steroids with or without oral immunosuppressants are often effective in inducing remission.[64] However, in severe cases of eczema, cessation of the anti-TNF may be necessary.[27,56,63]

Hypersensitivity Reactions

Rarely, type IV hypersensitivity reactions may occur and can range in severity from localized erythema multiforme to life-threatening Stevens Johnson syndrome and toxic epidermal necrolysis. Most cases reported to the FDA have been in female patients with underlying RA. The classic findings include erythema, blisters, erosions, and bullae involving the mucus membranes.[27]

Miscellaneous Dermatologic Reactions

Less commonly, nonspecific dermatologic reactions have been described in patients on anti-TNF therapy. These case reports have included dermatomyositis, lichen planus, alopecia, rosacea, oral ulcers, gingivitis, tongue discoloration, and rarely, cutaneous sarcoidosis.[27,32,65] Other rare dermatologic conditions reported include pyoderma gangrenosum, pustular folliculitis, erythema multiforme, lichenoid reaction, interface dermatitis, granuloma annulare, neutrophilic eccrine hidradenitis, and Sweet syndrome.[1,32] It remains unknown if there is a clear association between these reactions and the anti-TNF therapy.

NEUROLOGIC COMPLICATIONS

The true prevalence of neurologic complications associated with anti-TNF is unclear, as IBD alone carries an increased risk of neurologic complications.[53,66] The most commonly reported conditions are optic neuritis (80% of cases), multiple sclerosis, multiple sclerosis–like disorders, and peripheral neuropathies.[37,67–70]

Neurologic disorders can affect the CNS or the peripheral nervous system (PNS). Disorders affecting the CNS reported to occur on anti-TNF include multiple sclerosis, multiple sclerosis-like disorders, optic neuritis, and acute transverse myelitis. Neurologic disorders associated with anti-TNF that affect the PNS include Guillain-Barre syndrome, Miller Fisher syndrome, chronic inflammatory demyelinating polyneuropathy, mononeuritis multiplex, axonal sensorimotor polyneuropathy, Lewis-Sumner syndrome, and multifocal motor neuropathy with conduction block.[2,67,69–71]

Demyelinating Disorders

Epidemiology
The true prevalence of demyelinating CNS disorders following initiation of anti-TNF is unknown, as IBD itself carries an increased risk of demyelinating disease.[53,66] Gupta and colleagues[66] reported using the General Practice Research Database with 7988 patients with Crohn disease and 12,185 with ulcerative colitis, that both Crohn and ulcerative colitis had a higher odds ratio (Crohn, 1.54; 95% CI, 1.03–2.32; ulcerative colitis, 1.75; 95% CI, 1.28–2.39) compared with age-matched controls of developing demyelinating disease. The reported occurrence of demyelinating disease on anti-TNF therapy ranges from 0.05% to 0.2%.[2,69] In a Danish anti-TNF IBD cohort, 4 of 651 (0.6%) patients developed demyelinating disease, with only 1 (0.15%) confirmed case of multiple sclerosis.[72] Similarly, a large Spanish registry (21,425 patient-years) of biologic therapies in rheumatic diseases reported only 9 cases of demyelinating disease.[73] The overall incidence rate was 0.65 per 1000 patient-years for demyelinating diseases and 0.05 for the incidence of multiple sclerosis.[73] This incidence is similar to that reported for new-onset multiple sclerosis in the general population in Spain.[73–76]

Demyelinating disease can occur at any time but usually develops early on in the treatment, with a mean of 5 months after initiation of therapy (range, 1–15 months).[71]

Pathophysiology
The cause of anti-TNF-mediated multiple sclerosis is unknown, but multiple theories have been postulated. One theory is that the immune suppression may allow an infection to develop, resulting in the downstream cascade of events triggering multiple sclerosis. This triggering is based on the theory that anti-TNF itself does not cause demyelination but may bring out latent disease. Other theories hypothesize that anti-TNF agents are a direct trigger of multiple sclerosis.[2,69]

Symptoms
Symptoms of demyelination are nonspecific and include confusion, ataxia, dysesthesia, visual disturbances, gait disturbances, and parathesias.[34,71] Examination findings may include nerve palsies, optic neuritis, ascending motor neuropathy, and hemiparesis.

Treatment
When demyelinating conditions are strongly suspected, cessation of anti-TNF therapy is warranted. In most cases, symptoms improve with discontinuation of anti-TNF therapy.[71] Once a demyelinating condition develops, anti-TNF therapy should not be restarted.[71,77]

Other Neurologic Complications

Also reported in the literature to occur with anti-TNF, but without any clear causality, are seizures and encephalitis.[1,34]

LIVER COMPLICATIONS

Although anti-TNF-associated hepatotoxicity is rare, a study by Ghabril and colleagues[78] reported on 34 cases of drug-induced liver injury (DILI) secondary to infliximab (n = 26), etanercept (n = 4), and adalimumab (n = 6). Given the presence of DILI associated with multiple anti-TNF agents, the authors conclude that DILI may be a class effect of anti-TNF agents. A recent study of the most common causes of DILI found anti-TNF agents to be the third most common cause, occurring in 1 in 148 patients treated with anti-TNF.[79]

There have also been cases of autoimmune hepatitis reported with anti-TNF agents.[2,80–85] Treatment of autoimmune hepatitis includes steroids, immunosuppressive agents, and/or cessation of anti-TNF. In some cases, changing anti-TNF agents may result in resolution of autoimmune hepatitis and can be considered.[82–84] However, because autoimmune hepatitis has been associated with infliximab, adalimumab, and etanercept, it may represent a class effect.[81–83,85]

Given the potential complications resulting from hepatic injury, episodic monitoring of liver function tests has been advocated to identify early signs of rising transaminases.

HEMATOLOGIC COMPLICATIONS

Hematologic dyscrasias are rarely associated with anti-TNF therapy. Interestingly, most cases involve patients with rheumatologic conditions and not IBD.

Neutropenia

Neutropenia is the most commonly reported hematologic complication. Manufacturer data from clinical trials in IBD report neutropenia rates ranging from 0.6% to 0.9% for adalimumab, and 1.1% to 5.7% for infliximab.[86] Rates of neutropenia may be higher with etanercept and have been noted in 16% of patients.[87] In contrast, Hastings and colleagues[88] reported on 367 patients with inflammatory arthritis who were treated with etanercept (73%), infliximab (19%), and adalimumab (8%), and showed the development of neutropenia in 19% of patients. Severe neutropenia ($<1.5 \times 10^9$/L) occurred in 9% of cases, and less than 1% of patients with arthritis developed profound neutropenia ($<0.5 \times 10^9$/L).[88] In most cases, neutropenia is mild and transient.[1,88] Risk factors reported in the rheumatologic literature for neutropenia include patients who have a history of neutropenia or who developed neutropenia with other biologics or immunosuppressive agents.[1,86] The pathogenesis of this complication is unclear, but theories include antigranulocyte antibodies, increased peripheral consumption, direct bone marrow suppression, or suppression of neutrophil precursors.[86]

Treatment of persistent neutropenia and drug discontinuation is rarely necessary. Given the potentially higher rates of neutropenia reported in the rheumatologic literature, episodic monitoring of a patient's blood counts is recommended.

Thrombocytopenia

Thrombocytopenia associated with anti-TNF agents is rare. Bessissow and colleagues[86] reported 19 cases of thrombocytopenia mostly related to infliximab, but no cases resulted in any serious complications. Manufacturer data from clinical trials indicate an incidence of thrombocytopenia of 0.5%–1.9% of patients on infliximab and 0.1% of patients on adalimumab.[86] The pathogenesis of this complication is unclear, but theories include development of antiplatelet antibodies, increased platelet aggregation, accelerated platelet destruction, or direct bone marrow suppression.[86]

The reported cases of thrombocytopenia have been mild and of little clinical significance. Cessation of anti-TNF or additional therapies to treat the thrombocytopenia have not been reported as necessary.[89]

Pancytopenia and Aplastic Anemia

Although pancytopenia and aplastic anemia have been reported with etanercept and infliximab, these patients were all on combination therapy with immunosuppressive agents.[86] The exact association with anti-TNF is very unclear, but nonetheless, if aplastic anemia develops, drug cessation is indicated.[86]

Thrombosis

Although thrombotic events have been reported in patients treated with anti-TNF agents, a direct effect is difficult to establish. Most conditions in which anti-TNF agents are used are also prothrombotic conditions.[90–92] Bessissow and colleagues[86] identified 69 cases of venous thrombosis and 20 cases of arterial thrombosis in patients on anti-TNF. Timing of thrombosis in relation to anti-TNF therapy ranged from less than 1 week to nearly 3 years.[86] Although these cases were reported to be associated with anti-TNF, the underlying disease remains the more likely culprit. At this time, patients who develop a thrombosis on anti-TNF do not need to stop therapy unless recommended by a hematologist.

Miscellaneous Hematologic Complications

A hypereosinophilic state has been associated with anti-TNF therapy, but is of unclear significance.[86] There has also been one case report of idiopathic thrombocytopenic purpura with anti-TNF.[93]

OPHTHALMOLOGIC COMPLICATIONS

There are reports that anti-TNF may lead to inflammatory ocular disease, although causation is not clear. Reported complications include uveitis, scleritis, endogenous endophthalmitis, and rarely, sarcoidosis.[2,37,94] Optic neuritis is the most frequently seen ophthalmologic complication associated with anti-TNF. Wendling and colleagues[95] reported that most new-onset uveitis resolved without cessation of anti-TNF, which supports the theory that anti-TNF was not the culprit.

PULMONARY COMPLICATIONS

Several uncommon pulmonary adverse events have been reported with anti-TNF therapy.

Sarcoidosis

Case reports of new-onset sarcoidosis associated with etanercept, infliximab, and adalimumab have been reported in the rheumatology literature.[94,96–99] Initial symptoms are nonspecific, including dyspnea, nonproductive cough, erythema nodosum, parotid enlargement, and neuro-ocular manifestations.[94,97] Radiologically, the most common findings are mediastinal and hilar adenopathy, and less frequently, upper lobe opacities. The diagnosis is confirmed histologically by the presence of well-formed nonnecrotizing granulomas. Ultimately, sarcoidosis is a diagnosis of exclusion, once all infectious causes have been ruled out. Treatment includes discontinuation of anti-TNF therapy with or without systemic steroids.[97]

Interstitial Lung Disease

There have been several case reports of anti-TNF-induced interstitial lung disease.[48,100,101] However, many of these patients were treated with methotrexate or had rheumatologic conditions that have also been associated with interstitial lung disease. Recently, a large retrospective study of patients with immune-mediated inflammatory disorders did not demonstrate an increase in interstitial lung disease in patients on anti-TNF.[102] Based on this large review, it seems unlikely that interstitial lung disease is a significant complication of anti-TNF therapy.

Miscellaneous Pulmonary Complications

Case reports have been published that detail pulmonary hemorrhage, granulomatous lung disease, and bronchiolitis obliterans organizing pneumonia occurring during anti-TNF therapy, but no larger studies have shown such an association.[103]

CARDIAC COMPLICATIONS

Cardiac complications related to anti-TNF therapy are extremely rare. In fact, a meta-analysis by Barnabe and colleagues[104] indicated that patients with RA treated with anti-TNF were less likely to have cardiovascular events (ie, myocardial infarction, congestive heart failure, cerebrovascular accident) compared with those who were not treated with anti-TNF agents.

Congestive Heart Failure

Heart failure was reported as a possible adverse event of anti-TNF based on trials using these agents as a therapy for heart failure. A trial of etanercept and one of infliximab suggested that the medications may worsen underlying heart failure and increase the risk of mortality.[105,106] Based on these trials, anti-TNF is contraindicated in patients with New York Heart Association class III or IV congestive heart failure.[34] Interestingly, in RA, in which the risk of developing heart failure is higher, those treated with anti-TNF were less likely to develop heart failure than those not receiving anti-TNF (3.1% vs 3.8%).[107]

Miscellaneous Cardiac Complications

Anti-TNF agents have also been associated with both hypertension and hypotension, although the potential mechanism is unknown and any true causal relationship is unclear. In addition, there are case reports of pericarditis developing secondary to infliximab usage, but evidence to support a causal relationship is lacking.[108,109]

SUMMARY

The overall risk of developing nonmalignant, noninfectious complications to anti-TNF therapy is rare. Aside from infusion reactions, injection site reactions, eczema, and psoriasis, the risk of developing a significant reaction from anti-TNF therapy is unusual. In fact, it is still unclear how many of the reported side effects of anti-TNF therapy are a true drug effect versus an incidental finding associated with the underlying disease process. Causality has not been proven despite many reported potential associations. The anti-TNF medications are safe but need to be administered with prudent clinical judgment and with a clear discussion with the patient regarding the potential risks and benefits associated with the drug. Patients on anti-TNF should be monitored closely for any possible adverse events.

REFERENCES

1. Perez-Alvarez R, Pérez-de-Lis M, Ramos-Casals M. Biologics-induced autoimmune diseases. Curr Opin Rheumatol 2013;25:56–64.

2. Ramos-Casals M, Diaz-Lagares C, Cuadrado MJ, et al. Autoimmune diseases induced by biological agents: a double-edged sword? Autoimmun Rev 2010; 9:188–93.
3. Cheifetz A, Smedley M, Martin S, et al. The incidence and management of infusion reactions to infliximab: a large center experience. Am J Gastroenterol 2003; 98:1315–24.
4. Vermeire S, Noman M, Van Assche G, et al. Effectiveness of concomitant immunosuppressive therapy in suppressing the formation of antibodies to infliximab in Crohn's disease. Gut 2007;56:1226–31.
5. Kapetanovic MC, Larsson L, Truedsson L, et al. Predictors of infusion reactions during infliximab treatment in patients with arthritis. Arthritis Res Ther 2006;8: R131.
6. Steenholdt C, Svenson M, Bendtzen K, et al. Severe infusion reactions to infliximab: aetiology, immunogenicity and risk factors in patients with inflammatory bowel disease. Aliment Pharmacol Ther 2011;34:51–8.
7. Schaible TF. Long term safety of infliximab. Can J Gastroenterol 2000;14(Suppl C):29C–32C.
8. Colombel J-F, Loftus EV Jr, Tremaine WJ, et al. The safety profile of infliximab in patients with Crohn's disease: the Mayo clinic experience in 500 patients. Gastroenterology 2004;126:19–31.
9. Rutgeerts P, Sandborn WJ, Feagan BG, et al. Infliximab for induction and maintenance therapy for ulcerative colitis. N Engl J Med 2005;353:2462–76.
10. Fidder H, Schnitzler F, Ferrante M, et al. Long-term safety of infliximab for the treatment of inflammatory bowel disease: a single-centre cohort study. Gut 2009;58:501–8.
11. Lichtenstein GR, Feagan BG, Cohen RD, et al. Serious infection and mortality in patients with Crohn's disease: more than 5 years of follow-up in the TREAT™ registry. Am J Gastroenterol 2012;107:1409–22.
12. Kugathasan S, Levy MB, Saeian K, et al. Infliximab retreatment in adults and children with Crohn's disease: risk factors for the development of delayed severe systemic reaction. Am J Gastroenterol 2002;97:1408–14.
13. Baert F, Noman M, Vermeire S, et al. Influence of immunogenicity on the long-term efficacy of infliximab in Crohn's disease. N Engl J Med 2003;348: 601–8.
14. Sany J, Kaiser M, Jorgensen C, et al. Study of the tolerance of infliximab infusions with or without betamethasone premedication in patients with active rheumatoid arthritis. Ann Rheum Dis 2005;64:1647–9.
15. Wasserman MJ, Weber DA, Guthrie JA, et al. Infusion-related reactions to infliximab in patients with rheumatoid arthritis in a clinical practice setting: relationship to dose, antihistamine pretreatment, and infusion number. J Rheumatol 2004;31:1912–7.
16. Hanauer SB, Feagan BG, Lichtenstein GR, et al. Maintenance infliximab for Crohn's disease: the ACCENT I randomised trial. Lancet 2002;359:1541–9.
17. Kavanaugh A, Keenan G, DeWoody K, et al. Long-term follow-up of patients treated with remicade (infliximab) in clinical trials. Arthritis Rheum 2001; 44(Suppl):S81.
18. Lequerré T, Vittecoq O, Klemmer N, et al. Management of infusion reactions to infliximab in patients with rheumatoid arthritis or spondyloarthritis: experience from an immunotherapy unit of rheumatology. J Rheumatol 2006;33:1307–14.
19. Uthman I, Touma Z, El-Sayyad J, et al. Successful retreatment with infliximab in patients with prior severe infusion reactions. Clin Rheumatol 2006;25:540–1.

20. Han PD, Cohen RD. Managing immunogenic responses to infliximab. Drugs 2004;64:1767–77.
21. Schnitzler F, Fidder H, Ferrante M, et al. Long-term outcome of treatment with infliximab in 614 patients with Crohn's disease: results from a single-centre cohort. Gut 2009;58:492–500.
22. Colombel JF, Sandborn WJ, Rutgeerts P, et al. Adalimumab for maintenance of clinical response and remission in patients with Crohn's disease: the CHARM trial. Gastroenterology 2007;132:52–65.
23. Sandborn WJ, Hanauer SB, Rutgeerts P, et al. Adalimumab for maintenance treatment of Crohn's disease: results of the CLASSIC II trial. Gut 2007;56: 1232–9.
24. Sandborn WJ, Feagan BG, Marano C, et al. Subcutaneous golimumab maintains clinical response in patients with moderate-to-severe ulcerative colitis. Gastroenterology 2014;146:96–109.e1.
25. Sandborn WJ, Feagan BG, Marano C, et al. Subcutaneous golimumab induces clinical response and remission in patients with moderate-to-severe ulcerative colitis. Gastroenterology 2014;146:85–95.
26. Sandborn WJ, Feagan BG, Stoinov S, et al. Certolizumab pegol for the treatment of Crohn's disease. N Engl J Med 2007;357:228–38.
27. Moustou AE, Matekovits A, Dessinioti C, et al. Cutaneous side effects of anti-tumor necrosis factor biologic therapy: a clinical review. J Am Acad Dermatol 2009;61:486–504.
28. Kerbleski JF, Gottlieb AB. Dermatological complications and safety of anti-TNF treatments. Gut 2009;58:1033–9.
29. Janssen Simponi Perscribing Information. Available at: https://www.simponi.com/prescribing-information.pdf. Accessed March 4, 2014.
30. Schreiber S, Khaliq-Kareemi M, Lawrance IC, et al. Maintenance therapy with certolizumab pegol for Crohn's disease. N Engl J Med 2007;357:239–50.
31. Zeltser R, Valle L, Tanck C, et al. Clinical, histological, and immunophenotypic characteristics of injection site reactions associated with etanercept: a recombinant tumor necrosis factor α receptor: Fc fusion protein. Arch Dermatol 2001; 137:893–9.
32. Mocci G, Marzo M, Papa A, et al. Dermatological adverse reactions during anti-TNF treatments: focus on inflammatory bowel disease. J Crohns Colitis 2013; 7(10):769–79.
33. Vermeire S, Noman M, Van Assche G, et al. Autoimmunity associated with anti-tumor necrosis factor α treatment in Crohn's disease: a prospective cohort study. Gastroenterology 2003;125:32–9.
34. Desai SB, Furst DE. Problems encountered during anti-tumour necrosis factor therapy. Best Pract Res Clin Rheumatol 2006;20:757–90.
35. Lin J, Ziring D, Desai S, et al. TNFα blockade in human diseases: an overview of efficacy and safety. Clin Immunol 2008;126:13–30.
36. Beigel F, Schnitzler F, Paul Laubender R, et al. Formation of antinuclear and double-strand DNA antibodies and frequency of lupus-like syndrome in anti-TNF-α antibody-treated patients with inflammatory bowel disease. Inflamm Bowel Dis 2011;17:91–8.
37. Fiorino G, Danese S, Pariente B, et al. Paradoxical immune-mediated inflammation in inflammatory bowel disease patients receiving anti-TNF-α agents. Autoimmun Rev 2014;13:15–9.
38. Puertas-Abreu E, Polanco ER, Azocar M, et al. Onset of lupus like syndrome in patients with spondyloarthritis treated with anti-TNF-a. Int Arch Med 2012;5:7.

39. Jonsdottir T, Forslid J, van Vollenhoven A, et al. Treatment with tumour necrosis factor alpha antagonists in patients with rheumatoid arthritis induces anticardiolipin antibodies. Ann Rheum Dis 2004;63:1075–8.

40. Sellam J, Allanore Y, Batteux F, et al. Autoantibody induction in patients with refractory spondyloarthropathy treated with infliximab and methotrexate. Joint Bone Spine 2005;72:48–52.

41. Ramos-Casals M, Brito-Zerón P, Soto MJ, et al. Autoimmune diseases induced by TNF-targeted therapies. Best Pract Res Clin Rheumatol 2008;22:847–61.

42. Wilkerson E, Hazey MA, Bahrami S, et al. Golimumab-exacerbated subacute cutaneous lupus erythematosus. Arch Dermatol 2012;148:1186–90.

43. De Bandt M, Sibilia J, Le Loët X, et al. Systemic lupus erythematosus induced by anti-tumour necrosis factor alpha therapy: a French national survey. Arthritis Res Ther 2005;7:R545.

44. Schiff MH, Burmester GR, Kent J, et al. Safety analyses of adalimumab (HUMIRA) in global clinical trials and US postmarketing surveillance of patients with rheumatoid arthritis. Ann Rheum Dis 2006;65:889–94.

45. Yanai H, Shuster D, Calabrese E, et al. The incidence and predictors of lupus-like reaction in patients with IBD treated with anti-TNF therapies. Inflamm Bowel Dis 2013;19:2778–86.

46. Subramanian S, Yajnik V, Sands BE, et al. Characterization of patients with infliximab-induced lupus erythematosus and outcomes after retreatment with a second anti-TNF agent. Inflamm Bowel Dis 2011;17:99–104.

47. Wetter DA, Davis MD. Lupus-Like Syndrome Attributable to Anti-Tumor Necrosis Factor α Therapy in 14 Patients During an 8-Year Period at Mayo Clinic. Mayo Clin Proc 2009;84(11):979–84.

48. Ramos-Casals M, Brito-Zerón P, Munoz S, et al. Autoimmune diseases induced by TNF-targeted therapies: analysis of 233 cases. Medicine 2007;86:242–51.

49. Mohan N, Edwards ET, Cupps TR, et al. Leukocytoclastic vasculitis associated with tumor necrosis factor-alpha blocking agents. J Rheumatol 2004;31:1955–8.

50. Sokumbi O, Wetter DA, Makol A, et al. Vasculitis associated with tumor necrosis factor-α inhibitors. Mayo Clinic Proceedings 2012;87:739–45.

51. Saint Marcoux B, De Bandt M. Vasculitides induced by TNFα antagonists: a study in 39 patients in France. Joint Bone Spine 2006;73:710–3.

52. Simms R, Kipgen D, Dahill S, et al. ANCA-associated renal vasculitis following anti-tumor necrosis factor α therapy. Am J Kidney Dis 2008;51:e11–4.

53. Bernstein CN, Wajda A, Blanchard JF. The clustering of other chronic inflammatory diseases in inflammatory bowel disease: a population-based study. Gastroenterology 2005;129:827–36.

54. Ko JM, Gottlieb AB, Kerbleski JF. Induction and exacerbation of psoriasis with TNF-blockade therapy: a review and analysis of 127 cases. J Dermatolog Treat 2009;20:100–8.

55. Harrison MJ, Dixon WG, Watson KD, et al. Rates of new-onset psoriasis in patients with rheumatoid arthritis receiving anti-tumour necrosis factor α therapy: results from the British Society for Rheumatology Biologics Register. Ann Rheum Dis 2009;68:209–15.

56. Rahier JF, Buche S, Peyrin–Biroulet L, et al. Severe skin lesions cause patients with inflammatory bowel disease to discontinue anti-tumor necrosis factor therapy. Clin Gastroenterol Hepatol 2010;8:1048–55.

57. Fiorino G, Allez M, Malesci A, et al. Review article: anti TNF-α induced psoriasis in patients with inflammatory bowel disease. Aliment Pharmacol Ther 2009;29:921–7.

58. Denadai R, Teixeira FV, Steinwurz F, et al. Induction or exacerbation of psoriatic lesions during anti-TNF-α therapy for inflammatory bowel disease: a systematic literature review based on 222 cases. J Crohns Colitis 2013;7:517–24.

59. Steinwurz F, Denadai R, Saad-Hossne R, et al. Infliximab-induced psoriasis during therapy for Crohn's disease. J Crohns Colitis 2012;6:610–6.

60. Cullen G, Kroshinsky D, Cheifetz A, et al. Psoriasis associated with anti-tumour necrosis factor therapy in inflammatory bowel disease: a new series and a review of 120 cases from the literature. Aliment Pharmacol Ther 2011;34:1318–27.

61. Wollina U, Hansel G, Koch A, et al. Tumor necrosis factor-α inhibitor-induced psoriasis or psoriasiform exanthemata. Am J Clin Dermatol 2008;9:1–14.

62. Sfikakis P, Iliopoulos A, Elezoglou A, et al. Psoriasis induced by anti-tumor necrosis factor therapy: a paradoxical adverse reaction. Arthritis Rheum 2005; 52:2513–8.

63. Flendrie M, Vissers W, Creemers M, et al. Dermatological conditions during TNF-alpha-blocking therapy in patients with rheumatoid arthritis: a prospective study. Arthritis Res Ther 2005;7:R666–76.

64. Vestergaard C, Deleuran M, Kragballe K. Two cases of atopic dermatitis-like conditions induced in psoriasis patients treated with infliximab. J Eur Acad Dermatol Venereol 2007;21:1272–4.

65. Klein R, Rosenbach M, Kim EJ, et al. Tumor necrosis factor inhibitor-associated dermatomyositis. Arch Dermatol 2010;146:780–4.

66. Gupta G, Gelfand JM, Lewis JD. Increased risk for demyelinating diseases in patients with inflammatory bowel disease. Gastroenterology 2005;129:819–26.

67. Stübgen JP. Tumor necrosis factor-α antagonists and neuropathy. Muscle Nerve 2008;37:281–92.

68. Nozaki K, Silver RM, Stickler DE, et al. Neurological deficits during treatment with tumor necrosis factor-alpha antagonists. Am J Med Sci 2011;342:352–5.

69. Kaltsonoudis E, Voulgari PV, Konitsiotis S, et al. Demyelination and other neurological adverse events after anti-TNF therapy. Autoimmun Rev 2014;13:54–8.

70. Bosch X, Saiz A, Ramos-Casals M. Monoclonal antibody therapy-associated neurological disorders. Nat Rev Neurol 2011;7:165–72.

71. Mohan N, Edwards ET, Cupps TR, et al. Demyelination occurring during anti-tumor necrosis factor α therapy for inflammatory arthritides. Arthritis Rheum 2001;44:2862–9.

72. Andersen NN, Caspersen S, Jess T, et al. Occurrence of demyelinating diseases after anti-TNFα treatment of inflammatory bowel disease: a Danish Crohn Colitis Database study. J Crohns Colitis 2008;2:304–9.

73. Cruz Fernandez-Espartero M, Perez-Zafrilla B, Naranjo A, et al. Demyelinating disease in patients treated with TNF antagonists in rheumatology: data from BIOBADASER, a pharmacovigilance database, and a systematic review. Semin Arthritis Rheum 2011;41:524–33.

74. Benito-León J, Martin E, Vela L, et al. Multiple sclerosis in Mostoles, central Spain. Acta Neurol Scand 1998;98:238–42.

75. Casquero P, Villoslada P, Montalban X, et al. Frequency of multiple sclerosis in Menorca, Balearic Islands, Spain. Neuroepidemiology 2001;20:129–33.

76. Pardo PM, Latorre MP, López A, et al. Prevalence of multiple sclerosis in the province of Teruel, Spain. J Neurol 1997;244:182–5.

77. Cisternas M, Gutiérrez M, Jacobelli S. Successful rechallenge with anti-tumor necrosis factor α for psoriatic arthritis after development of demyelinating nervous system disease during initial treatment: comment on the article by Mohan et al. Arthritis Rheum 2002;46:3107–8.

78. Ghabril M, Bonkovsky HL, Kum C, et al. Liver injury from tumor necrosis factor-α antagonists: analysis of thirty-four cases. Clin Gastroenterol Hepatol 2013;11: 558–64.e3.

79. Björnsson ES, Bergmann OM, Björnsson HK, et al. Incidence, presentation, and outcomes in patients with drug-induced liver injury in the general population of Iceland. Gastroenterology 2013;144:1419–25.e3.

80. Czaja AJ. Drug-induced autoimmune-like hepatitis. Dig Dis Sci 2011;56:958–76.

81. Adar T, Mizrahi M, Pappo O, et al. Adalimumab-induced autoimmune hepatitis. J Clin Gastroenterol 2010;44:e20–2.

82. Goldfeld DA, Verna EC, Lefkowitch J, et al. Infliximab-induced autoimmune hepatitis with successful switch to adalimumab in a patient with Crohn's disease: the index case. Dig Dis Sci 2011;56:3386–8.

83. Grasland A, Sterpu R, Boussoukaya S, et al. Autoimmune hepatitis induced by adalimumab with successful switch to abatacept. Eur J Clin Pharmacol 2012;68: 895–8.

84. Becker H, Willeke P, Domschke W, et al. Etanercept tolerance in a patient with previous infliximab-induced hepatitis. Clin Rheumatol 2008;27:1597–8.

85. Fathalla BM, Goldsmith DP, Pascasio JM, et al. Development of autoimmune hepatitis in a child with systemic-onset juvenile idiopathic arthritis during therapy with etanercept. J Clin Rheumatol 2008;14:297–8.

86. Bessissow T, Renard M, Hoffman I, et al. Review article: non-malignant haematological complications of anti-tumour necrosis factor alpha therapy. Aliment Pharmacol Ther 2012;36:312–23.

87. Bathon JM, Martin RW, Fleischmann RM, et al. A comparison of etanercept and methotrexate in patients with early rheumatoid arthritis. N Engl J Med 2000;343: 1586–93.

88. Hastings R, Ding T, Butt S, et al. Neutropenia in patients receiving anti-tumor necrosis factor therapy. Arthritis Care Res (Hoboken) 2010;62:764–9.

89. Chen M, Holland MJ, Mir MR, et al. Frequency of thrombocytopenia in psoriasis patients treated with tumor necrosis factor-a inhibitors. J Drugs Dermatol 2011; 10:280–4.

90. Matta F, Singala R, Yaekoub AY, et al. Risk of venous thromboembolism with rheumatoid arthritis. Thromb Haemost 2009;101:134–8.

91. Nguyen GC, Sam J. Rising prevalence of venous thromboembolism and its impact on mortality among hospitalized inflammatory bowel disease patients. Am J Gastroenterol 2008;103:2272–80.

92. Solem CA, Loftus EV, Tremaine WJ, et al. Venous thromboembolism in inflammatory bowel disease. Am J Gastroenterol 2004;99:97–101.

93. Selby LA, Hess D, Shashidar H, et al. Crohn's disease, infliximab and idiopathic thrombocytopenic purpura. Inflamm Bowel Dis 2004;10:698–700.

94. Fonollosa A, Artaraz J, Les I, et al. Sarcoid intermediate uveitis following etanercept treatment: a case report and review of the literature. Ocul Immunol Inflamm 2012;20:44–8.

95. Wendling D, Paccou J, Berthelot JM, et al. New onset of uveitis during anti-tumor necrosis factor treatment for rheumatic diseases. Semin Arthritis Rheum 2011; 41(3):503–10.

96. Dhaille F, Viseux V, Caudron A, et al. Cutaneous sarcoidosis occurring during anti-TNF-alpha treatment: report of two cases. Dermatology 2010;220:234–7.

97. Massara A, Cavazzini L, La Corte R, et al. Sarcoidosis appearing during anti-tumor necrosis factor α therapy: a new "class effect" paradoxical phenomenon. Two case reports and literature review. Semin Arthritis Rheum 2010;39(4):313–9.

98. Tong D, Manolios N, Howe G, et al. New onset sarcoid-like granulomatosis developing during anti-TNF therapy: an under-recognised complication. Intern Med J 2012;42:89–94.

99. Toussirot E, Pertuiset E, Kantelip B, et al. Sarcoidosis occuring during anti-TNF-alpha treatment for inflammatory rheumatic diseases: report of two cases. Clin Exp Rheumatol 2008;26:471.

100. Perez-Alvarez R, Perez-de-Lis M, Diaz-Lagares C, et al. Interstitial lung disease induced or exacerbated by TNF-targeted therapies: analysis of 122 cases. Semin Arthritis Rheum 2011;41(2):256–64.

101. Panopoulos ST, Sfikakis PP. Biological treatments and connective tissue disease associated interstitial lung disease. Curr Opin Pulm Med 2011;17:362–7.

102. Herrinton LJ, Harrold LR, Liu L, et al. Association between anti-TNF-α therapy and interstitial lung disease. Pharmacoepidemiol Drug Saf 2013;22(4):394–402.

103. Ramos-Casals M, Perez-Alvarez R, Perez-de-lis M, et al. Pulmonary disorders induced by monoclonal antibodies in patients with rheumatologic autoimmune diseases. Am J Med 2011;124:386–94.

104. Barnabe C, Martin BJ, Ghali WA. Systematic review and meta-analysis: anti-tumor necrosis factor α therapy and cardiovascular events in rheumatoid arthritis. Arthritis Care Res 2011;63:522–9.

105. Mann DL, McMurray JJ, Packer M, et al. Targeted anticytokine therapy in patients with chronic heart failure results of the Randomized Etanercept Worldwide Evaluation (RENEWAL). Circulation 2004;109:1594–602.

106. Chung ES, Packer M, Lo KH, et al. Randomized, double-blind, placebo-controlled, pilot trial of infliximab, a chimeric monoclonal antibody to tumor necrosis factor-α, in patients with moderate-to-severe heart failure results of the anti-TNF Therapy Against Congestive Heart failure (ATTACH) Trial. Circulation 2003;107:3133–40.

107. Wolfe F, Michaud K. Heart failure in rheumatoid arthritis: rates, predictors, and the effect of anti-tumor necrosis factor therapy. Am J Med 2004;116:305–11.

108. Burke J, Kelleher B, Ramadan S, et al. Pericarditis as a complication of infliximab therapy in Crohn's disease. Inflamm Bowel Dis 2008;14:428–9.

109. Harney S, O'Shea F, FitzGerald O. Peptostreptococcal pericarditis complicating anti-tumour necrosis factor α treatment in rheumatoid arthritis. Ann Rheum Dis 2002;61:653–4.

Pharmacokinetics of Biologics and the Role of Therapeutic Monitoring

Kirk Lin, MD, MA, Uma Mahadevan, MD*

KEYWORDS

- Pharmacokinetics • Biologics • Inflammatory bowel disease
- Therapeutic drug monitoring

KEY POINTS

- Therapeutic drug monitoring (TDM) is an evidence-based strategy for managing biologic therapies in inflammatory bowel disease (IBD) after the loss of clinical response.
- Clinicians' understanding of the pharmacokinetics of biologic therapy and the application of TDM is instrumental in the optimal management of moderate-to-severely active IBD.
- The newest assays for monitoring anti-TNF therapy consistently demonstrate that serum drug and antidrug antibodies (ADA) levels correlate with endoscopic and biomarkers of disease activity, and furthermore predict sustained remission versus later loss of response.
- More data are necessary to determine the cost-effectiveness and clinical use of proactive TDM to optimize the induction and maintenance phases of therapy.

INTRODUCTION

Biologic therapies, including the anti–tumor necrosis factor (TNF)-α and cell adhesion molecule inhibitor (CAMi) drugs, have revolutionized the treatment of moderate-to-severe inflammatory bowel disease (IBD). Monoclonal antibodies are designed to inhibit inflammatory pathways instrumental in the pathophysiology of IBD, but not all patients respond to biologic therapy and many lose response over time. Clinical trials report that primary nonresponse to anti-TNF therapies occurs in 20% to 40% of patients with IBD, and loss of response (LOR) to anti-TNF therapy ranges from 10% to 50% per year.[1] Since the introduction of anti-TNF therapies, the strategy of empiric dose-escalation, either increasing the dose or frequency of administration, has been used to recapture clinical response in IBD. Clinical trials and series suggest that 60% to 90% will initially respond to dose-escalation, but 40% to 50% will again

UCSF Center for Colitis and Crohn's Disease, Division of Gastroenterology, Department of Medicine, University of California, San Francisco, 1701 Divisadero Street, San Francisco, CA 94115, USA
* Corresponding author.
E-mail address: uma.mahadevan@ucsf.edu

Gastroenterol Clin N Am 43 (2014) 565–579
http://dx.doi.org/10.1016/j.gtc.2014.05.007
0889-8553/14/$ – see front matter © 2014 Elsevier Inc. All rights reserved.

gastro.theclinics.com

lose response to therapy over the next 12 months.[2] Disparate clinical outcomes have been linked to serum drug and antidrug antibody (ADA) levels. Therapeutic drug monitoring (TDM) has emerged as a framework for understanding and responding to the variability in clinical response and remission.

ANTI-TNF BIOLOGIC AGENTS
Pharmacokinetics

TNF-α is a proinflammatory cytokine that mediates gut recruitment of neutrophils, procoagulation, and fibrinolytic cascades, and promotes granuloma formation. Given the pivotal role of TNF-α in the pathogenesis of IBD, the available array of anti–TNF-α biologics continues to expand. Infliximab (IFX; Remicade; Janssen, Malvern, PA), the earliest and most well-studied TNF-α inhibitor, is an intravenously (IV) administered chimeric monoclonal antibody comprised of a human constant region IgG$_1\kappa$ light chain linked to a mouse variable region. IFX exhibits linear pharmacokinetics, with a direct relation between administered doses and the maximum serum concentration and area under the concentration-time curve. Conversely, volume of distribution at steady state and clearance are independent of dose. At standard dosing (5 mg/kg) the median half-life is 7.7 to 9.5 days. Steady state is achieved by week 14 of treatment, and maintenance dosing does not demonstrate systemic accumulation.[3]

There are three subcutaneously (SC) administered anti-TNF biologic therapies for IBD: adalimumab (ADL) and certolizumab pegol (CZP) for Crohn disease (CD), and ADL and golimumab (GOL) for ulcerative colitis (UC). Similar to IFX, each demonstrates linear dose pharmacokinetics. ADL (Humira; Abbvie, Abbott Park, IL) is a recombinant IgG$_1$ antibody comprised of both a human constant region IgG$_1\kappa$ and human heavy and light chain variable regions. The drug distributes primarily in the extracellular space, with a bioavailability of 64% and half-life (T$_{1/2}$) of roughly 2 weeks.[4] CZP (Cimzia; UCB, Smyrna, GA) is a humanized Fab' fragment linked to polyethylene glycol resulting in high-affinity binding of TNF-α without an Fc region. It has a bioavailability of 80% after SC administration and T$_{1/2}$ of roughly 14 days.[5] GOL (Simponi; Janssen, Radnor, PA), the latest anti-TNF biologic, is a fully human IgG$_1$ antibody that in vitro has demonstrated higher affinity for soluble human TNF-α than its predecessors, IFX and ADL.[6] The reported median T$_{1/2}$ ranges from 7 to 20 days, with a volume of distribution that is body weight–dependent.[7] Although all anti-TNF therapies exhibit linear pharmacokinetics, there is substantial interindividual variability in serum drug concentration across biologics, even with weight-based and IV dosing.[4]

Assay technology

Traditional serum testing for anti-TNF drug and ADA concentrations has been performed with radioimmunoassay, solid-phase enzyme-linked immunosorbent assay, and bridging enzyme-linked immunosorbent assay technologies.[8] The older assay technology has notable limitations. First, false-negative results for ADA presence and underestimation of ADA levels may occur in the setting of drug interference. Second, distinguishing specific ADA binding of TNF-α from nonspecific binding of serum IgG requires incubation with enzyme-labeled antidrug idiotype antibodies.[9] The recent development of novel assays incorporating high-performance liquid chromatography and acid dissociation technology has enabled quantification of drug-complexed ADA in addition to "free" or excess ADA, thereby increasing overall diagnostic accuracy over prior solid-phase assays.[10] Newer assays also demonstrate marked blocking of nonspecific binding serum IgG without the application of antidrug idiotype antibodies. Despite technologic advances, the absence of a universal assay across studies has been implicated in the discrepant findings regarding the association between ADAs and clinical outcomes.

Mechanisms of drug clearance

The mechanisms of anti-TNF drug clearance have not been fully elucidated, but there is increasing appreciation that disease severity accelerates drug clearance. Direct proteolytic catabolism of anti-TNF drug within the reticuloendothelial system (RES) is believed to be a primary route of drug clearance.[11] Monoclonal antibodies cross-linked by antigen may undergo phagocytosis in the RES by receptors (Fc-γ) for the Fc portion of the IgG, with resultant lysosomal degradation. Increased protein catabolism within the RES is observed with increased systemic inflammation. In addition to clearance from systemic circulation, antibody clearance may also occur directly by membrane-bound antigen. TNF-α exists in soluble and membrane-bound form, with upregulation of serum and mucosal concentrations in active IBD. The concept of an "antigen sink" has been proposed, whereby circulating drug IgG becomes bound to membrane antigen, internalized into the cell, and degraded in lysosomes. Severe inflammation and diffuse ulcerative disease, marked by elevated C-reactive protein (CRP) and hypoalbuminemia, correlates with decreased serum drug concentration. A positive correlation between CRP levels and drug clearance has been demonstrated with IFX and ADL.[12] Baseline serum hypoalbuminemia has been linked to low serum IFX concentrations in severe hospitalized UC[13] and increased IFX clearance in CD.[14] Albumin and IgG_1 antibodies may compete for RES-mediated drug clearance by FcRn receptors; thus, increased FcRn receptor binding and drug clearance may occur in the setting of hypoalbuminemia. Low albumin levels may also be a surrogate marker of high TNF-α and severe inflammation, a disease phenotype marked by extensive ulceration and massive weeping of protein and electrolytes. Disease phenotype, in addition to severity, has been implicated to mediate drug clearance. Whereas IV administered IFX and SC administered ADL exhibit comparable efficacy in CD,[15] IV IFX induces higher remission rates than SC ADL in UC.[16,17] Comparatively, a higher proportion of patients with UC than CD exhibit undetectable IFX trough levels.[18,19] In a small study of patients with either severe CD or UC, elevated fecal IFX levels predicted low serum IFX levels.[20] Thus, it is plausible that the pharmacokinetic differences observed between CD and UC may be conceptually explained by a phenotype characterized by extensive inflammation.

Disease-independent patient factors including age, body mass index, and genetics also affect drug clearance. In rheumatoid arthritis (RA), body weight has been positively associated with ADL clearance, whereas age has been negatively associated with ADL clearance.[21] Increased body weight predicts earlier LOR to IFX in IBD,[22] and the reduction of clinical efficacy seems more pronounced with ADL, which is not dosed by body weight.[23] In a prospective study of patients with IBD treated with ADL, high body mass index predicted the need for dose escalation in a multivariate analysis.[24] Further investigation is necessary to clarify whether obesity alters the bioavailability of anti-TNF therapy, or if increased mesenteric adiposity itself is a proinflammatory condition that augments TNF burden.[25]

Intolerance to the anti-TNF biologic results in the development of ADA, which interferes with targeted antigen-binding and accelerates drug clearance by the RES. Factors that may affect immunogenicity include administration schedule, concomitant therapies, and individual pharmacogenetics. In patients with CD treated with IFX, the incidence of antibody formation has been reported between 36% and 61% with episodic therapy, and 5% and 18% with maintenance therapy.[26] Immunotolerance to the monoclonal antibody seems to be promoted by scheduled infusions and maintenance of therapeutic drug concentrations. One prospective study of patients with CD treated with IFX suggests that low drug concentration after induction (IFX trough levels <2.5 μg/mL at 4 weeks postinitial infusion) predicts subsequent development of high-titer ADAs (positive predictive value, 86%).[27] Fewer data are available regarding ADA formation with respect to the SC anti–TNF-α biologics, but available studies have reported a similar prevalence of ADA formation among patients with CD treated with ADL (9.2%–22%) and CZP (12%).[28,29]

Concomitant immunomodulator (IMM) therapy with azathioprine or methotrexate may increase anti–TNF-α drug levels, presumably inhibiting ADA formation by altering RES clearance or impairing B-cell antibody development. A post hoc analysis of four randomized controlled trials administering maintenance IFX (5 mg/kg) with concomitant IMM therapy demonstrated a higher prevalence of ADAs with monotherapy (8%–23% vs 2%–7%).[30] In the SONIC trial, ADA development was 15% with IFX monotherapy compared with less than 1% with concomitant azathioprine.[31] In a recent 50-week randomized controlled trial of 126 patients with CD, IFX monotherapy, compared with IFX with concomitant methotrexate, was associated with an increased development of ADAs (20% vs 4%; $P = .01$) and a trend toward lower serum IFX trough (3.75 μg/mL vs 6.35 μg/mL; $P = .08$), but there was no difference in clinical remission between treatment groups.[32] Lastly, in select cases, patient genotype may influence the development of ADA. Polymorphisms in interleukin-10 and the HLA-DR1 locus have been associated with a higher prevalence of ADA to ADL in patients with RA and IFX in patients with CD, respectively.[33,34] Furthermore, polymorphisms of the rs1143634C allele of interleukin-1β and the TNF promoter region have been associated with nonresponse to IFX in CD and UC.[35]

Serum Drug Concentration and Clinical Response

An abundance of literature has demonstrated that serum drug levels correlate with clinical response and endoscopic disease activity in CD and UC. In CD, high serum anti-TNF trough levels positively correlate with sustained response, fistula response, and mucosal healing,[19,28,31,36–39] but low and undetectable levels are associated with elevated inflammatory markers, and predict LOR.[40–43] Similarly, higher serum anti-TNF trough levels are positively correlated with clinical remission and mucosal healing in UC,[44–46] but undetectable trough levels predict colectomy (**Table 1**).[18]

Immunogenicity and Clinical Response

The formation of antibodies to anti-TNF biologics increases drug clearance and impairs binding of the target antigen, resulting in low or undetectable serum anti-TNF concentrations and clinical LOR. In a meta-analysis of 13 studies totaling 1378 patients with IBD treated with IFX, Nanda and colleagues[47] determined a pooled risk ratio (RR) of 3.2 (95% confidence interval [CI], 2.0-4.9; $P<.001$) for loss of clinical response among patients with IBD with antibodies against IFX. Three of 13 studies (N = 243) also reported on serum IFX levels, which were uniformly lower in the presence of IFX ADA.

In patients with IBD treated with ADL maintenance therapy, multiple studies[28,48,49] have demonstrated an inverse relation between the presence of detectable ADA (range, 9%–47%) and serum trough ADL concentrations, and a positive relation between ADAs and LOR. Yarur and colleagues[48] reported a significant association between the presence of ADAs and lower serum ADL trough levels (odds ratio, 8.6; 95% CI, 2.3-31), higher CRP, mucosal inflammation on colonoscopy (odds ratio, 3.8; 95% CI, 1.1-13), and steroid use (odds ratio, 3.7; 95% CI, 1.1-13). Similarly, a prospective study of 113 patients with IBD (11 UC) by Velayos and colleagues[49] reported lower median serum ADL concentration (4.78 μg/mL) among those with detectable ADA compared with those without (9.11 μg/mL). Moreover, detectable ADAs predicted worse clinical symptoms and higher CRP levels independent of serum ADL concentration. The presence of ADAs has also been shown to negate the effect of therapeutic IFX concentrations (>3 μg/mL) to control inflammation as measured by CRP level.[50] Such findings suggest that significant immunogenicity disrupts drug efficacy beyond its direct effects on drug concentration. The clinical relevance of antibodies to CZP has been less studied, and a CZP assay is not commercially available. In the PRECISE 1 and 2 trials, ADAs against CZP was detected in 8% to 9% of patients with CD.[51,52] The presence of ADA was mitigated by concurrent immunosuppressive therapy (4% vs 10%). Although ADA to CZP has not been demonstrated to decrease clinical efficacy in CD, the presence of ADA has been associated with decreased serum CZP levels and decreased clinical efficacy in RA randomized-controlled trials.[53]

ADAs may also increase the risk for infusion reactions. In a systematic review by Chaparro and colleagues,[54] the presence of ADAs was associated with a higher incidence of infusion reactions in six of eight studies. Among a consecutive cohort[55] of 128 patients with IBD (105 CD, 23 UC) receiving IFX reinfusion after a median drug holiday of 15 months, 20% experienced an acute or delayed infusion reaction. Detectable ADA predicted the development of infusion reaction after reinfusion (hazard ratio, 7.7; 95% CI, 1.88–31.3; P = .004), but concomitant IMM therapy with retreatment attenuated ADA formation and predicted short-term response (hazard ratio, 6; 95% CI, 1.3–27; P = .019). In a prospective French trial,[56] after discontinuation of IFX in patients with CD on IMM therapy, 39 (98%) of 40 patients who experienced relapse regained clinical response with retreatment, and none had detectable ADAs.

The presence of ADAs has not uniformly predicted LOR. In the pivotal ACCENT I trial,[26] 67% of patients with detectable ADA still had a clinical response at week 54. Some studies have demonstrated successful dose escalation in the presence of ADAs.[57,58] Heterogeneity in pharmacometrics across studies (assay technology, timing of measurement, unit of measurement, and cut-off level) may partially explain the inconsistency in the literature. LOR may be from noninflammatory causes of symptoms, there may be a lag-time between detection of ADA and later LOR, ADAs may be heterogeneous in their drug clearance and neutralizing effects, and alternative pathways of inflammation may emerge to circumvent anti-TNF therapy and thereby mitigate the relevance of ADA levels.

An emerging concept is that the clinical relevance of ADAs may be titer- and time-dependent. Although clinical response may occur in the setting of detectable ADA, higher median ADA titers significantly predict LOR.[8] In a prospective study by Ungar and colleagues[59] of 125 patients with IBD treated with IFX, 90% of patients who developed persistent ADA did so within the first 12 months of therapy (median, 22 weeks), and persistent ADA preceded clinical LOR by a median delay of 2 months. Transient ADA could be detectable at any time during the course of therapy and was without clinical relevance. In a retrospective study of 90 patients with IBD, Vande Casteele and colleagues[60] reported detection of ADA at a median of 16 weeks after the start of IFX therapy (ie, after four infusions). Persistent ADAs exhibited significantly higher titer levels (median, 22 U/mL) than transient ADAs (median, 17 U/mL), and conferred a five times higher risk for discontinuation of IFX therapy because of LOR or hypersensitivity reaction compared with transient ADAs. ADA development was mitigated by concomitant IMM therapy; patients receiving IFX monotherapy during the first 6 months of treatment had an almost two-fold higher risk for ADA compared with those receiving combination therapy (RR, 1.8; 95% CI, 1.2–2.6; P = .0025).

Table 1
Clinical impact of serum anti-TNF-α levels

Reference	Study Design	Subjects (N)	Anti-TNF-α	Follow-up	Clinical Impact of Serum Anti-TNF-α Drug Level
Crohn Disease					
Cornillie et al,[36] 2014	Post hoc analysis of ACCENT I	147	IFX	54 wk	Week 14 serum TL >3.5 μg/mL associated with higher rates of remission
Fasanmade et al,[37] 2003	Subanalysis of ACCENT II	282	IFX	30 wk	Higher serum TL correlated with complete fistula response
Bortlik et al,[40] 2013	Retrospective	84	IFX	25 mo	Week 14 or 22 serum TL >3 μg/mL associated with sustained clinical response
Van Moerkercke et al,[38] 2010	Prospective	210	IFX	N/A	TL quartile positively predicted degree of mucosal healing (absence, partial, and complete)
Maser et al,[19] 2006	Retrospective	90	IFX	23 mo	Detectable serum drug levels associated with remission, lower CRP, and endoscopic improvement
Colombel et al,[31] 2010	Prospective, SONIC	338	IFX	46 wk	Higher serum TL correlated with clinical remission
Imaeda et al,[39] 2014	Prospective	45	IFX	30 d	Higher serum TL required for mucosal healing (4 μg/mL) than for normalization of CRP, albumin, and fecal calprotectin
Li et al,[41] 2010	Subanalysis, CLASSIC I/II	258	ADL	4, 24, 56 wk	Week 4 serum TL predicted clinical remission in CLASSIC I, but no dose-exposure-response relationship identified in CLASSIC II

Study	Study type	N	Drug	Timepoint	Findings
Karmiris et al,[28] 2009	Prospective	168	ADL	20.3 mo (median)	Low serum TL predicted LOR
Mazor et al,[42] 2013	Retrospective	121	ADL	N/A	Serum TL >5 µg/mL associated with higher clinical remission rates and normal CRP
Sandborn et al,[43] 2012	Subanalysis, PRECISE (open-label study)	203	CZP	6 wk	Drug plasma concentrations positively correlated with clinical remission
Ulcerative Colitis					
Seow et al,[18] 2010	Prospective	108	IFX	13.9 mo (median)	Detectable serum TL predicted clinical remission and endoscopic improvement; undetectable TL levels predicted colectomy
Roblin et al,[44] 2014	Cross-sectional	40 CD/UC	ADL	—	Higher serum TL (median 6.5 µg/mL) associated with clinical remission and mucosal healing
Sandborn et al,[45] 2014	Prospective, PURSUIT	625 (110)	GOL	6 wk	Drug concentration quartile at week 6 positively predicted improvement in Mayo score and rates of clinical response and remission
Sandborn et al,[46] 2014	Prospective, PURSUIT	157	GOL	30, 54 wk	Drug concentration quartile positively predicted higher rates of clinical remission

Abbreviations: N/A, not available; TL, Trough level.
 Data from Refs.[18,19,28,31,36,37,39–46]

NATALIZUMAB

Natalizumab (NAT), a forerunner of the emerging class of selective adhesion molecule inhibitors, is a recombinant monoclonal antibody (95% human and 5% murine) directed against the α_4 subunit of the integrins $\alpha_4\beta_1$ and $\alpha_4\beta_7$ expressed on the surface of lymphocytes and monocytes. It is an IV biologic administered every 4 weeks (weeks 0, 4, 8 induction), and most patients have detectable serum NAT levels (mean, 0.99 μg/ mL) at 4 weeks after their first infusion.[3] Possibly because of higher levels of circulating leukocytes expressing α_4, the mean plasma $T_{1/2}$ of NAT (3 mg/kg) is shorter in patients with CD than in healthy volunteers (4.8 vs 8.7 days).[61] In a meta-analysis of five clinical trials, NAT has been shown to be efficacious in the induction and maintenance of response and remission in moderate to severe CD.[62]

Although humanized, NAT is immunogenic like all protein-based biologic therapies. A variety of enzyme-linked immunosorbent assays have been used to detect NAT antibodies.[63] In the ENACT 1 and 2 trials[64] (N = 1040), 9% of patients with CD treated with NAT developed ADAs. In ENACT 1, the presence of ADA compared with undetectable ADA was associated with a trend toward decreased clinical response at week 12 (53% vs 62%; P = .18). In ENACT 2, antibodies against NAT were serially measured and categorized as transient versus persistent; none of the patients with persistent ADAs maintained clinical response through week 60, whereas 75% of patients with transient ADAs maintained clinical response. In both trials, ADAs positively predicted acute infusion and hypersensitivity reactions. In multiple sclerosis, the incidence of ADAs against NAT is also reported at 9%,[65] and persistent ADAs predict lower serum NAT concentrations and higher rates of relapse and disease progression. High-titer ADA levels on a first-positive sample in patients with multiple sclerosis predict ADA persistence such that cut-off values have been generated to advise discontinuation of NAT at 3 months.[66] Data from the recently published CD and UC trials of vedolizumab (antibody to α4β7-integrin) induction and maintenance therapy suggest that antibody formation against vedolizumab may be less prevalent, with single test ADA positivity rates of approximately 4%, and persistently positive ADA rates of less than or equal to 1% in both trials.[67,68]

TDM IN CLINICAL PRACTICE

The clinical efficacy of biologic therapies, whether anti–TNF-α or CAMi, depends on optimally titrating serum drug concentrations to effectively saturate proinflammatory targets. Dosing adjusted to maintain therapeutic drug levels over time promotes sustained clinical remission and may help to minimize the development of persistent antibodies. TDM respects that a given patient's serum drug levels temporally evolve depending on disease activity, drug clearance, and immunotolerance to monoclonal antibody treatment. In IBD, the clinical application of TDM has focused on the anti-TNF therapies, but the optimal use of biologics as a class, as suggested by the NAT literature, seems to obey the same general principles.

Routinely, TDM has been performed to evaluate and respond to LOR. Low drug troughs during the induction phase predict ADA formation,[60] which commonly occurs early in the course of maintenance therapy. Maintaining optimal serum drug levels from the outset may help suppress the development of persistent antibodies, and concurrent IMM therapy during the first 6 to 12 months enhances serum drug levels and reduces immunogenicity. Clinical response may be maintained or recaptured by dose escalation in response to low serum drug trough with undetectable ADA or in the presence of transient, low-titer ADA. The resultant increase in serum drug level after dose escalation, or "delta-anti-TNF," is predictive of recaptured clinical response and mucosal healing.[28,69] If the patient was previously on anti-TNF monotherapy, the addition of an IMM may also help restore clinical response by decreasing ADA formation while increasing serum drug troughs.[70] However, high-titer ADAs should prompt a switch to an alternative anti-TNF biologic, because further dose escalation is unlikely to recapture clinical response and poses an increased risk for an adverse drug reaction. Persistent inflammation despite therapeutic drug levels should warrant a switch to an alternative mechanism of therapy.[71] Finally, in regards to reinitiation of therapy, prospective studies demonstrate that preemptively assessing for ADAs to IFX after a drug holiday exceeding 12 months duration is of low yield,[56,72] but undetectable serum IFX levels and detectable ADAs before the second or third infusion indicate that retreatment is futile, if not potentially harmful.[55]

A recent prospective trial[73] substantiated the utility and cost-effectiveness of a test-based algorithm in 69 patients with CD with LOR to IFX. Patients were randomized to either empiric dose escalation or a test-based algorithm whereby dose escalation was performed for ADA-negative low trough IFX (TLI), switch to ADL for ADA-positive low TLI, or discontinuation of anti–TNF-α therapy for high TLI with or without ADA positivity. Treatment guided by a test-based algorithm resulted in a cost-reduction of 56% compared with empiric dose escalation, without compromise of clinical care (**Fig. 1**).

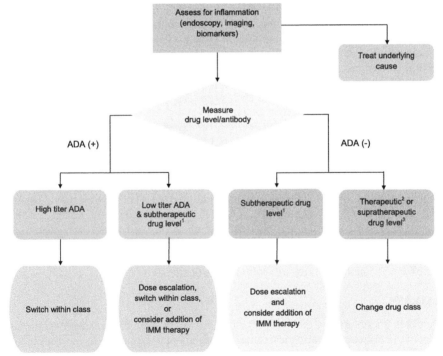

Fig. 1. Therapeutic drug monitoring to manage loss of response to anti–TNF-α therapy. Trough levels: (1) IFX, <3 μg/mL; ADL, <5 μg/mL; CZP, <27.5 μg/mL. (2) IFX, 3–7 μg/mL (midpoint level≥12 μg/mL); ADL, ≥5 μg/mL; CZP, ≥27.5 μg/mL. (3) IFX, >7 μg/mL. Optimal cut-off values for ADL and CZP are not well-established. (*Adapted from* Ordas I, Feagan BG, Sandborn WJ. Therapeutic drug monitoring of tumor necrosis factor antagonists in inflammatory bowel disease. Clin Gastroenterol Hepatol 2012;10:1084, with permission; and Yanai H, Hanauer SB. Assessing response and loss of response to biological therapies in IBD. Am J Gastroenterol 2011;106:685–9.)

FUTURE RESEARCH

There is a clear role for TDM to guide treatment decisions in the setting of LOR, but the cost-effectiveness and clinical use of proactive TDM to dose-optimize clinically well patients in the maintenance phase of therapy are less well-studied. Emerging data in this population suggest that lower serum troughs may be associated with endoscopic disease activity despite normal biomarkers, and increase risk for ADA formation.[39,60] In the Trough Level Adapted Infliximab Treatment trial,[74] 263 patients with IBD on IFX maintenance therapy were randomized to dose optimization based on clinical symptoms and CRP level versus a drug level–based algorithm (goal trough level between 3 and 7 μg/mL). Only 43% of responders on maintenance IFX therapy had optimal IFX trough levels: 26% had supratherapeutic levels, 22% had subtherapeutic levels, and 9% had an undetectable level. During the dose optimization phase, drug level–based dosing led to dose intensification and better disease control in patients with subtherapeutic levels. In those with supratherapeutic drug levels, dose reduction led to decreased drug exposure and costs. Compared with drug level–based dosing, clinically based dosing was more likely to result in undetectable IFX levels (RR, 3.7; 95% CI, 1.7–8.0; $P<.001$) and ADA formation (RR, 3.3; 95% CI, 1.4–7.7; $P<.01$), but there was no difference between treatment groups in rate of clinical remission at 1-year follow-up.

There are few data regarding the clinical application of TDM during induction therapy, but there is compelling evidence that primary nonresponse in severe, acute disease may be attributable to accelerated drug clearance and inadequate saturation of upregulated TNF-α. In acute UC, high levels of fecal IFX and low levels of serum IFX are predictive of failure to induction therapy and subsequent colectomy.[20,75] Immediate postinfusion IFX levels have correlated with LOR in patients with CD on maintenance therapy,[76] but there are no data regarding the measurement of peak IFX levels in the severe, hospitalized patient with the presumed "antigen sink." Early TDM may help risk-stratify patients who require higher than standard dosing for successful induction. The initiation of anti-TNF therapy in combination with an IMM increases serum drug levels and reduces antibody formation, but further investigation is necessary to clarify the optimal duration of combination therapy in light of the risks associated with long-term IMM exposure. Cut-off norms for serum drug and ADA concentrations have not been uniformly established, and TDM is not yet readily available for more recently introduced anti–TNF-α and CAMi biologic therapies. Specific patient characteristics (eg, obesity) and pharmacogenetics may accelerate drug clearance, increase immunogenicity, or even predict nonresponse; however, whether such data may be incorporated into a dose-adjustment model or be of clinical use above and beyond routine TDM requires further investigation.

SUMMARY

Clinicians' understanding of the pharmacokinetics of biologic therapy and the application of TDM is instrumental in the optimal management of moderate-to-severely active IBD. Significant interindividual variability exists with regards to disease activity, drug bioavailability and clearance, and immunotolerance. This variability manifests in the differential magnitude and duration of response to biologic therapies among patients. Within a given individual, the dose-response may evolve temporally during the course of disease, continued drug-exposure, and with the adjustment of concurrent immunosuppressive medications. Historically, primary nonresponse and LOR have been managed with empiric adjustment of biologic therapy. TDM provides a means of individually tailoring therapy to optimally "treat to target."[77] The newest assays for monitoring anti-TNF therapy consistently demonstrate that serum drug and ADA levels correlate with endoscopic and biomarkers of disease activity, and furthermore predict sustained remission versus later LOR. Targeted dose-escalation, with or without IMM therapy, may re-establish therapeutic drug levels and mitigate immunogenicity to restore clinical response and remission. After a prolonged drug holiday, assessing drug levels and the presence of ADAs during early retreatment may identify patients most likely to respond safely and successfully. TDM provides a rational framework for guiding these treatment decisions, reducing the cost of patient care and the risks associated with unnecessary drug exposure. The potential of TDM to improve care may extend beyond its established role in the evaluation of LOR, but more data are necessary to determine the cost-effectiveness and clinical use of proactive TDM to optimize the induction and maintenance phases of therapy.

REFERENCES

1. Ben-Horin S, Kopylov U, Chowers Y. Optimizing anti-TNF treatments in inflammatory bowel disease. Autoimmun Rev 2014;13(1):24–30.
2. Katz L, Gisbert JP, Manoogian B, et al. Doubling the infliximab dose versus halving the infusion intervals in Crohn's disease patients with loss of response. Inflamm Bowel Dis 2012;18(11):2026–33.
3. Kozuch PL, Hanauer SB. General principles and pharmacology of biologics in inflammatory bowel disease. Gastroenterol Clin North Am 2006;35:757–73.
4. Garimella TPJ, Beck K, Noertersheuser P, et al. Pharmacokinetics of adalimumab in a long-term investigation of the induction and maintenance of remission in patients with Crohn's disease (CLASSIC I and CLASSIC II). Gastroenterology 2006;130(4 Suppl 2):A481.
5. Certolizumab pegol (CDP870): pharmacology. Smyrna (GA): UCB; 2006.
6. Shealy D, Cia A, Staquet K, et al. Characterization of golimumab, a human monoclonal antibody specific for human tumor necrosis factor α. MAbs 2010; 2(4):428–39.
7. Zhou H, Jang H, Fleischmann RM. Pharmacokinetics and safety of golimumab, a fully human anti-TNF-alpha monoclonal antibody, in subjects with rheumatoid arthritis. J Clin Pharmacol 2007;47(3):383–96.
8. Ainsworth MA, Bendtzen K, Brynskov J. Tumor necrosis factor-alpha binding capacity and anti-infliximab antibodies measured by fluid-phase radioimmunoassays as predictors of clinical efficacy of infliximab in Crohn's disease. Am J Gastroenterol 2008;103:944–8.
9. Imaeda H, Takahashi K, Fujimoto T. Clinical utility of newly developed immunoassays for serum concentrations of adalimumab and anti-adalimumab antibodies in patients with Crohn's disease. J Gastroenterol 2014;49(1):100–9.
10. Wang S, Hauenstein S, Ohrmund L, et al. Monitoring of adalimumab and antibodies-to-adalimumab levels in patient serum by the homogenous mobility shift assay. J Pharm Biomed Anal 2013;78–79:39–44.
11. Mould D, Green B. Pharmacokinetics and pharmacodynamics of monoclonal antibodies: concepts and lessons for drug development. BioDrugs 2010;24: 23–39.
12. Fasanmade AA, Adedokun OJ, Ford J, et al. Population pharmacokinetic analysis of infliximab in patients with ulcerative colitis. Eur J Pharmacol 2009;65:1211–28.
13. Kevans D, Murthy S, Iaccono A, et al. Accelerated clearance of serum infliximab during induction therapy for acute ulcerative colitis is associated with treatment failure. Gastroenterology 2012;142(Suppl 1):S384–5.

14. Fasanmade AA, Adedokun OJ, Blank M, et al. Pharmacokinetic properties of infliximab in children and adults with Crohn's disease: a retrospective analysis of data from 2 phase III clinical trials. Clin Ther 2011;33:946–64.

15. Colombel JF, Sandborn WJ, Rutgeerts P, et al. Adalimumab for maintenance of clinical response and remission in patients with Crohn's disease: the CHARM trial. Gastroenterology 2007;132:52–65.

16. Reinisch W, Sandborn WJ, Hommes DW, et al. Adalimumab for induction of clinical remission in moderately to severely active ulcerative colitis: results of a randomized controlled trial. Gut 2011;60:780–7.

17. Rutgeerts P, Sandborn WJ, Feagan BG, et al. Infliximab for induction and maintenance therapy for ulcerative colitis. N Engl J Med 2005;353:2462–76.

18. Seow CH, Newman A, Irwin SP, et al. Trough serum infliximab: a predictive factor of clinical outcome for infliximab treatment in acute ulcerative colitis. Gut 2010; 59:49–54.

19. Maser EA, Villela R, Silverberg MS, et al. Association of trough serum infliximab to clinical outcome after scheduled maintenance treatment for Crohn's disease. Clin Gastroenterol Hepatol 2006;4:1248–54.

20. Brandse J, Wildenberg ME, Bruyn JR, et al. Fecal loss of infliximab as a cause of lack of response in severe inflammatory bowel disease. Digestive Disease Week. May 18, 2013; abstract 157.

21. Weisman MH, Moreland LW, Furst DE, et al. Efficacy, pharmacokinetic, and safety assessment of adalimumab, a fully human anti-tumor necrosis factor-alpha monoclonal antibody, in adults with rheumatoid arthritis receiving concomitant methotrexate: a pilot study. Clin Ther 2003;25:1700–21.

22. Harper JW, Sinanan MN, Zisman TL. Retrospective studies report that increased body mass index is associated with earlier time to loss of response to infliximab in patients with inflammatory bowel disease. Inflamm Bowel Dis 2013;19(10):2118–24.

23. Bhalme M, Sharma A, Kled R, et al. Does weight-adjusted anti-tumour necrosis factor treatment favour obese patients with Crohn's disease? Eur J Gastroenterol Hepatol 2013;25(5):543–9.

24. Bultman E, de Haar C, van Liere-Baron A, et al. Predictors of dose escalation of adalimumab in a prospective cohort of Crohn's disease patients. Aliment Pharmacol Ther 2012;35:335–41.

25. Ordas I, Feagan BG, Sandborn WJ. Therapeutic drug monitoring of tumor necrosis factor antagonists in inflammatory bowel disease. Clin Gastroenterol Hepatol 2012;10:1079–87.

26. Hanauer SB, Wagner CL, Bala M, et al. Incidence and importance of antibody responses to infliximab after maintenance or episodic treatment in Crohn's disease. Clin Gastroenterol Hepatol 2004;2:542–3.

27. Vermeire S, Noman M, Van Assche G, et al. Effectiveness of concomitant immunosuppressive therapy in suppressing the formation of antibodies to infliximab in Crohn's disease. Gut 2007;56:1226–31.

28. Karmiris K, Paintaud G, Noman M, et al. Influence of trough serum levels and immunogenicity on long-term outcome of adalimumab therapy in Crohn's disease. Gastroenterology 2009;137:1628–40.

29. Schreiber S, Rutgeerts P, Fedorak RN, et al. A randomized, placebo-controlled trial of certolizumab pegol (CDP870) for treatment of Crohn's disease. Gastroenterology 2005;129:807–18.

30. Lichtenstein GR, Diamond RH, Wagner CL, et al. Clinical trial: benefits and risks of immunomodulators and maintenance infliximab for IBD-subgroup analyses across four randomized trials. Aliment Pharmacol Ther 2009;30(3):210–26.

31. Colombel JF, Sandborn WJ, Reinisch W. Infliximab, azathioprine, or combination therapy for Crohn's disease. N Engl J Med 2010;7(2):86–92.
32. Feagan BG, McDonald JW, Panaccione R, et al. Methotrexate in combination with infliximab is no more effective than infliximab alone in patients with Crohn's disease. Gastroenterology 2014;146:681–8.e1.
33. Bartelds GM, Wijbrandts CA, Nurmohamed MT, et al. Anti-adalimumab antibodies in rheumatoid arthritis patients are associated with interleukin-10 gene polymorphisms. Arthritis Rheum 2009;60:2541–2.
34. Magira E, Lind C, Baldassano R, et al. The HLA DRβ313 residue is associated with the development of human anti-chimeric antibody in some Crohn's patients treated with infliximab. Hum Immunol 2009;70:131.
35. Lacruz-Guzman D, Torres-Moreno D, Pedrero F, et al. Influence of polymorphisms and TNF and IL1β serum concentration on the infliximab response in Crohn's disease and ulcerative colitis. Eur J Clin Pharmacol 2013;69(3):431–8.
36. Cornillie F, Hanauer SB, Diamond RH, et al. Postinduction serum infliximab trough level and decrease of C-reactive protein level are associated with durable sustained response to infliximab: a retrospective analysis of the ACCENT I trial. Gut 2014. [Epub ahead of print].
37. Fasanmade AA, Marsters P, Munsanje E, et al. Infliximab pharmacokinetics and improvement in fistulizing Crohn's disease. Gastroenterology 2003; 124(4 Suppl 1):A61.
38. Van Moerkercke W, Ackaert C, Compernolle G, et al. High infliximab trough levels are associated with mucosal healing in Crohn's disease. Gastroenterology 2010;138(5):S60.
39. Imaeda H, Bamba S, Takahashi K, et al. Relationship between serum infliximab trough levels and endoscopic activities in patients with Crohn's disease under scheduled maintenance treatment. J Gastroenterol 2014;49:674–82.
40. Bortlik M, Duricova D, Malickova K, et al. Infliximab trough levels may predict sustained response to infliximab in patients with Crohn's disease. J Crohns Colitis 2013;7:736–43.
41. Li J, Chiu Y, Robinson A, et al. Evaluation of potential correlations between serum adalimumab concentration and remission in patients with Crohn's disease in CLASSIC I and II. J Crohns Colitis 2010;4:S73.
42. Mazor Y, Kopylov U, Ben Hur D, et al. Evaluating adalimumab drug and antibody levels as predictors of clinical and laboratory response in Crohn's disease patients. Gastroenterology 2013;144(5):S-778.
43. Sandborn WJ, Hanauer SB, Pierre-Louis B, et al. Certolizumabpegol plasma concentration and clinical remission in Crohn's disease. Gastroenterology 2012;142:S-563.
44. Roblin X, Marotte H, Rinaudo M, et al. Association between pharmacokinetics of adalimumab and mucosal healing in patients with inflammatory bowel diseases. Clin Gastroenterol Hepatol 2014;12(1):80–4.
45. Sandborn WJ, Feagan BG, Marano C, et al. Subcutaneous golimumab induces clinical response and remission in patients with moderate-to-severe ulcerative colitis. Gastroenterology 2014;146:85–95.
46. Sandborn WJ, Feagan BG, Marano C, et al. Subcutaneous golimumab maintains clinical response in patients with moderate-to-severe ulcerative colitis. Gastroenterology 2014;146:96–109.
47. Nanda KS, Cheifetz AS, Moss AC. Impact of antibodies to infliximab on clinical outcomes and serum infliximab levels in patients with inflammatory bowel disease (IBD): a meta-analysis. Am J Gastroenterol 2013;108:40–7.

48. Yarur AJ, Deshpande AR, Sussman DA, et al. Serum adalimumab levels and antibodies correlate with endoscopic intestinal inflammation and inflammatory markers in patients with inflammatory bowel disease. Abstract presented at: Digestive Disease Week. Orlando (FL), May 18–21, 2013.

49. Velayos F, Sheibani S, Lockton S, et al. Prevalence of antibodies to adalimumab (ATA) and correlation between ATA and low serum drug concentration on CRP and clinical symptoms in a prospective sample of IBD patients. Gastroenterology 2013;144:S-490.

50. Feagan BG, Singh S, Lockton S, et al. Novel infliximab and antibody-to-infliximab assays are predictive of disease activity in patients with Crohn's disease. Gastroenterology 2012;142:S114.

51. Sandborn WJ, Feagan BG, Stoinov S, et al. Certolizumab pegol for the treatment of Crohn's disease. N Engl J Med 2007;357(3):228–38.

52. Schreiber S, Khaliq-Kareemi M, Lawrance IC, et al. Maintenance therapy with certolizumab pegol for Crohn's disease. N Engl J Med 2007;357(3):239–50.

53. Prescribing information, certolizumab. Smyrna (GA): UCB; 2006.

54. Chaparro M, Guerra I, Munoz-Linares P, et al. Systematic review: antibodies and anti-TNF-α levels in inflammatory bowel disease. Aliment Pharmacol Ther 2012; 35:971–86.

55. Baert FJ, Drobne D, Gils A, et al. Early trough levels and antibodies to infliximab predict safety and success of re-initiation of infliximab therapy. Clin Gastroenterol Hepatol 2014. [Epub ahead of print].

56. Louis E, Mary JV, Vernier-Massouille G, et al. Maintenance of remission among patients with Crohn's disease on antimetabolite therapy after infliximab therapy is stopped. Gastroenterology 2012;142:63–70.

57. Vermeire S, Gabriels F, Ballet V, et al. The effect of dose escalation on trough levels in patients who lost response to infliximab. Gut 2010;59(Suppl III):A81.

58. Ternant D, Aubourg A, Magdelaine-Beuzelin C, et al. Infliximab pharmacokinetics in inflammatory bowel disease patients. Ther Drug Monit 2008;30:523–9.

59. Ungar B, Chowers Y, Yavzori M, et al. The temporal evolution of antidrug antibodies in patients with inflammatory bowel disease treated with infliximab. Gut 2013. [Epub ahead of print].

60. Vande Casteele N, Gils A, Singh S, et al. Antibody response to infliximab and its impact on pharmacokinetics can be transient. Am J Gastroenterol 2013;108(6): 962–71.

61. Gordon FH, Lai CW, Hamilton MI, et al. A randomized placebo-controlled trial of a humanized monoclonal antibody to alpha4 integrin in active Crohn's disease. Gastroenterology 2001;121:268–74.

62. Ford AC, Sandborn WJ, Khan KJ, et al. Efficacy of biological therapies in inflammatory bowel disease: systematic review and meta-analysis. Am J Gastroenterol 2011;106(4):644.

63. Lundkvist M, Engdahl E, Holmen C, et al. Characterization of anti-natalizumab antibodies in multiple sclerosis patients. Mult Scler 2012;19(6):757–64.

64. Sandborn WJ, Colombel JF, Enns R, et al. For the international Efficacy of Natalizumab as Active Crohn's Therapy (ENACT-1) and the Evaluation of Natalizumab as Continuous Therapy (ENACT-2) trial groups. Natalizumab induction and maintenance therapy for Crohn's disease. N Engl J Med 2005;353: 1912–25.

65. Calabresi PA, Giovannoni G, Confavreux C, et al. The incidence and significance of anti-natalizumab antibodies: results from AFFIRM and SENTINEL. Neurology 2007;69(14):1391–403.

66. Jensen PR, Koch-Henriksen N, Sellebjerg F, et al. Prediction of antibody persistency from antibody titres to natalizumab. Mult Scler 2012;18(10):1493–9.
67. Sandborn WJ, Feagan BG, Rutgeerts P, et al. Vedolizumab as induction and maintenance therapy for Crohn's disease. N Engl J Med 2013;369:711–21. Supplementary appendix.
68. Feagan BG, Rutgeerts P, Sands BE, et al. Vedolizumab as induction and maintenance therapy for ulcerative colitis. N Engl J Med 2013;369:699–710. Supplementary appendix.
69. Paul S, Del Tedesco E, Marotte H, et al. Therapeutic drug monitoring of infliximab and mucosal healing in inflammatory bowel disease: a prospective study. Inflamm Bowel Dis 2013;19(12):2568–76.
70. Ben-Horin S, Waterman M, Kopylov U, et al. Addition of an immunomodulator to infliximab therapy eliminates antidrug antibodies in serum and restores clinical response of patients with inflammatory bowel disease. Clin Gastroenterol Hepatol 2013;11(4):444–7.
71. Afif W, Loftus EV Jr, Faubion WA, et al. Clinical utility of measuring infliximab and human anti-chimeric antibody concentrations in patients with inflammatory bowel disease. Am J Gastroenterol 2010;105:1133–9.
72. Ben-Horin S, Mazor Y, Yanai H, et al. The decline of anti-drug antibody titres after discontinuation of anti-TNFs: implications for predicting re-induction outcome in IBD. Aliment Pharmacol Ther 2012;35:714–22.
73. Steenholdt C, Brynskov J, Thomsen OO, et al. Individualised therapy is more cost-effective than dose intensification in patients with Crohn's disease who lose response to anti-TNF treatment: a randomised, controlled trial. Gut 2014; 63:919–27.
74. Vande Casteele N, Gils A, Ballet V, et al. Randomised controlled trial of drug levels versus clinically based dosing of infliximab maintenance therapy in IBD: final results of the TAXIT study. Presented at UEG Week. Berlin, October 15, 2013 [abstract: UEG13-ABS-2468].
75. Murthy S, Kevans D, Seow CH, et al. Association of serum infliximab and antibodies to infliximab to long-term clinical outcome in acute ulcerative colitis. Presented at Digestive Disease Week. San Diego (CA), May 19–22, 2012 [abstract: Sa2047].
76. Yamada A, Sono K, Hosoe N, et al. Monitoring functional serum antitumor necrosis factor antibody level in Crohn's disease patients who maintained and those who lost response to anti-TNF. Inflamm Bowel Dis 2010;16(11):1898–904.
77. Bouguen G, Levesque BG, Feagan BG, et al. Treat to target: a proposed new paradigm for the management of Crohn's disease. Clin Gastroenterol Hepatol 2013. [Epub ahead of print].

Lymphocyte Homing Antagonists in the Treatment of Inflammatory Bowel Diseases

Masayuki Saruta, MD, PhD[a], Konstantinos A. Papadakis, MD, PhD[b],*

KEYWORDS

- Natalizumab • Vedolizumab • Etrolizumab • Integrins • Chemokine receptors
- Inflammatory bowel disease • Ulcerative colitis • Crohn disease

KEY POINTS

- Inhibiting the interactions between adhesion molecules expressed on inflamed intestinal endothelium and lymphocyte integrins has proved to be a successful therapeutic strategy for the management of chronic inflammatory bowel disease (IBD).
- Targeting specifically the MAdCAM-1/$\alpha 4 \beta 7$ interactions with vedolizumab and, possibly, AMG 181 is likely to be effective and safe treatment approach for refractory IBD patients.
- Future studies need to address the use of these agents in the treatment of fistulizing Crohn disease phenotypes and extraintestinal manifestation of IBD.
- Subgroup analysis may identify genetic, serologic, and clinical parameters that may predict response to adhesion molecule inhibition and the best timing for therapeutic intervention.
- Combination therapeutic strategies with immunomodulators or even anti–tumor necrosis factor agents in a selective refractory group of IBD patients should also be entertained.

INTRODUCTION

Inflammatory bowel diseases (IBD) comprise a heterogeneous group of intestinal inflammatory disorders characterized by periods of disease exacerbation and remission, and are broadly classified into ulcerative colitis (UC) and Crohn disease (CD). Their pathogenesis is still unknown, but they are thought to develop as a result of a dysregulated immune response to certain gut bacterial antigens in the context of

Financial Disclosure: None.

[a] Division of Gastroenterology and Hepatology, Department of Internal Medicine, The Jikei University School of Medicine, 3 Chome-25-8 Nishishinbashi, Minato, Tokyo 105-0003, Japan; [b] Division of Gastroenterology and Hepatology, Mayo Clinic, 200 1st Street Southwest, Rochester, MN 55905, USA
* Corresponding author.
E-mail address: Papadakis.Konstantinos@mayo.edu

genetic susceptibility, certain environmental triggers, and gut dysbiosis.[1–3] Histopathologically, IBD is characterized by the extent and distribution of mucosal architectural abnormality, the cellularity of the lamina propria, and the cell types present, but with significant overlap between the 2 diseases.[4] Disease activity can be reflected by neutrophil granulocyte infiltration and epithelial cell damage.[4] Characteristics of disease that could interfere with response to medical therapy, whether to traditional medications or to biological agents (including adhesion molecule inhibitors), include early disease or long-standing disease, which could reflect differences in inflammatory cell infiltrate and their immunologic characteristics.[4]

Traditional therapies of IBD, such as 5-aminosalicylic acid, corticosteroids, and immunomodulators, have been shown to modulate the intestinal immune responses to some degree in a nonspecific manner.[5,6] The introduction of biological agents for the treatment of IBD has targeted specific pathways of inflammation, including proinflammatory cytokines such as tumor necrosis factor (TNF)-α, with remarkable long-term beneficial effects that may alter the natural history of IBD.[7] Such treatment approaches include the introduction of monoclonal antibodies targeting TNF-α, such as infliximab, adalimumab, certolizumab pegol, and golimumab.[7,8] However, despite the remarkable effectiveness of these agents, they may lose efficacy over time or rarely produce treatment-related side effects. Therefore, alternative therapeutic agents with a different mode of action are urgently needed.

Active IBD is characterized by the recruitment of large numbers of granulocytes, lymphocytes, and macrophages into the gastrointestinal mucosa.[9] The recruitment of leukocytes to peripheral tissues is a highly coordinated, multistep process (**Fig. 1**). As they circulate at high speed through the postcapillary vessels, a highly coordinated sequential adhesion pathway is activated, which consists of the capture/tethering, rolling, activation, adhesion, and migration through the vascular wall, and eventual transmigration to the tissue.[10] These infiltrating leukocytes may perpetuate the inflammatory process through the secretion of proinflammatory cytokines, further endothelial cell activation, and upregulation of adhesion molecules and enhancement of inflammatory cell recruitment. Further tissue damage may result from the release of proteases by the infiltrating leukocytes.[9] The process of intestinal leukocyte infiltration is regulated by the expression of integrins and chemokine receptors on leukocytes, and adhesion molecules such as intercellular adhesion molecule 1 (ICAM-1), vascular cell adhesion molecule 1 (VCAM-1), and mucosal addressin cell adhesion molecule 1 (MAdCAM-1) expressed on endothelial cells (see **Fig. 1**).[11–13]

Integrins comprise a family of α, β heterodimeric transmembrane receptors that are constitutively expressed and mediate the attachment of cells to the extracellular matrix (ECM), but can also take part in specialized cell-cell interactions.[14,15] The integrin family consists of at least 24 different forms representing the combination of 18 α subunits and 8 β subunits.[16] These integrins are expressed on the surface of leukocytes and require activation to bind their own specific ligand. The α subunit determines integrin ligand specificity, and the β subunit connects to the cytoskeleton and affects multiple signaling pathways.[16] Integrins involved in the T-cell migration include leukocyte function–associated antigen 1 (LFA-1 or $\alpha 2\beta 2$) and the 2 $\alpha 4$ integrins ($\alpha 4\beta 1$ and $\alpha 4\beta 7$).[17] LFA-1 is expressed on neutrophils, and interacts with ICAM-1, which is expressed on leukocytes, dendritic cells, fibroblasts, epithelial cells, and endothelial cells.[18,19] The $\alpha 4\beta 1$ integrin is expressed on most leukocytes but not on neutrophils, and interacts with VCAM-1.[20] The $\alpha 4\beta 7$ integrin is expressed on the lymphocytes in the gut-associated lymphoid tissue, and interacts with MAdCAM-1.[21] This ligand is expressed on endothelial venules in the small intestine and the colon, especially in the Peyer patches.[22]

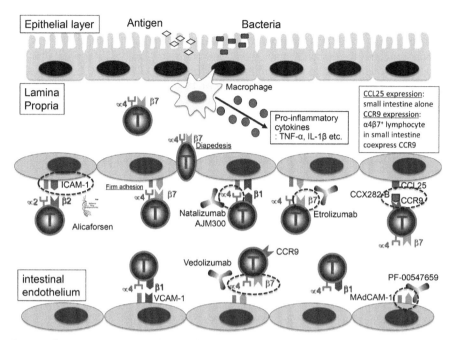

Fig. 1. Adhesion molecules and chemokine receptors in the recruitment of immune cells in the intestinal endothelium. In the intestine, the adhesion molecule MAdCAM-1 functions as docking site for integrins α4β1 and α4β7 expressed by T cells.[69] By contrast, the adhesion molecule VCAM-1 also acts as docking molecule for α4β1. Natalizumab inhibits α4 integrins, therefore blocking the adhesion of T cells to the entire intestinal mucosa and extramucosal tissues (eg, brain). Vedolizumab, an α4β7 integrin inhibitor, inhibits the adhesion of T cells to the intestinal mucosa only, and thus does not limit immune surveillance of the central nervous system while dampening the inflammatory response.[69] In the endothelium of the small intestine, the chemokine CCL25 is constitutively expressed and upregulated during inflammation. It acts as a ligand for the chemokine receptor 9 (CCR9) on T cells. The inhibitor CCX282-B, or vercirnon, blocks the CCL25-CCR9 interaction, thus inhibiting T-cell adhesion to the small intestinal mucosa. Phase 3 trials of CCX282-B are currently on hold. ICAM, intercellular adhesion molecule; IL, interleukin; MAdCAM, mucosal addressin cell adhesion molecule; TNF, tumor necrosis factor; VCAM, vascular cell adhesion molecule.

Proinflammatory cytokines such as TNF-α and interleukin (IL)-1β upregulate the expression of gut-expressed adhesion molecules such as MAdCAM-1, ICAM-1, and VCAM-1. These adhesion molecules are overexpressed in IBD, especially in the active phase of the disease. Cultured supernatants from colonic biopsies taken from UC and CD patients induce upregulation of ICAM-1 and E-selectin,[23] and there is increased expression of various endothelial adhesion molecules by immunohistochemistry from colonic biopsies in patients with IBD.[24–26] Moreover, it has been shown that the proportion of venular endothelium within the lamina propria that expresses MAdCAM-1 at inflammatory foci associated with UC and CD is increased compared with normal tissues, and MAdCAM-1 is not detected in most normal or inflamed extraintestinal tissues, including those at other mucosal surfaces.[22] Similarly, VCAM-1 is also overexpressed in the colonic IBD mucosa in comparison with normal controls by immunohistochemistry.[24]

PREVENTING LEUKOCYTE INFILTRATION BY BLOCKING ADHESION RECEPTORS

Inhibition of leukocyte trafficking to the gut mucosa during the inflammatory process in IBD has become the second major therapeutic target of biological agents after the introduction of anticytokine agents in the development of IBD therapeutics.[13] Several critical steps outlined in **Fig. 1** that are involved in the recruitment of inflammatory cells to the intestinal mucosa can be targeted for therapeutic purposes. The $\alpha 4\beta 7$ integrin is highly expressed on a subpopulation of $CD4^+CD45RA^-$ memory T cells, which have been shown to preferentially home to the gut.[27,28] The ligand mediating $\alpha 4\beta 7$ T-cell gut-homing is MAdCAM-1, which is selectively expressed in the gut endothelium and is upregulated in the chronically inflamed small and large intestines of patients with IBD.[22,29]

The predominant targets of the novel biological agents in this group are the integrins $\alpha 4\beta 1$, $\alpha 4\beta 7$, and $\alpha 2\beta 2$, which interact with VCAM-1, MAdCAM-1, and ICAM-1, respectively, to mediate the interactions between leukocytes and endothelial cells.[12,13] The agents that target the integrins include the monoclonal antibodies natalizumab (anti-$\alpha 4$ integrin), vedolizumab (MLN-02, anti-$\alpha 4\beta 7$ integrin), AMG181 (anti-$\alpha 4\beta 7$ integrin), etrolizumab (RG7413, rhuMAb $\beta 7$, anti-$\beta 7$ integrin), which targets both $\alpha 4\beta 7$ and $\alpha E\beta 7$, and PF-00547659 (anti-MAdCAM-1). AJM-300 (Ajinomoto Pharmaceuticals, Tokyo, Japan) is a small-molecule inhibitor of the $\alpha 4$ integrin subunit. Other molecules that aim to prevent leukocyte infiltration include alicaforsen (ISIS-2302), an antisense oligonucleotide against ICAM-1 messenger RNA. Vercirnon (CCX282-B, GSK-1605786) is a small molecule that targets the chemokine receptor CCR9, the key chemokine receptor in the targeting of leukocytes to the intestinal mucosa (see **Fig. 1**, **Table 1**).[30,31]

CURRENT ANTIADHESION THERAPIES FOR IBD
Antiadhesion Therapies for IBD

Natalizumab
Natalizumab (Tysabri; Biogen-Idec, Cambridge, MA, USA) is a humanized immunoglobulin G4 (IgG4) monoclonal antibody against $\alpha 4$ integrins.[32] Previous randomized studies have suggested that natalizumab may be effective as induction therapy for patients with moderately to severely active CD.[33–35] The first study of natalizumab was reported by Gordon and colleagues,[34] and focused on the evaluation of the safety and efficacy of natalizumab in patients with mildly to moderately active CD.

Ghosh and colleagues[33] conducted a double-blind, placebo-controlled trial of natalizumab in 248 patients with moderate to severe CD. Patients were randomly assigned to receive 1 of 4 treatments: 2 infusions of placebo; 1 infusion of 3 mg natalizumab per kg body weight, followed by placebo; 2 infusions of 3 mg natalizumab per kg; or 2 infusions of 6 mg natalizumab per kg. The highest remission rate was 44% and the highest response rate was 71% at week 6 in the group given 2 infusions of 3 mg/kg.

Patients with moderate to severe disease (Crohn Disease Activity Index [CDAI] scores ≥ 220 to ≤ 450) were enrolled in the phase 3 induction trial, Efficacy of Natalizumab as Active Crohn Therapy (ENACT-1) (N = 905), and received 3 infusions of natalizumab (300 mg) or placebo over 8 weeks.[35] Response was defined as a reduction of 70 or more points from week 0 in the CDAI score, whereas remission was defined as a CDAI score of less than 150 points. A clinical response at week 10 was observed in 56% of patients treated with natalizumab and 49% of patients with placebo (P = .051), and remission obtained at week 10 in 37% of natalizumab-treated patients and 30% of patients with placebo (P = .124). Although there were no significant differences among the 2 treatment groups, analysis in subgroups of patients,

Table 1
Selected leukocyte trafficking modulators for inflammatory bowel disease

Drug	Description	Developer	Target	Indication	Clinical Status
Tysabri	Humanized IgG4 mAb	Biogen Idec (Cambridge, MA)	$\alpha4\beta1$ integrin, $\alpha4\beta7$ integrin	Multiple sclerosis, Crohn disease	Approved (FDA)
Entyvio	Humanized IgG1 mAb	Takeda Pharmaceuticals (Deerfield, IL)	$\alpha4\beta7$ integrin	Crohn disease	Registration (in USA)
AMG-181	Fully human IgG2 mAb	AstraZeneca (London, UK)/Amgen (Thousand Oaks, CA)	$\alpha4\beta7$ integrin	Crohn disease, ulcerative colitis	Phase 2
Etrolizumab (rhuMAb $\beta7$, RG7413)	Humanized IgG1 mAb	Genentech (South San Francisco, CA)	$\alpha4\beta7$ integrin, $\alpha E\beta7$ integrin	Ulcerative colitis	Phase 2
PF-00547659	Fully human IgG2k mAb	Pfizer (New York, NY, USA)	MAdCAM-1	Crohn disease, ulcerative colitis	Phase 2
AJM300	Oral small-molecule prodrug	Ajinomoto Pharmaceuticals (Tokyo, Japan)	$\alpha4$ integrin	Ulcerative colitis, Crohn disease	Phase 2
Vercirnon (CCX282-B)	Oral small molecule	ChemoCentryx (Mountain View, CA)/GSK (Brentwood, Middlesex, UK)	CCR9	Crohn disease	Phase 3 (on hold)

Data sources: Company Web sites; PubMed.
Abbreviations: FDA, Food and Drug Administration; IgG, immunoglobulin G; mAb, monoclonal antibody.
Adapted from Sheridan C. First integrin inhibitor since Tysabri nears approval for IBD. Nat Biotechnol 2014;32:206; with permission.

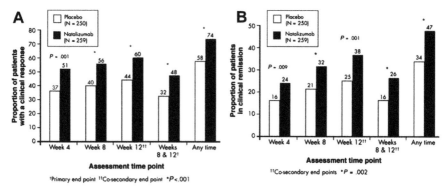

†Primary end point ††Co-secondary end point *P<.001

Fig. 2. Efficacy of Natalizumab in Crohn's disease Response and Remission (ENCORE) trial. The primary end point was induction of response (≥70-point decrease from baseline Crohn's Disease Activity Index [CDAI] score) at week 8 that was sustained through week 12. (*A*) Proportion of patients with a clinical response (≥70-point decrease from baseline CDAI score). The secondary end points were induction of remission (CDAI score<150) at week 8 that was sustained through week 12 and the proportion of patients in response or remission at week 12. (*B*) Proportion of patients in clinical remission (CDAI score<150). (*From* Targan SR, Feagan BG, Fedorak RN, et al. Natalizumab for the treatment of active Crohn's disease: results of the ENCORE Trial. Gastroenterology 2007;132:1677; with permission.)

including those with active inflammation and a baseline C-reactive protein (CRP) concentration above the upper limit of normal range (>2.87 mg/L), demonstrated clinically and statistically significant differences in response and remission rates. Among the patients in the ENACT-1 trial with CRP concentrations above the upper limit of normal (n = 660; 73% of the total registered patients), 58% of natalizumab-treated patients and 45% of patients with placebo had a clinical response at week 10 (*P* = .007) while 40% and 28%, respectively, had clinical remission (*P* = .014).

Targan and colleagues[32] performed a randomized, placebo-controlled trial that evaluated the efficacy of natalizumab induction therapy in patients with moderately to severely active CD and active inflammation characterized by elevated CRP concentrations (Efficacy of Natalizumab in Crohn's Disease Response and Remission [ENCORE] trial). In this trial, 509 patients with moderately to severely active CD were enrolled; 48% of natalizumab-treated patients had a sustained response at week 8 through week 12 compared with 32% of patients treated with placebo (*P*<.001), while 26% and 16%, respectively, had sustained remission (**Fig. 2**) (*P* = .002).

The Evaluation of Natalizumab as Continuous Therapy (ENACT-2) trial evaluated the efficacy of natalizumab to maintain clinical response. In ENACT-2, 339 patients who had a response to natalizumab in the ENACT-1 trial were randomly reassigned to receive 300 mg of natalizumab or placebo every 4 weeks through week 56. The primary outcome was a sustained response through week 36. A secondary outcome was disease remission (CDAI score<150). Continuing natalizumab in the second trial resulted in higher rates of sustained response (61% vs 28%, *P*<.001) and remission (44% vs 26%, *P* = .003) through week 36 than did switching to placebo.[35]

A pilot study evaluating the efficacy of natalizumab in UC patients was reported in 2002.[36] A significant decrease in the median Powell-Tuck score was observed at 2 and 4 weeks postinfusion (7.5 and 6, respectively) compared with the median baseline score of 10. Five of 10 patients achieved a good clinical response at 2 weeks and 1 more patient by 4 weeks, defined by a Powell-Tuck score of 5 or less. Significant improvements in quality-of-life scores were found at week 4. The median CRP at 2 weeks

(6 mg/L) was also lower than that pretreatment (16 mg/L); however, rescue medication was required by 2 (20%), 3 (30%), and 8 (80%) patients by weeks 2, 4, and 8, respectively (median, 34 days; range, 8–43 days).[36]

Safety of natalizumab The main serious adverse event that has been reported with the use of natalizumab in multiple sclerosis (MS) and CD studies and postmarketing experience is the development of progressive multifocal leukoencephalopathy (PML), a demyelinating disease of the white matter of the brain caused by lytic infection of oligodendrocytes with the human polyomavirus, John Cunningham virus (JCV).[30] Although most PML cases occur in severely immunosuppressed individuals, with human immunodeficiency virus 1 infection as the predominant factor, PML has been increasingly diagnosed in patients treated with biological therapies such as anti–LFA-1 (efalizumab [Raptiva] for severe forms of plaque psoriasis) that prevents extravasation of inflammatory T cells into tissues, or anti-CD20 (rituximab [Rituxan] for hematologic malignancies and rheumatoid arthritis) that depletes peripheral circulating B cells.[30] Mutations of JCV capsid viral protein 1 (VP1), the capsid protein involved in binding to sialic acid cell receptors, might favor PML onset.[37] JCV is often acquired during childhood. Most adults have been infected with JCV but do not develop the disorder. The virus seems to remain inactive until immune suppression allows it to be reactivated and start to multiply. During clinical trials of natalizumab in more than 2000 MS and 1000 CD patients, PML was diagnosed in 2 MS patients and one CD patient in 2005.[38] As of April 3, 2014, among approximately 123,000 patients who have received natalizumab worldwide in the postmarketing setting, 454 have developed PML, and the estimated incidence of PML is 3.6 per 1000 patient-years (Biogen Idec, personal communication, 2014). Three factors that are known to increase the risk of PML in natalizumab-treated patients have been identified: (1) longer treatment duration, especially beyond 2 years; (2) prior treatment with an immunosuppressive agent; and (3) the presence of anti-JCV antibodies. Patients who are anti-JCV antibody positive have a higher risk for developing PML (**Table 2**).

AJM300 (anti-α4 integrin)
AJM300 (Ajinomoto Pharmaceuticals) is an orally available, highly specific α4-integrin inhibitor shown to be effective in a murine model of colitis.[39] Takazoe and colleagues[40]

Table 2
Estimated United States incidence of PML stratified by risk factor

Anti-JCV Antibody Negative[a]	Tysabri Exposure (mo)[b]	Anti-JCV Antibody Positive[c]	
		No Prior Immunosuppressant Use	Prior Immunosuppressant Use
<1/1000	1–24	<1/1000	1/1000
	25–48	3/1000	13/1000
	49–72	7/1000	9/1000

The anti-JCV antibody status was determined using an anti-JCV antibody test (enzyme-linked immunosorbent assay) that has been analytically and clinically validated, and is configured with detection and inhibition steps to confirm the presence of JCV-specific antibodies with an analytical false-negative rate of 3%.

[a] Calculation based on 2 cases of anti-JCV antibody negative PML in patients exposed for at least 1 month of therapy as of September 3, 2013. Data for anti-JCV antibody negative patients reflects worldwide exposure.

[b] Data beyond 6 years of treatment are limited.

[c] Based on United States postmarketing PML data as of September 3, 2013, and Tysabri use data as of August 31, 2013.

reported the efficacy, safety, and dose response of AJM300 in patients with CD in a randomized, double-blind, placebo-controlled multicenter trial. In this study, 71 active CD patients with CDAI scores of at least 150 and elevated CRP concentrations were randomized to receive placebo, AJM300 40 mg 3 times daily, 120 mg 3 times daily, or 240 mg 3 times daily orally for 8 weeks. The primary efficacy end point was the decrease of CDAI score from baseline to final evaluation at week 4 or later. A secondary efficacy end point was clinical response, defined as a reduction of at least 70 points in the CDAI. In the AJM300 groups, the decreases of CDAI (mean $\pm$ standard deviation: 40 mg, 19.9 $\pm$ 74.1; 120 mg, 25.5 $\pm$ 61.3; 240 mg, 21.6 $\pm$ 84.9) were higher than in the placebo group (5.2 $\pm$ 71.0).[40] Although no significant difference in clinical response was observed between AJM300 groups and the placebo group, in the patients who had CDAI scores of 200 or higher at week 0, the decreases in CDAI from baseline were 41.5 $\pm$ 57.5 in the 120-mg group (P = .0485, paired t-test) and 41.6 $\pm$ 94.1 in the 240-mg group, and the clinical response rate in the 240-mg group was 50% at the final evaluation. In the 240-mg group, mean CRP decreased from 19.7 mg/L (at week 0) to 9.6 mg/L (at week 8) (P = .0220, paired t-test). AJM300 was safe, well tolerated, and effective to active CD at doses of 120 and 240 mg 3 times daily.

Watanabe and colleagues[41] also recently reported on a randomized, double-blind, placebo-controlled phase 2A trial of AJM300 in 102 Japanese patients with moderately active UC. The primary end point of the trial (clinical response at week 8) was 62.7% versus 25.5% in the AJM300 group and placebo group, respectively (odds ratio [OR] 5.35; 95% confidence interval [CI] 2.23–12.82; P = .0002). The secondary end points, clinical remission at week 8, was 23.5% versus 3.9% (OR 7.81; 95% CI 1.64–37.24; P = .0099), and mucosal healing at week 8 was 58.8% versus 29.4% (OR 4.65; 95% CI 1.81–11.90; P = .0014) in the AJM300 group and placebo group, respectively. Neither serious adverse events (including PML) nor serious infection were observed during the trial. The conclusion of the study (presented only in abstract form) was that AJM300 was well tolerated and significantly effective in patients with moderately active UC.[41]

Vedolizumab (anti-$\alpha 4\beta 7$ integrin)

Vedolizumab (Entyvio; Takeda Pharmaceuticals, Deerfield, IL, USA and Osaka, Japan) is a humanized monoclonal IgG1 antibody that recognizes the integrin $\alpha 4\beta 7$.[42] Feagan and colleagues[42] first reported on a multicenter, double-blind, placebo-controlled trial of 181 active UC patients who were treated with intravenous infusion of 0.5 mg/kg MLN0002, 2.0 mg/kg MLN0002, or placebo. Each patient received an intravenous infusion of study drug on days 1 and 29. This study showed that week 6 clinical remission rates were 33%, 32%, and 14% for the group receiving 0.5 mg/kg MLN0002, 2.0 mg/kg MLN0002, and placebo, respectively (P = .03). The corresponding proportions of patients who improved by at least 3 points on the UC clinical score were 66%, 53%, and 33% (P = .002). Twenty-eight percent of patients receiving 0.5 mg/kg and 12% of those receiving 2.0 mg/kg had endoscopically evident remission, compared with 8% of those receiving placebo (P = .007). In this short-term study, MLN0002 was more effective than placebo for the induction of clinical and endoscopic remission in patients with active UC. For the minority of patients in whom an MLN0002 antibody titer was greater than 1:125, incomplete saturation of the $\alpha 4\beta 7$ receptor on circulating lymphocytes was observed, and no benefit of treatment was identified.[41]

A phase 2 randomized, double-blind, controlled trial assessed the efficacy and safety of MLN0002 in patients with active CD.[43] Patients with CD were randomized to receive MLN0002 2.0 mg/kg (n = 65), MLN0002 0.5 mg/kg (n = 62), or placebo (n = 58) by intravenous infusion on days 1 and 29. The primary efficacy end point was clinical response (>70-point decrement in the CDAI score) on day 57. Secondary end points were the proportions of patients with clinical remission (CDAI score<150) and with an enhanced clinical response (>100-point decrement in CDAI). Clinical response rates at day 57 were 53%, 49%, and 41% in the MLN0002 2.0 mg/kg, MLN0002 0.5 mg/kg, and placebo groups, respectively. Clinical remission rates at day 57 were 37%, 30%, and 21%, respectively ($P = .04$ for the 2.0 mg/kg vs placebo comparison). At day 57, 12% and 34% of patients in the 2.0- and 0.5-mg/kg groups had clinically significant human antihuman antibody levels (titers>1:125). There was one infusion-related hypersensitivity reaction reported.[43]

Vedolizumab has completed several phase 3 clinical trials for CD and UC (GEMINI I, GEMINI II, and GEMINI III) that demonstrate vedolizumab to be an effective and well-tolerated drug. The results of the GEMINI I and GEMINI II randomized, placebo-controlled, multicenter trials of induction and maintenance therapy in CD and UC have been recently published (**Fig. 3**).[44,45]

Feagan and colleagues[44] reported the GEMINI I clinical trial, comprising 2 integrated randomized, double-blind, placebo-controlled trials of vedolizumab as induction and maintenance therapy for UC (see **Fig. 3**). In the trial of induction therapy, 374 patients received vedolizumab (300 mg) or placebo intravenously at weeks 0 and 2, and 521 patients received open-label vedolizumab at weeks 0 and 2, with disease evaluation at week 6. In the trial of maintenance therapy, patients in either cohort who had a response to vedolizumab at week 6 were randomly assigned to continue receiving vedolizumab every 8 or 4 weeks or to switch to placebo for up to 52 weeks. A response was defined as a reduction in the Mayo Clinic score (range 0–12, with higher scores indicating more active disease) of at least 3 points and a decrease of at least 30% from baseline, with an accompanying decrease in the rectal bleeding subscore of at least 1 point or an absolute rectal bleeding subscore of 0 or 1. Response rates at week 6 were 47.1% and 25.5% among patients in the vedolizumab group and placebo group, respectively (difference with adjustment for stratification factors, 21.7 percentage points; 95% CI 11.6–31.7; $P<.001$). At week 52, 41.8% of patients who continued to receive vedolizumab every 8 weeks and 44.8% of patients who continued to receive vedolizumab every 4 weeks were in clinical remission (Mayo Clinic score ≤2 and no subscore >1), compared with 15.9% of patients who switched to placebo (adjusted difference, 26.1 percentage points for vedolizumab every 8 weeks vs placebo [95% CI 14.9–37.2; $P<.001$], and 29.1 percentage points for vedolizumab every 4 weeks vs placebo [95% CI 17.9–40.4; $P<.001$]). The frequency of adverse events was similar in the vedolizumab and placebo groups.[44]

Sandborn and colleagues[45] reported the GEMINI II clinical trial, which was an integrated trial of vedolizumab as induction and maintenance therapy for CD (**Fig. 4**). In the induction trial, 368 patients were randomly assigned to receive vedolizumab or placebo at weeks 0 and 2, and 747 patients received open-label vedolizumab at weeks 0 and 2; disease status was assessed at week 6. In the maintenance trial, 461 patients who had had a response to vedolizumab were randomly assigned to receive placebo or vedolizumab every 8 or 4 weeks until week 52. At week 6, a total of 14.5% of the patients in the blinded cohort who received vedolizumab and 6.8% who received placebo were in clinical remission (CDAI≤150) ($P = .02$); a total of 31.4% and 25.7% of the patients, respectively, had a CDAI-100 response (≥100 points in the CDAI) ($P = .23$). Among patients who had a response to induction therapy, 39.0% and 36.4% of those assigned to vedolizumab every 8 weeks and every 4 weeks, respectively, were in clinical remission at week 52, compared with 21.6% assigned to placebo ($P<.001$ and $P = .004$ for the 2 vedolizumab groups, respectively, vs placebo).

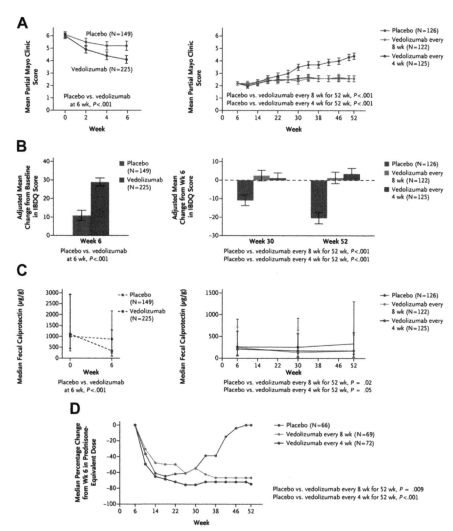

Fig. 3. Exploratory outcomes in the trials of vedolizumab as induction and maintenance therapy in ulcerative colitis. (*A*) Partial Mayo Clinic scores, which range from 0 to 9, with higher scores indicating more active disease. (*B*) Scores on the Inflammatory Bowel Disease Questionnaire (IBDQ), which range from 0 to 224, with higher scores indicating a better quality of life. Vertical bars in *A* and *B* indicate standard errors. (*C*) Median fecal calprotectin concentrations. Vertical bars indicate the interquartile range. (*D*) Median change from week 6 in prednisone-equivalent doses. Patients receiving placebo during the trial of maintenance therapy received 2 doses of vedolizumab during the trial of induction therapy. For patients who withdrew early, the last observation was carried forward (*A, B* [graph at *right*], *C* [graph at *right*], and *D*). (*From* Feagan BG, Rutgeerts P, Sands BE, et al. Vedolizumab as induction and maintenance therapy for ulcerative colitis. N Engl J Med 2013;369:706; with permission.)

Antibodies against vedolizumab developed in 4.0% of the patients. Nasopharyngitis occurred more frequently, and headache and abdominal pain less frequently, in patients receiving vedolizumab than in those receiving placebo. In comparison with placebo, vedolizumab was associated with a higher rate of serious adverse events

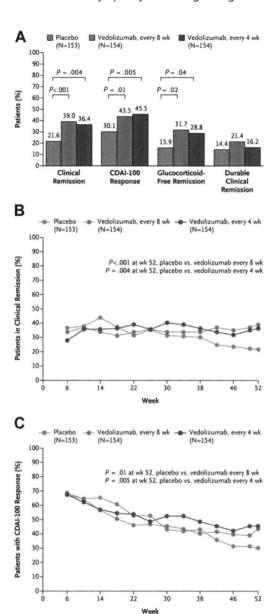

Fig. 4. End points in the trial of vedolizumab maintenance therapy in Crohn disease. (*A*) Proportions of patients, among those who had had clinical remission at week 6, who were still in clinical remission at week 52, who had a CDAI-100 response at week 52, and who had glucocorticoid-free remission (ie, clinical remission without glucocorticoid therapy) at week 52 (with data for this end point available for 82 patients receiving placebo, 82 patients receiving vedolizumab every 8 weeks, and 80 patients receiving vedolizumab every 4 weeks), and the proportion of patients who had a durable clinical remission (defined as a clinical remission at ≥80% of study visits, including the final visit) at week 52. (*B*) Proportions of patients who were in clinical remission from week 6 to week 52. (*C*) Proportions of patients who had a CDAI-100 response from week 6 to week 52. (*From* Sandborn WJ, Feagan BG, Rutgeerts P, et al. Vedolizumab as induction and maintenance therapy for Crohn's disease. N Engl J Med 2013;369:717; with permission.)

(24.4% vs 15.3%), infections (44.1% vs 40.2%), and serious infections (5.5% vs 3.0%). Vedolizumab-treated patients with active CD were more likely than patients receiving placebo to have a remission, but not a CDAI-100 response, at week 6; patients with a response to induction therapy who continued to receive vedolizumab (rather than switching to placebo) were more likely to be in remission at week 52. Adverse events were more common with vedolizumab.

GEMINI III addressed the efficacy and safety of vedolizumab as induction therapy in CD patients who had prior anti-TNF failure.[46] In a phase 3 study, patients with moderately to severely active CD (CDAI 220–400) and failure or intolerance to prior therapy were randomized 1:1 to receive intravenous vedolizumab 300 mg or placebo at weeks 0, 2, and 6. The primary end point was clinical remission (CDAI≤150) at week 6 in patients with prior anti-TNF failure. Secondary end points included clinical remission at week 6 in the overall population, clinical remission at week 10 in anti-TNF failure and overall populations, sustained clinical remission (CDAI≤150 at weeks 6 and 10) in both populations, and CDAI-100 response (≥100-point decrease from baseline in CDAI) in the anti-TNF failure population.[46] Clinical remission rates at week 6 were not statistically significant between the vedolizumab and placebo groups (15.2% vs 12.1%; P = .4332). However, greater proportions of vedolizumab-treated patients had CDAI-100 response at week 6 (39.2% vs 22.3%; P = .0011) and were in clinical remission by week 10 (26.6% vs 12.1%; P = .0012) versus placebo in the anti-TNF failure population.[46] In the overall population, more patients in the vedolizumab group had sustained clinical remission in comparison with placebo (15.3% vs 8.2%; P = .0249). Treatment-related adverse events were reported in 56% of vedolizumab-treated patients versus 60% of placebo patients; serious adverse events were reported in 6% versus 8%, respectively, with no deaths.

Based on these positive trial results of vedolizumab in IBD, the Committee for Medicinal Products for Human Use recommended granting a marketing authorization for vedolizumab in March 2014, and the US Food and Drug Administration approved vedolizumab for the treatment of both moderate to severe UC and CD in May 2014.

Safety of vedolizumab Vedolizumab has the advantage of being able to specifically bind and neutralize the integrin α4β7 expressed primarily by intestinal-homing lymphocytes and, therefore, inhibit α4β7-MAdCAM-1 adhesive interactions between gut-homing effector lymphocytes and inflamed endothelium without interfering with brain immunosurveillance. Indeed, in the phase 2 trial of MLN0002 in CD,[43] there were no opportunistic infections (PML or otherwise) reported. In addition, there were no reported cases of PML in the GEMINI I trial in approximately 3000 patients exposed to vedolizumab for a median of 18.8 months (mean, 20.9 months; range, 4–67). At present, it is believed that vedolizumab does not carry a significant risk of PML; however, close postmarketing monitoring is important.

AMG181 (anti-α4β7 integrin)

AMG 181 (anti-α4β7 integrin; Amgen, Thousand Oaks, CA, USA) is a fully human antibody specific to the α4β7 heterodimer. AMG 181 binds α4β7, but does not bind either α4β1 or αEβ7. AMG 181 specifically inhibits MAdCAM-1 binding, but not VCAM-1 binding, to α4β7.[47] AMG181 does not cross-react with murine or rat α4β7 and, therefore, no studies on the efficacy of AMG181 in murine or rat models of IBD have been performed. AMG 181 had relative bioavailabilities ranging from 80% to 95% after subcutaneous administration.[47] AMG 181 has reported in vitro pharmacology, and pharmacokinetic/pharmacodynamic and safety characteristics in cynomolgus monkeys that were suitable for further investigation in humans.[47] AMG 181 is currently being evaluated in phase 1 and 2 trials in subjects with IBD (http://www.clinicaltrials.gov). Given its similarity to vedolizumab for the specificity to $\alpha4\beta7$ heterodimer, it is anticipated that it will likely carry a lower risk of PML development, if any.

Anti-MAdCAM-1/PF-00547659

PF-00547659 (anti-MAdCAM-1; Pfizer, New York, NY, USA) is a monoclonal IgG2 antibody directed against MAdCAM-1. The mechanism of action for this medication is the inhibition of adhesive interactions mediated through MAdCAM-1 (see **Fig. 1**). PF-00547659 bound with high affinity to mouse and human MAdCAM-1 and blocked the adhesion of $\alpha4\beta7^+$ leukocytes to MAdCAM-1 with similar potency.[48] PF-00547659 induced a similar, dose-dependent 2- to 3-fold increase in circulating populations of $\beta7^+$ memory T cells in the mouse and macaque; without affecting the $\beta7^-$ populations. PF-00547659 therefore has potential utility in the treatment of IBD by blocking tissue homing of activated $\alpha4\beta7$ leukocytes.[48]

Vermeire and colleagues[49] conducted a randomized, double-blind, placebo-controlled study of 80 patients with active UC who received single or multiple (3 doses, 4-week intervals) doses of PF-00547659, 0.03 to 10 mg/kg intravenously/subcutaneously, or placebo. In this study, exploratory efficacy analyses were based on Mayo Clinic score and endoscopic responder rates at weeks 4 and 12. Fecal calprotectin was quantified as a measure of disease activity, and the number of $\alpha4\beta7$ lymphocytes was measured to demonstrate drug activity. This study demonstrated no obvious drug-related side effects in the PF-00547659 group, although patient numbers, especially those fully exposed, were small. Overall response/remission rates at 4 and 12 weeks were 52%/13% and 42%/22%, respectively, with combined PF-00547659 doses compared with 32%/11% and 21%/0%, respectively, with placebo.[49] Equivalent endoscopic responder rates were 50% and 42% versus 26% and 29%, respectively. Fecal calprotectin levels decreased to a greater extent with PF-00547659 than with placebo (week 4: 63% vs 18%). Despite variability, there was a trend for an increase in $\alpha4\beta7$ lymphocytes in patients receiving PF-00547659.[49]

Recently, phase 2 trials of PF-00547659 on induction (OPERA) and maintenance (OPERA II) in CD, and phase 2 trials on induction (TURANDOT) and maintenance (TUR-ANDOT II) in UC are in progress (http://www.clinicaltrials.gov/).

Safety of PF-00547659/anti-MAdCAM-1 Given the risk of PML development with some class of adhesion molecule inhibitors (natalizumab), the TOSCA study was developed to address potential effects of anti–MAdCAM-1 inhibition in cerebrospinal fluid (CSF) cellularity. This study was presented at the European Crohn's and Colitis Organisation congress of 2014.[50] Patients with moderate to severe CD (Harvey-Bradshaw Index >8 and highly sensitive CRP >5.0 mg/L or active lesions on endoscopy or imaging) and prior treatment with anti-TNF and immunosuppressants underwent a lumbar puncture (LP) followed by subcutaneous injections of 225 mg PF-00547659 every 4 weeks for 3 doses. Two weeks after the last dose of PF-00547659, a second LP was performed. CSF was analyzed by flow cytometry for enumeration of lymphocytes and T-cell subsets. Twenty-four subjects were enrolled with similar baseline characteristics. Twelve subjects had a second LP after treatment. The number of first LP lymphocytes was 471 cells/mL (132% compared with that of pretreatment) and that of second LP lymphocytes was 626 cells/mL (185%). In the anti-TNF and immunosuppressant experienced patients with moderate to severe CD, a full induction course of the highest clinical dose of PF-00547659 did not affect CSF lymphocytes.[50] The results of the TOSCA study support the gut selectivity and the central nervous system–sparing mechanism proposed for PF-00547659.

Etrolizumab (anti-β7)

Etrolizumab (RG7413, rhuMAb β7, anti-β7 integrin; Genentech, South San Francisco, CA, USA) is a humanized IgG1 monoclonal antibody that targets the β7 subunit of the α4β7[51,52] and αEβ7[53] integrins with high affinity, blocking binding to their ligands, MAdCAM-1 and E-cadherin, respectively. Murine and primate studies indicate that etrolizumab provides selective targeting of lymphocyte homing to mucosal sites, with limited to no effects on migration to nonmucosal tissues.[54] Amelioration of IBD in nonclinical models is associated with downmodulation and/or disappearance of α4β7 and αEβ7 cells from the inflamed mucosa.[42,43,48,49,55,56]

A randomized phase 1 study evaluated the safety and pharmacology of etrolizumab in patients with moderate to severe UC.[54] In this single ascending dose (SAD) stage, etrolizumab (0.3, 1.0, 3.0, 10 mg/kg intravenously, 3.0 mg/kg subcutaneously, or placebo) was administered 4:1 (n = 25) in each cohort. In the multiple dose (MD) stage, new patients received monthly etrolizumab 0.5 mg/kg subcutaneously (n = 4), 1.5 mg/kg subcutaneously (n = 5), 3.0 mg/kg subcutaneously (n = 4), 4.0 mg/kg intravenously (n = 5), or placebo (n = 5). The pharmacokinetics were studied and Mayo Clinic score evaluated at baseline, day 29 (SAD), and days 43 and 71 (MD). In the SAD stage, there were no dose-limiting toxicities, infusion, or injection-site reactions. Two serious adverse events, which included impaired wound healing, occurred in 2 patients receiving etrolizumab. In the MD stage, there were no dose-limiting toxicities, and no infusion or injection-site reactions. Headache was the most common adverse event, occurring more often in etrolizumab patients. Anti-etrolizumab antibodies were detected in 2 subjects. The duration of β7-receptor full occupancy was dose-related. A clinical response was observed in 12 of 18 patients, and clinical remission in 3 of 18 patients treated with etrolizumab in the MD stage, compared with 4 of 5 and 1 of 5 placebo patients, respectively.[57] More recently, Vermeire and colleagues[58] reported on a double-blind, placebo-controlled, randomized phase 2 study of etrolizumab in the treatment of patients with moderately to severely active UC who had not responded to conventional therapy. Eligible patients (aged 18–75 years; Mayo Clinic score of 5 of higher [or ≥6 in United States]; and disease extending 25 cm or more from anal verge) were randomized (1:1:1) to 1 of 2 dose levels of subcutaneous etrolizumab (100 mg at weeks 0, 4, and 8, with placebo at week 2; or 420-mg loading dose [LD] at week 0 followed by 300 mg at weeks 2, 4, and 8), or matching placebo.[58] The primary end point was clinical remission at week 10, defined as Mayo Clinic score of 2 or less (with no individual subscore of >1). One hundred twenty-four patients were randomly assigned to receive etrolizumab 100 mg (n = 39 patients), etrolizumab 300 mg plus LD (n = 39 patients), or placebo (n = 41 patients). No patients in the placebo group had clinical remission at week 10, compared with 8 (21% [95% CI 7–36]) patients in the etrolizumab 100-mg group ($P = .0040$) and 4 (10% [95% CI 2–24]) patients in the 300-mg plus LD group ($P = .048$).[58] The investigators concluded that etrolizumab was more likely to lead to clinical remission at week 10 than was placebo, and was well tolerated in moderate to severe UC. Further investigations are ongoing.[58]

Targeting the Chemokine and Chemokine Receptor Pathway

Vercirnon (anti-CCR9)

The chemokine receptor system represents a diverse group of G-protein–coupled receptors responsible for orchestrating cell recruitment under both homeostatic and inflammatory conditions.[59] CCR9 is a chemokine receptor known to be central for migration of immune cells into the intestine.[60] Its only ligand, CCL25, is expressed at the mucosal surface of the intestine and is known to be elevated in intestinal inflammation.[61] Vercirnon (CCX282-B, GSK1605786A; ChemoCentryx, Mountain View, CA and GlaxoSmithKline, Brentwood, Middlesex, UK) is a small-molecule, orally bioavailable, selective, and potent antagonist of human CCR9. Vercirnon has potent in vitro activity in inhibiting CCR9-mediated calcium mobilization and chemotaxis, and showed in vivo activity in a Crohn-like ileitis murine model.[31]

Recently a randomized, placebo-controlled trial was conducted to evaluate the safety and efficacy of vercirnon in 436 patients with CD.[62] Patients with active CD (CDAI scores between 250 and 450 and a CRP of >7.5 mg/L at study entry) were enrolled. The patients were randomized to receive placebo or vercirnon (250 mg once daily, 250 mg twice daily, or 500 mg once daily) for 12 weeks; they then received 250 mg vercirnon twice daily, open-label, through week 16. Subjects who had a clinical response ($\geq$70-point CDAI drop) at week 16 were randomly assigned to placebo or vercirnon (250 mg twice daily) for 36 weeks. Primary end points were clinical response at week 8 and sustained clinical response at week 52. During the 12-week induction period, the clinical response was highest in the group given 500 mg vercirnon once daily. Response rates at week 8 were 49% in the placebo group, 52% in the group given vercirnon 250 mg once daily (OR 1.12; $P = .667$ vs placebo), 48% in the group given vercirnon 250 mg twice daily (OR 0.95; $P = .833$), and 60% in the group given vercirnon 500 mg once daily (OR 1.53; $P = .111$). At week 12, response rates were 47%, 56% (OR 1.44; $P = .168$), 49% (OR 1.07; $P = .792$), and 61% (OR 1.74; $P = .039$), respectively. At the end of the maintenance period (week 52), 47% of subjects on vercirnon were in remission, compared with 31% on placebo (OR 2.01; $P = .012$); 46% showed sustained clinical responses, compared with 42% on placebo (OR 1.14; $P = .629$). Vercirnon was well tolerated. Encouraging results from this clinical trial led to initiation of phase 3 clinical trials in CD. Unfortunately, a recent press release indicated that vercirnon did not meet the primary end point of a phase 3 clinical trial evaluating its use in patients with moderate to severe CD. In the double-blind, international, multicenter SHIELD-1 trial, 608 patients with moderate to severe CD across 200 facilities were randomized to receive either placebo or 500 mg vercirnon once or twice daily for 12 weeks. All participants had not responded adequately to prior conventional therapy. The primary end point of the trial was clinical response, defined as a CDAI score decrease of 100 points or more after conclusion of therapy. A CDAI score lower than 150 points after 12 weeks of treatment was a key secondary end point. Serious adverse events and study withdrawal because of serious adverse events occurred at similar rates across the groups, but a dose-dependent increase in the incidence of overall adverse events was observed. Further recruitment and dosing has been suspended pending further review of the initial results (http://www.clinicaltrials.gov/). The trial was the first of a planned 4 studies (SHIELD 1–4) assessing the safety and efficacy of vercirnon in a total of more than 2500 patients with CD.

Alicaforsen (anti-ICAM-1)

Alicaforsen (ISIS 2302; ISIS Pharmaceuticals, Carlsbad, CA, USA) is a 20-base phosphorothioate oligodeoxynucleotide antisense molecule designed to downregulate messenger RNA for ICAM-1. The first placebo-controlled trial of alicaforsen was conducted by Yacyshyn and colleagues.[63] In this trial, 20 active steroid-treated CD patients were randomized (3:1, alicaforsen to placebo) to receive over 26 days 13 intravenous infusions of alicaforsen or placebo. This study showed that 47% of alicaforsen-treated patients achieved remission compared with 20% of placebo, and that alicaforsen was a well-tolerated and promising therapy for steroid-treated CD. The next double-blind, placebo controlled trial, however, did not show significant efficacy between 2- and 4-week alicaforsen groups compared with the placebo group (20.2% and 21.2% vs 18.8%).[64] Schreiber and colleagues[65] conducted a dose-interval, multicenter, placebo-controlled trial in 75 patients with steroid-refractory CD. The primary end point of this study was steroid-free remission (CDAI<150) at week 14. This study demonstrated that only 2 of 60 (3.3%) alicaforsen-treated and no placebo patients reached the primary end point, and steroid-free remission at week 26 (secondary end point) was reached in 8 of 60 (13.3%) active treatment and 1 of 15 (6.7%) placebo patients. This trial also did not prove clinical efficacy of alicaforsen based on the primary end point, although positive trends were observed in some of the secondary end points. The program of ICAM-1 antisense oligonucleotide for the treatment of CD was therefore terminated.

Van Deventer and colleagues[66] performed the first clinical evaluation of alicaforsen enemas in the treatment of UC. This study evaluated the acute and long-term safety and efficacy of 4 different doses of alicaforsen enema administered once a day for 28 consecutive days. It was a randomized, placebo-controlled, double-blind, escalating-dose multicenter study of 40 patients with mildly to moderately active distal UC (disease activity index [DAI] 4–10). Patients were assigned to 4 dosing cohorts of 10 patients each (8 active, 2 placebo). Each patient received 60 mL of alicaforsen enema (0.1, 0.5, 2, or 4 mg/mL or placebo) once daily for 28 consecutive days. Safety and efficacy (DAI and clinical activity index) scores were evaluated up to 6 months after initiation of dosing. At day 29, alicaforsen enemas resulted in dose-dependent improvement in DAI (overall $P = .003$). Alicaforsen 4 mg/mL improved DAI by 70% compared with the placebo response of 28% ($P = .004$). Alicaforsen 2 and 4 mg/mL improved DAI status by 72% and 68% compared with a placebo response of 11.5% at month 3 ($P = .016$ and 0.021, respectively). None of the patients in the 4-mg/mL group, compared with 4 of 8 placebo patients, required additional medical or surgical intervention over baseline during the 6-month period after starting the enema treatment. Alicaforsen enemas showed promising acute and long-term benefit in patients with mild to moderate UC.[66]

Atlantic Pharmaceuticals is currently developing alicaforsen for the treatment of UC, and currently supplies alicaforsen in response to physicians' requests under international Named Patient Supply regulations for patients with IBD. However, larger, randomized controlled clinical trials in UC are needed before its adoption in routine clinical practice.

DISCUSSION

The therapeutic approach to IBD has dramatically changed in the last decade with the introduction of anticytokine agents, the most successful examples being anti-TNF-α antibodies, such as infliximab, adalimumab, certolizumab pegol, and golimumab.[7] In clinical practice, however, clinicians are often faced with patients refractory to anti-TNF agents or with attenuated response to TNF-inhibition strategies. The introduction of therapeutic agents that target lymphocyte homing to the intestine in inflammatory conditions in UC and CD are likely to revolutionize the management of IBD.[12,67] The interactions of MAdCAM-1/α4β7 integrin, VCAM-1/α4β1 integrin, ICAM-1/LFA-1 or α2β2 integrin, and CCL25/CCR9 are potential targets to be exploited for effective inhibition of lymphocyte migration and homing to the intestine. Specifically, the inhibition of the MAdCAM-1/α4β7 integrin interaction with vedolizumab, AMG 181, or PF-00547659/anti-MAdCAM-1 may hold the most promise for effective and safe treatment of IBD, particularly UC. Given the specificity of MAdCAM-1/α4β7 integrin to intestinal lymphocyte homing, it can be envisaged that the risk of PML with these therapeutic agents will be minimal or nonexistent. The authors anticipate that such a therapeutic approach may also be effective and safe in CD, although the recruitment of effector cells in different layers of the intestine and the presence of transmural inflammation is likely more challenging to treat effectively with single antiadhesion molecules. Combination therapies may be more effective, but may carry the risk of significant toxicities. Because the MAdCAM-1/$\alpha4\beta7$ pathway is also used during homeostatic lymphocyte homing, potential toxicity concerns related to susceptibility to infections with enteric pathogens will require vigilance in postmarketing evaluation. Etrolizumab, in addition to inhibiting MAdCAM-1/$\alpha4\beta7$ interactions, interferes with E-cadherin/αE interactions, and may interfere with lymphocyte/epithelial or lymphocyte/dendritic cell interactions. Therefore, etrolizumab may induce more widespread effects in homeostatic or inflammatory mechanisms in peripheral tissues by affecting DC and T-cell pathways.[68]

In conclusion, inhibiting the interactions between adhesion molecules expressed on inflamed intestinal endothelium and lymphocyte integrins has proved to be a successful therapeutic strategy for the management of chronic IBD. Targeting specifically the MAdCAM-1/$\alpha4\beta7$ interactions with vedolizumab and, possibly, AMG 181 is likely to be an effective and safe treatment approach for refractory IBD patients. Incorporation of these agents into treatment algorithms in the context of the existing anti-TNF biologics and immunomodulators needs to be performed for both UC and CD, following carefully conducted therapeutic trials. Future studies need to address the use of these agents in the treatment of fistulizing CD phenotypes and extraintestinal manifestation of IBD. Subgroup analysis may identify genetic, serologic, and clinical parameters that may predict response to adhesion molecule inhibition and the best timing for therapeutic intervention. Combination therapeutic strategies with immunomodulators or even anti-TNF agents in a selective refractory group of IBD patients should also be entertained.

REFERENCES

1. Jostins L, Ripke S, Weersma RK, et al. Host-microbe interactions have shaped the genetic architecture of inflammatory bowel disease. Nature 2012;491: 119–24.
2. Shih DQ, Targan SR. Insights into IBD pathogenesis. Curr Gastroenterol Rep 2009;11:473–80.
3. Gevers D, Kugathasan S, Denson LA, et al. The treatment-naive microbiome in new-onset Crohn's disease. Cell Host Microbe 2014;15:382–92.
4. Langner C, Magro F, Driessen A, et al. The histopathological approach to inflammatory bowel disease: a practice guide. Virchows Arch 2014;464(5):511–27.
5. Dassopoulos T, Sultan S, Falck-Ytter YT, et al. American Gastroenterological Association Institute technical review on the use of thiopurines, methotrexate, and anti-TNF-alpha biologic drugs for the induction and maintenance of remission in inflammatory Crohn's disease. Gastroenterology 2013;145:1464–78.e1–5.
6. Plevy SE, Targan SR. Future therapeutic approaches for inflammatory bowel diseases. Gastroenterology 2011;140:1838–46.
7. D'Haens GR, Panaccione R, Higgins PD, et al. The London Position Statement of the World Congress of Gastroenterology on Biological Therapy for IBD with the European Crohn's and Colitis Organization: when to start, when to stop, which drug to choose, and how to predict response? Am J Gastroenterol 2011;106: 199–212 [quiz: 213].
8. Khanna R, Sattin BD, Afif W, et al. Review article: a clinician's guide for therapeutic drug monitoring of infliximab in inflammatory bowel disease. Aliment Pharmacol Ther 2013;38:447–59.

9. Yamada T, Grisham MB. Role of neutrophil-derived oxidants in the pathogenesis of intestinal inflammation. Klin Wochenschr 1991;69:988–94.

10. von Andrian UH, Mackay CR. T-cell function and migration. Two sides of the same coin. N Engl J Med 2000;343:1020–34.

11. Bevilacqua MP, Nelson RM, Mannori G, et al. Endothelial-leukocyte adhesion molecules in human disease. Annu Rev Med 1994;45:361–78.

12. Lobaton T, Vermeire S, Van Assche G, et al. Review article: anti-adhesion therapies for inflammatory bowel disease. Aliment Pharmacol Ther 2014;39:579–94.

13. Danese S. New therapies for inflammatory bowel disease: from the bench to the bedside. Gut 2012;61:918–32.

14. Sawada K, Kusugami K, Suzuki Y, et al. Leukocytapheresis in ulcerative colitis: results of a multicenter double-blind prospective case-control study with sham apheresis as placebo treatment. Am J Gastroenterol 2005;100:1362–9.

15. van der Flier A, Sonnenberg A. Function and interactions of integrins. Cell Tissue Res 2001;305:285–98.

16. Barczyk M, Carracedo S, Gullberg D. Integrins. Cell Tissue Res 2010;339: 269–80.

17. Hynes RO. Integrins: bidirectional, allosteric signaling machines. Cell 2002;110: 673–87.

18. Marlin SD, Springer TA. Purified intercellular adhesion molecule-1 (ICAM-1) is a ligand for lymphocyte function-associated antigen 1 (LFA-1). Cell 1987;51: 813–9.

19. Panes J, Granger DN. Leukocyte-endothelial cell interactions: molecular mechanisms and implications in gastrointestinal disease. Gastroenterology 1998;114: 1066–90.

20. Elices MJ, Osborn L, Takada Y, et al. VCAM-1 on activated endothelium interacts with the leukocyte integrin VLA-4 at a site distinct from the VLA-4/ fibronectin binding site. Cell 1990;60:577–84.

21. Tidswell M, Pachynski R, Wu SW, et al. Structure-function analysis of the integrin beta 7 subunit: identification of domains involved in adhesion to MAdCAM-1. J Immunol 1997;159:1497–505.

22. Briskin M, Winsor-Hines D, Shyjan A, et al. Human mucosal addressin cell adhesion molecule-1 is preferentially expressed in intestinal tract and associated lymphoid tissue. Am J Pathol 1997;151:97–110.

23. Pooley N, Ghosh L, Sharon P. Up-regulation of E-selectin and intercellular adhesion molecule-1 differs between Crohn's disease and ulcerative colitis. Dig Dis Sci 1995;40:219–25.

24. Koizumi M, King N, Lobb R, et al. Expression of vascular adhesion molecules in inflammatory bowel disease. Gastroenterology 1992;103:840–7.

25. Nakamura S, Ohtani H, Watanabe Y, et al. In situ expression of the cell adhesion molecules in inflammatory bowel disease. Evidence of immunologic activation of vascular endothelial cells. Lab Invest 1993;69:77–85.

26. Oshitani N, Campbell A, Bloom S, et al. Adhesion molecule expression on vascular endothelium and nitroblue tetrazolium reducing activity in human colonic mucosa. Scand J Gastroenterol 1995;30:915–20.

27. Campbell JJ, Haraldsen G, Pan J, et al. The chemokine receptor CCR4 in vascular recognition by cutaneous but not intestinal memory T cells. Nature 1999;400:776–80.

28. Rott LS, Rose JR, Bass D, et al. Expression of mucosal homing receptor alpha4-beta7 by circulating CD4+ cells with memory for intestinal rotavirus. J Clin Invest 1997;100:1204–8.

29. Arihiro S, Ohtani H, Suzuki M, et al. Differential expression of mucosal addressin cell adhesion molecule-1 (MAdCAM-1) in ulcerative colitis and Crohn's disease. Pathol Int 2002;52:367–74.
30. Major EO. Progressive multifocal leukoencephalopathy in patients on immuno-modulatory therapies. Annu Rev Med 2010;61:35–47.
31. Walters MJ, Wang Y, Lai N, et al. Characterization of CCX282-B, an orally bioavailable antagonist of the CCR9 chemokine receptor, for treatment of inflammatory bowel disease. J Pharmacol Exp Ther 2010;335:61–9.
32. Targan SR, Feagan BG, Fedorak RN, et al. Natalizumab for the treatment of active Crohn's disease: results of the ENCORE Trial. Gastroenterology 2007;132:1672–83.
33. Ghosh S, Goldin E, Gordon FH, et al. Natalizumab for active Crohn's disease. N Engl J Med 2003;348:24–32.
34. Gordon FH, Lai CW, Hamilton MI, et al. A randomized placebo-controlled trial of a humanized monoclonal antibody to alpha4 integrin in active Crohn's disease. Gastroenterology 2001;121:268–74.
35. Sandborn WJ, Colombel JF, Enns R, et al. Natalizumab induction and maintenance therapy for Crohn's disease. N Engl J Med 2005;353:1912–25.
36. Gordon FH, Hamilton MI, Donoghue S, et al. A pilot study of treatment of active ulcerative colitis with natalizumab, a humanized monoclonal antibody to alpha-4 integrin. Aliment Pharmacol Ther 2002;16:699–705.
37. Gorelik L, Reid C, Testa M, et al. Progressive multifocal leukoencephalopathy (PML) development is associated with mutations in JC virus capsid protein VP1 that change its receptor specificity. J Infect Dis 2011;204:103–14.
38. Van Assche G, Van Ranst M, Sciot R, et al. Progressive multifocal leukoencephalopathy after natalizumab therapy for Crohn's disease. N Engl J Med 2005;353:362–8.
39. Sugiura T, Kageyama S, Andou A, et al. Oral treatment with a novel small molecule alpha 4 integrin antagonist, AJM300, prevents the development of experimental colitis in mice. J Crohn's Colitis 2013;7:e533–42.
40. Takazoe M, Watanabe M, Kawaguchi T, et al. Oral alpha-4 integrin inhibitor (AJM300) in patients with active Crohn's disease-A randomized, double-blind, placebo-controlled trial. Gastroenterology 2009;136:A181.
41. Watanabe M, Yoshimura N, Motoya S, et al. AJM300, an oral alpha4 integrin antagonist for active ulcerative colitis: a multicenter, randomized, double-blind, placebo-controlled phase 2A study. Gastroenterology 2014;146(Suppl 1):S82.
42. Feagan BG, Greenberg GR, Wild G, et al. Treatment of ulcerative colitis with a humanized antibody to the alpha4beta7 integrin. N Engl J Med 2005;352:2499–507.
43. Feagan BG, Greenberg GR, Wild G, et al. Treatment of active Crohn's disease with MLN0002, a humanized antibody to the alpha4beta7 integrin. Clin Gastroenterol Hepatol 2008;6:1370–7.
44. Feagan BG, Rutgeerts P, Sands BE, et al. Vedolizumab as induction and maintenance therapy for ulcerative colitis. N Engl J Med 2013;369:699–710.
45. Sandborn WJ, Feagan BG, Rutgeerts P, et al. Vedolizumab as induction and maintenance therapy for Crohn's disease. N Engl J Med 2013;369:711–21.
46. Sands B, Feagan B, Rutgeerts P, et al. Vedolizumab induction therapy for patients with Crohn's disease and prior anti-tumour necrosis factor antagonist failure: a randomized, placebo-controlled, double-blind, multicentre trial [abstract]. J Crohn's Colitis 2013;7(Suppl 1):S5–6.
47. Pan WJ, Hsu H, Rees WA, et al. Pharmacology of AMG 181, a human anti-alpha4 beta7 antibody that specifically alters trafficking of gut-homing T cells. Br J Pharmacol 2013;169:51–68.

48. Pullen N, Molloy E, Carter D, et al. Pharmacological characterization of PF-00547659, an anti-human MAdCAM monoclonal antibody. Br J Pharmacol 2009;157:281–93.

49. Vermeire S, Ghosh S, Panes J, et al. The mucosal addressin cell adhesion molecule antibody PF-00547,659 in ulcerative colitis: a randomised study. Gut 2011; 60:1068–75.

50. D'Haens G, Vermeire S, Cataldi F, et al. Anti-MAdCAM monoclonal antibody PF-00547659 does not affect immune surveillance in the central nervous system of anti-TNF and immunosuppressant experienced Crohn's disease patients who are anti-TNF inadequate responders: results from the TOSCA study [abstract]. J Crohn's Colitis 2014;8(Suppl 1):S4–5.

51. Holzmann B, McIntyre BW, Weissman IL. Identification of a murine Peyer's patch–specific lymphocyte homing receptor as an integrin molecule with an alpha chain homologous to human VLA-4 alpha. Cell 1989;56:37–46.

52. Hu MC, Crowe DT, Weissman IL, et al. Cloning and expression of mouse integrin beta p(beta 7): a functional role in Peyer's patch-specific lymphocyte homing. Proc Natl Acad Sci U S A 1992;89:8254–8.

53. Cepek KL, Parker CM, Madara JL, et al. Integrin alpha E beta 7 mediates adhesion of T lymphocytes to epithelial cells. J Immunol 1993;150:3459–70.

54. Stefanich EG, Danilenko DM, Wang H, et al. A humanized monoclonal antibody targeting the beta7 integrin selectively blocks intestinal homing of T lymphocytes. Br J Pharmacol 2011;162:1855–70.

55. Hesterberg PE, Winsor-Hines D, Briskin MJ, et al. Rapid resolution of chronic colitis in the cotton-top tamarin with an antibody to a gut-homing integrin alpha 4 beta 7. Gastroenterology 1996;111:1373–80.

56. Picarella D, Hurlbut P, Rottman J, et al. Monoclonal antibodies specific for beta 7 integrin and mucosal addressin cell adhesion molecule-1 (MAdCAM-1) reduce inflammation in the colon of scid mice reconstituted with CD45RBhigh CD4+ T cells. J Immunol 1997;158:2099–106.

57. Rutgeerts PJ, Fedorak RN, Hommes DW, et al. A randomised phase I study of etrolizumab (rhuMAb beta7) in moderate to severe ulcerative colitis. Gut 2013; 62:1122–30.

58. Vermeire S, O'Byrne S, Keir M, et al. Etrolizumab as induction therapy for ulcerative colitis: a randomised, controlled, phase 2 trial. Lancet 2014. http://dx.doi. org/10.1016/S0140-6736(14)60661-9.

59. Papadakis KA, Targan SR. The role of chemokines and chemokine receptors in mucosal inflammation. Inflamm Bowel Dis 2000;6:303–13.

60. Papadakis KA, Prehn J, Nelson V, et al. The role of thymus-expressed chemokine and its receptor CCR9 on lymphocytes in the regional specialization of the mucosal immune system. J Immunol 2000;165:5069–76.

61. Papadakis KA, Prehn J, Moreno ST, et al. CCR9-positive lymphocytes and thymus-expressed chemokine distinguish small bowel from colonic Crohn's disease. Gastroenterology 2001;121:246–54.

62. Keshav S, Vanasek T, Niv Y, et al. A randomized controlled trial of the efficacy and safety of CCX282-B, an orally-administered blocker of chemokine receptor CCR9, for patients with Crohn's disease. PLoS One 2013;8:e60094.

63. Yacyshyn BR, Bowen-Yacyshyn MB, Jewell L, et al. A placebo-controlled trial of ICAM-1 antisense oligonucleotide in the treatment of Crohn's disease. Gastroenterology 1998;114:1133–42.

64. Yacyshyn BR, Chey WY, Goff J, et al. Double blind, placebo controlled trial of the remission inducing and steroid sparing properties of an ICAM-1 antisense

oligodeoxynucleotide, alicaforsen (ISIS 2302), in active steroid dependent Crohn's disease. Gut 2002;51:30–6.

65. Schreiber S, Nikolaus S, Malchow H, et al. Absence of efficacy of subcutaneous antisense ICAM-1 treatment of chronic active Crohn's disease. Gastroenterology 2001;120:1339–46.

66. van Deventer SJ, Tami JA, Wedel MK. A randomised, controlled, double blind, escalating dose study of alicaforsen enema in active ulcerative colitis. Gut 2004; 53:1646–51.

67. Ghosh S, Panaccione R. Anti-adhesion molecule therapy for inflammatory bowel disease. Therap Adv Gastroenterol 2010;3:239–58.

68. Sung SS, Fu SM, Rose CE Jr, et al. A major lung CD103 (alphaE)-beta7 integrin-positive epithelial dendritic cell population expressing Langerin and tight junction proteins. J Immunol 2006;176:2161–72.

69. Pedersen J, Coskun M, Soendergaard C, et al. Inflammatory pathways of importance for management of inflammatory bowel disease. World J Gastroenterol 2014;20:64–77.